"We wish we had this helpful, easy-to-read book when we gave birth to our children! New information and its readable style make this a valuable breastfeeding resource. Returning to work, breastfeeding for the first time or last—this book is for all mothers."

—JAN RIORDAN, EdD, F.A.A.N., IBCLC (WICHITA, KS)
KATHLEEN G. AUERBACH, PhD, IBCLC (FERNDALE, WA)
CO-AUTHORS, *BREASTFEEDING AND HUMAN LACTATION, 2ND EDITION*
(BOSTON: JONES AND BARTLETT, 1999)

"Eiger and Olds have done it again—a book on breastfeeding that is easy and enjoyable to read while accurate enough to survive the most rigorous academic challenge. It should be read by prospective, pregnant and postpartum moms, but especially by all of their health providers. Whether you are preparing for motherhood or breastfeeding your third child, or just curious about breastfeeding or the health of moms and kids, this book is worth the read."

—MIRIAM LABBOK
ADJUNCT ASSOCIATE PROFESSOR, JOHNS HOPKINS UNIVERSITY, BALTIMORE, MD
AND TULANE UNIVERSITY, NEW ORLEANS, LA
MEMBER, BOARD OF DIRECTORS, INTERNATIONAL BOARD OF
LACTATION CONSULTANT EXAMINERS (IBLCE)

"Breast may be best, but it doesn't always come naturally. Your odds for success can be significantly increased by the practical advice in, and warm support of, this valuable book."

—ARLENE EISENBERG AND HEIDI MURKOFF
AUTHORS OF *WHAT TO EXPECT WHEN YOU'RE EXPECTING*

"A very helpful book! This new edition includes the very latest information from the American Academy of Pediatrics and the most current research findings. It is now even more valuable to my nursing families than the previous editions!"

—ARNOLD L. TANIS, M.D., F.A.A.P., IBCLC
CLINICAL ASSOCIATE PROFESSOR, PEDIATRICS, UNIVERSITY OF MIAMI
PAST PRESIDENT, INTERNATIONAL BOARD OF LACTATION CONSULTANT EXAMINERS

"Human milk is the preferred feeding for all infants . . . with rare exceptions. Exclusive breastfeeding is ideal nutrition . . . for approximately the first 6 months after birth. . . . It is recommended that breastfeeding continue for at least 12 months, and thereafter for as long as mutually desired."

—*PEDIATRICS*. 1997; 100: 1035-1039 "BREASTFEEDING AND THE USE OF HUMAN MILK"

"The original text published more than two decades ago has been invaluable to generations of mothers. This new updated edition combines time tested advice and the latest scientific information for the perfect combination of traditional wisdom and expert guidance."

—LAURA J. BEST—MACIA, IBCLC
PRESIDENT AND CO-FOUNDER, WELLCARE, INC.

"Current research shows that breastfeeding has even more wide-ranging benefits than previously realized. This excellent book provides a superb blend of up-to-the-minute scientific information and warm, practical advice for nursing mothers."

—MIRIAM E. NELSON, PH.D. AND SARAH WERNICK, PH.D.
CO-AUTHORS OF *STRONG WOMEN STAY YOUNG* AND *STRONG WOMEN STAY SLIM*

"If you're thinking about breastfeeding, you definitely need this book. If you're thinking about NOT breastfeeding, you definitely need this book! This book saved *me* a number of times when I had what I thought were unanswerable questions. It also gives the nursing mother the validation that is sometimes needed in a mysterious and wondrous experience."

—KATIE DAVIS, MOTHER OF TWO BREASTFED CHILDREN AND
AUTHOR/ILLUSTRATOR OF *WHO HOPS?*

THE COMPLETE
BOOK OF
BREASTFEEDING

THIRD EDITION

THE COMPLETE BOOK OF BREASTFEEDING

by Marvin S. Eiger, M.D. & Sally Wendkos Olds

Photography by Roe Di Bona
Additional photography by Robin Holland
Illustrations by Wendy Wray

WORKMAN PUBLISHING, NEW YORK

Library of Congress Cataloging-in-Publications Data
Eiger, Marvin S.
The complete book of breastfeeding/ by Marvin S. Eiger and Sally Wendkos Olds; photographs by
Roe Di Bona and Robin Holland; illustrations by Wendy Wray. — 3rd ed.
p. cm.
Includes bibliographical references and index.
ISBN 0-7611-0902-1 (pbk.)
1. Breast feeding. 2. Mothers—Health and hygiene. I. Olds, Sally Wendkos. II. Title.
RJ216.E34 1999   98-38879
649'.33—dc21   CIP

Book design: Susan Aronson Stirling
Cover photograph: Roe Di Bona
Book photographs: Roe Di Bona and Robin Holland
Book illustrations: Wendy Wray

Workman Publishing Company, Inc.
708 Broadway
New York, NY 10003-9555

Manufactured in the United States of America

First printing January 1999
10 9 8 7 6 5 4

To our children,
who have taught us so much
and from whom we keep learning:

Nancy and Dorri Olds
Jennifer Olds Möbus
Michael and Pamela Eiger

THANKS FROM THE AUTHORS

We want to express our appreciation to the many friends, colleagues, and family members who generously gave of their expertise and time, who contributed the fruits of their research, and who offered valuable suggestions to aid us in making this edition of our book as helpful as possible to nursing mothers.

First, we want to acknowledge our spouses. Their consistent support, helpful suggestions, and flexibility in accommodating their schedules to ours made our task easier and more pleasurable. So, our thanks to Carol Eiger and David Mark Olds.

We are grateful to the following persons who reviewed various parts of the manuscript for the third edition and whose evaluations and suggestions were enormously helpful: Elizabeth Baldwin, Esq., Jane Balkam, Cheston M. Berlin, Jr., M.D., Rona Cohen, Brenda Dobson, M.S., R.D., L.D., Lawrence Gartner, M.D., Sue Huml, IBCLC, Miriam H. Labbok, M.D., M.P.H., Jennifer Möbus, David S. Newburg, Ph.D., Dorri Olds, Nancy Olds, Ph.D., Judith Roepke, Ph.D., Julianna Simon, Rifka Stern, M.D., and Arnold L. Tanis, M.D.

We owe a very special debt to three people who put their expertise, their time, and their eyesight to our service to read *all* of the manuscript for this edition. The book is better for the many questions, comments, and suggestions of Kathleen G. Auerbach, Ph.D., IBCLC (co-author of *Breastfeeding and Human Lactation*); Betty Crase, IBCLC (formerly Director of the Center for Breastfeeding Information at La Leche League International and currently Program Manager, Breastfeeding Promotion in Pediatric Office Practices, at the American Academy of Pediatrics); and Sarah Wernick, Ph.D. (co-author of *Strong Women Stay Young* and *Strong Women Stay Slim*).

We received valuable information and help from the following organizations and agencies: American Academy of Pediatrics, American Cancer Society, American College of Obstetricians and Gynecologists, American Dental Association, American Medical Association, American Public Health Association, Human Lactation Center, Ltd., International Board of Lactation Consultant Examiners (IBLCE), International

Childbirth Education Association, La Leche League International, Melpomene Institute for Women's Health Research, National Institute of Child Health and Human Development, New York Academy of Medicine, Port Washington Public Library, United Nations Fund for Children (UNICEF), World Health Organization (WHO), Maternity Center Association, and Wellcare, Inc.

We also received important help from the following individuals: Helen Armstrong, M.D., Judith Elder, Esq., Carolyn Longay, and, of course, to the many mothers and fathers who shared with us their thoughts and feelings about breastfeeding. We are especially grateful to Laura Best–Macia, IBCLC, President of Wellcare, Inc., for the expertise she so graciously offered us in many ways, including her able supervision of the photo program for this third edition.

And we are still indebted to those whose research and thinking helped us shape the first and second editions, especially Jimmie Lynne Avery, Harry Bakwin, M.D., Saul Blatman, M.D., T. Berry Brazelton, M.D., Michael J. Brennan, M.D., Nathaniel S. Cooper, D.D.S., Mary Cossman, Lois Dwyer, Paul Elber, Sylvia Feldman, Ph.D., Christopher R. Fletcher, M.D., Samuel J. Fomon, M.D., Florence Fralin, Vincent Freda, M.D., Helen Rosengren Freedman, Barbara Goodheart, Frank R. Greer, M.D., Elizabeth Hormann, Derrick B. Jelliffe, M.D., Tobe Joffe, Alice Ladas, Ed.D., Charlotte Lee–Carrihill, Philip Lipsitz, M.D., Toni Littlejohn, Michael Newton, M.D., Niles Newton, Ph.D., Kathleen O'Regan, R.N., Frank A. Oski, M.D., Judith Palsgraf, R.N., Alice Rossi, Ph.D., Asoka Roy, R.N., C.N.M., M.S., Richard Saphir, M.D., Benjamin Segal, M.D., Concepcion G. Sia, M.D., Barbara Silver, R.N., Christopher Springman, Frances Stout, M.S., R.D., Samuel Stone, M.D., Frank W. Summers, M.D., Maurice Teitel, M.D., Evelyn B. Thoman, Ph.D., Edith Tibbetts, M.Ed., Marian Tompson, Reginald C. Tsang, M.D., Elaine S. Turner, M.D., Tilla Vahanian, Ed.D., Eleanor R. Williams, Ph.D., Jan Yager, Ph.D., the staffs of the Departments of Pediatrics at Beth Israel Hospital Medical Center and New York University Medical Center and of the Newborn Service at University Hospital.

Our very special thanks to Ari and Michael Aster; Lori, Eric, and Samuel Baumel; Yaa and Kofi Brinkley; Jane, Ron and Peter Brown; Dolores DeLuise; Bobbi Lurie; Amy Manso and Kira Manso Brown; Ariel and Carl Pellman; Margaret, Tom, and Julia Preston; Craig and Dalva Senna; Natalie Weinstein; Katharine, Benjamin, and Joshua Zalusky;

Tami Coyne; Victoria Jordan; Tanya Johnson; Sin Yung Lo and Kwon Bor Ng; and Shirley Brown and Ezekiel Alleyne.

We thank all of the above for their help, but we take full responsibility for the book you hold in your hands. We hope you find it helpful.

Finally, we want to express our gratitude to our agent, Carolyn Krupp at the Julian Bach–IMG Literary Agency, and to our publishers. We owe a huge debt of gratitude to Peter Workman, president of Workman Publishing Company, who saw the need for this book so many years ago and who has supported it consistently through every edition. Our editors, Suzanne Rafer and Carrie Schoen, have shepherded the book through with sensitive and sensible care. We appreciate Maureen Clark's skillful and conscientious copy editing, as well as Penelope Hull's careful proofreading. Among the others at Workman who have contributed to the book's success are Natsumi Uda in the art department and Ellen Morgenstern in publicity. At Bantam Books we are grateful for the interest and abilities of Toni Burbank and Robin Michaelson. Right from the start, through the lives of the first and second editions and into this third edition, our partners in publishing have given us the kind of enthusiastic support that nurtures and strengthens both books and authors.

Contents

CHAPTER THREE

CHAPTER FOUR

CHAPTER FIVE

CHAPTER SIX

CHAPTER SEVEN

CHAPTER EIGHT

CHAPTER NINE

CHAPTER TEN

CHAPTER FIFTEEN

CHAPTER SIXTEEN

CHAPTER SEVENTEEN

CHAPTER EIGHTEEN

RESOURCE APPENDIX:

Introduction

If you were living at some other time or in some other place, you might not need this book. You might even wonder about its purpose, since you would be getting much of the information in these pages from your mother, your aunts, your older sisters, and your neighbors. They would share with you their breastfeeding experiences and those of their mothers before them. As you saw them suckling their infants, you would pick up the "tricks of the trade" without even realizing it. It would never occur to you that you would not nurse your baby, because every baby that you had ever seen would have been fed at his mother's breast—except in the extremely rare case when a mother was too ill to nurse.

The paragraph you have just read appeared as the introduction to the original edition of this book, published in 1972. It is one of the very few paragraphs that were carried over to the second edition, published in 1987, and once again into this edition.

Much has changed in the twenty-six years since *The Complete Book of Breastfeeding* was first conceived. The year 1971 (when the first edition of this book was being researched and written) marked the lowest rate of breastfeeding in the history of this country: Only one in four women even *began* to breastfeed their babies. By 1987, well over half of all American mothers were nursing their newborn infants, and among well-educated middle-class women, the incidence was even higher. There was a slight dip in the prevalence of breastfeeding in the early 1990s, but that reversal has been righted, and the rates of breastfeeding are climbing again.

Over these years we, the authors (a pediatrician who has cared for hundreds of breastfed babies and a medical writer who nursed her own three children), have been delighted to see an explosion of research into the properties of breast milk, the value of nursing for both mothers and babies, and the practices that enhance or hinder the course of breastfeeding.

We have applauded professional organizations like the American Academy of Pediatrics, which in its December 1997 policy statement on breastfeeding acknowledged its great importance and urged doctors to help mothers and babies follow practices to ensure healthy nursing experiences. The Canadian Paediatric Society and the World Health Organization have also issued strong statements urging mothers to nurse and urging medical professionals to help mothers breastfeed their babies.

We've been happy to note that today's physicians learn more about breastfeeding in medical school and are less likely to believe that formula is "just as good" as breast milk, and that more hospitals are instituting more policies that promote breastfeeding rather than interfere with it.

Today, then, if you have questions about breastfeeding, you're more likely to have sources to go to—the doctors, nurses, and midwives who help you in childbirth, the friends and neighbors who are nursing or have nursed their own children, and a wealth of published material. Still, depending on where you live and where you have your baby, the information you get may or may not be helpful.

In too many places you're still likely to hear outdated, incorrect advice. Some medical professionals have not kept up with new research findings about the nutritional and immunological advantages of human milk for infants. Some laypersons, especially those from a generation more familiar with bottle-fed babies, are still convinced of the myths and superstitions they heard in a less enlightened time.

Breastfeeding is easy; there is nothing complicated about it. And there is no single best way to do it. Still, it is a skill that you have to learn, and it is an activity whose success depends on the kind of information and support that you get. Nursing a baby may fulfill an instinctual drive, but both you and your baby need to learn the actual procedures for breastfeeding and need to be reassured while you're learning.

Some mothers intuitively know what to do, puzzled by no questions and troubled by no problems. Most new mothers, however, have questions about all aspects of infant care. Sometimes a lack of information about breastfeeding makes a woman hesitate to embark upon an adventure that seems strange and bewildering. Other times, women reluctantly switch to the bottle when, had their questions been answered and their problems solved, they would have much preferred to continue being part of a nursing couple.

To help you do what you want to do and to make the most of what may be among the most memorable and enjoyable experiences of your entire life, we have once again updated and revised this book. It is very exciting for us to realize that many of the women who are reading this edition of our book are the grown children of our first readers, now nursing *their* babies. It is always a thrill to have so many women—some of them grandmothers—come up to us at meetings and tell us, "Your book was my bible."

While we thought our book was quite complete when the first edition came out, it included much more in the second edition, and has even more in this third edition: the findings from the most up-to-date scientific research and the results of what so many nursing mothers have learned works well for them. It also addresses a number of lifestyle issues that are increasingly important to contemporary mothers.

Thus, you'll see more in this edition about diet and fitness, about breastfeeding for the working mother (including the best ways to express or pump and store breast milk), about breastfeeding as a sexual passage in the life of the mother, about nursing in public and legal issues related to this and other aspects of breastfeeding, and about nursing in a variety of special situations.

A Note About Language

Since babies come in two sexes, we write about them accordingly, alternating gender pronouns throughout the book. This seems to be the fairest solution to a problem that plagues most writers sensitive to the bias implicit in the English language.

We made another linguistic decision by alternating references to "your husband," "your partner," and "your baby's father." It's likely that most readers of this book are married, but that quite a few are not. You may be living with an adult who is neither your husband nor your baby's father. Or you may be raising your child alone; in this case, you may not be able to get the kind of help that a life partner can provide, and you may need to reach out for help to family members, friends, and members of your community. No matter what your personal situation may be, you can still breastfeed your baby and you can still benefit from most of the suggestions in these pages.

Although there is, as we said, no one "best way" to breastfeed, there are certain practices that seem to make the course of nursing go more smoothly for most mothers and babies, and it's these practices that we describe and recommend in these pages. However, every baby is unique, every mother is unique, and every family situation is unique. You may find that you and your baby do better by changing some of our recommendations. If it works for you, do it—and more power to you!

We're really happy that you're beginning this journey, which may be among the most exhilarating of your life, and we hope that this book will help you navigate it smoothly.

The three essential tools for successful breastfeeding are (1) knowing what to do, (2) feeling confident that you're doing the right thing for your baby and yourself, and (3) being determined to persist in the face of any minor setbacks that may come your way.

As authors who've learned much more about our subject since we wrote our first book—and then still more since the publication of its second edition—we hope that this newest edition will help you develop all three of these tools.

Marvin S. Eiger, M.D.   Sally Wendkos Olds
New York, New York   Port Washington, New York

Will You or Won't You?

The best times are when babies come.

—*Melanie, in* Gone With the Wind

Only in relatively recent times has there been any question at all as to whether or not a baby would be breastfed. In earlier days, if a mother was either unable or unwilling to nurse her baby herself, she had to find another woman to do it. Early in the twentieth century, however, the advent of dependable refrigeration and pasteurization and the development of ways to modify cow's milk for infant consumption meant that babies could be fed a specially formulated product that was both digestible and nutritious.

Today you have a choice in the way you feed your baby. You can decide whether you want to feed your baby with the milk produced by your own body the way mothers have done from time immemorial—or whether you want to provide your baby's nourishment in a bottle. Many factors will enter into your decision: the customs of your community; the attitudes of your doctor, your husband or life partner, your friends and family; your lifestyle, including your work commitments; your personality; your feelings about mothering; and how much emotional support you receive.

We hope that once you read this chapter and see all the benefits that breastfeeding holds for you, your baby, and the world you live in, you'll give nursing a try. You might look on it as a thirty-day money-back guarantee. You will most likely find it gratifying for both you and your baby and go on to nurse well beyond those initial thirty days.

But suppose you begin to nurse your baby and you feel that you must stop. You haven't lost anything; you haven't invested in anything; you can always stop. The stores will always have those bottles, nipples, sterilizers, and formulas. You haven't made a lifelong commitment. You can easily change your mind.

Meanwhile, you have given your baby the wonderful substance of colostrum, which, as you'll see, is like giving your child an injection of antibodies at the most vulnerable time of his or her life, right after birth. And while exclusive breastfeeding for at least the first six months confers the most benefits on you and your child, some breastfeeding is better than no breastfeeding.

However, if you decide to bottle-feed right away, it's much harder, and sometimes impossible, to change your mind later on. Initiating breastfeeding after only a week has gone by requires a great deal of determination, persistence, and patience. It *has* been done by mothers who found that their babies needed breast milk to survive and by women who discovered that bottle-feeding has its own problems, but it is not easy.

WHY BREASTFEED?

For many years in the United States, the nursing mother was the nonconformist, a member of a minority group. By 1971, formula feeding had become the norm in this country, with only 25 percent of women (only one in four) nursing. Since then, however, the long-term trend away from breastfeeding has been reversed,* so that today 60 percent of new mothers nurse their babies. (This book was first published in 1972, and we like to think that the advice and encouragement it offered helped to accelerate the trend toward the rediscovery of breastfeeding!)

You probably have heard many of the reasons why breastfeeding is good for babies, most of which we'll talk about in this chapter. You may not be as aware of all the benefits it can hold for you, which we'll also talk about in this chapter. One of the prime benefits for the mother is the all-around good feeling you're likely to derive from the experience.

In talking about their breastfeeding experiences, women often emphasize how good it feels (or felt)—emotionally, physically, and intellectually.

---

*There was one dip in the years 1984 through 1989. This decline was greater among younger women, those receiving federal supplemental food benefits, full-time workers, first-time mothers, and women living in certain regions of the United States. However, by 1995 breastfeeding rates rose sharply again, especially among these groups of women. At this writing it is at its highest rate in this country since 1982.

One proof of the enjoyment many women get from this aspect of mothering can be seen in the fact that when a woman has breastfed one baby, she almost always nurses the next.

Women who have bottle-fed one baby and nursed another tend to feel closer to their nursing infants in the early months of life. One mother told us, "I never knew what I was missing by not nursing my first baby. I loved him and I enjoyed him, yes, but I never got so many of the 'extras' that I get from this one—that little hand that touches my skin as she's nursing, the way she'll pull away from the breast, smile at me, and go right back again, the happiness that I feel at being able to give her what she wants."

The "nursing pair"—mother and baby—forge an especially close and interdependent relationship. Your baby depends upon you for sustenance and comfort, and you look forward to feeding times to gain a pleasurable sense of closeness with your infant. If a feeding time is too long delayed, both of you become distressed—your baby because of hunger and you because of uncomfortably full breasts. Each of you needs the other, yearns for the other, is intimate with the other in a very special way. Because of this unique symbiotic relationship, many women consider the period of nursing among the most fulfilling times of their lives.

In addition, nursing can be an intensely pleasurable, sensuous activity. And finally, knowing all the health benefits that breastfeeding confers on both mother and baby affirms a woman's conviction that she is making the best possible decision for herself and her baby. Let's see what some of these benefits are.

BENEFITS FOR THE BABY

Nutrition

Human breast milk is the ultimate health food for human infants. For at least the first six months, it is the *only* food most babies need. Even after other foods are introduced in the latter half of the first year, breast milk continues to supply such important nutrients as essential fatty acids, lactose (the predominant sugar in milk) for proper growth of brain cells, and the correct balance of proteins. (See Chapter 3 for more about this ideal food.)

In recent years nutritionists have voiced concern about overly high levels of protein in the American diet. Since cow's milk contains about twice as much protein as human milk, formula-fed babies usually receive more protein than they need (much of it in the form of the less digestible casein). The stools of formula-fed babies are so bulky because the babies cannot ab-

A Mother's Enjoyment

When I (Sally Olds) was nursing my first baby, I was struck by how much information was available about the benefits breastfeeding conferred on babies, but I felt I had really discovered something when I realized how many advantages it held for mothers. My first published article, "Nursing Is Good for Mothers Too," appeared in a small-circulation baby-care magazine.

Nancy, my first baby, is now a mother herself (who nursed her own daughter), but my memories of Nancy's infancy are still vivid. I remember so clearly hearing her lusty cry, picking her up and holding her next to my heart, inhaling her incredibly sweet new-baby fragrance, feeling the tingling in my breasts that told me my milk was letting down for her, and looking down with a heart full of joy as she suckled eagerly.

I thought—and wrote in that first article—"There's something very right about a system that makes one human being so happy about being responsible for another. I could never have the same good feeling of accomplishment by relying on the neighborhood store or the dairy for my baby's milk. Knowing that I was giving her something no one else could give her created a tie between us that became one of my deepest joys."

As I watched Nancy's little legs become chubby and dimpled, and as I laughed at the little-old-lady look that her double chin gave her, any doubts about the quality of "my formula" vanished. In those days I knew very little about breastfeeding—I knew only that both Nancy and I loved it.

sorb so much protein, and excrete the excess in their stool, whereas breast-fed babies absorb virtually 100 percent of the protein in human milk.

In the United States today, there's a new awareness of the serious problem of overnutrition and of the problems caused by overweight. Bottle-fed babies tend to be fatter than breastfed babies. One reason for this may stem from the fact that bottle-feeding mothers who see milk left in the bottle tend to encourage their babies to drain the last drop, while breastfeeding mothers usually assume that their babies know when they have had enough. When the baby stops suckling, the mother takes her off the breast.

Another way that nursing may discourage overfeeding lies in the difference between the high-protein milk produced at the beginning of a feeding (fore milk) and the high-fat milk produced at the end (hind milk). The richness of the hind milk may make the baby feel full and send a signal that mealtime is over.

Breastfed children like vegetables better than do formula-fed infants when they're first introduced to them, probably because breastfed babies become more familiar with the varied tastes and smells that come through the milk of their vegetable-eating mothers. Thus, by encouraging a diverse and healthy diet, breastfeeding can offer health protection later, when babies will be more receptive to new foods.

In fact, research has shown that even before birth your baby becomes familiar with different tastes and smells in the amniotic fluid; the variety of tastes and smells that then come through your milk accustoms your child to the foods of your particular culture. While your breast milk varies from day to day, depending on what you have eaten, commercial formula tastes and smells the same, day after unvarying day. Consequently, the formula-fed baby misses out on the rich and varied sensory experiences transmitted through a mother's milk.

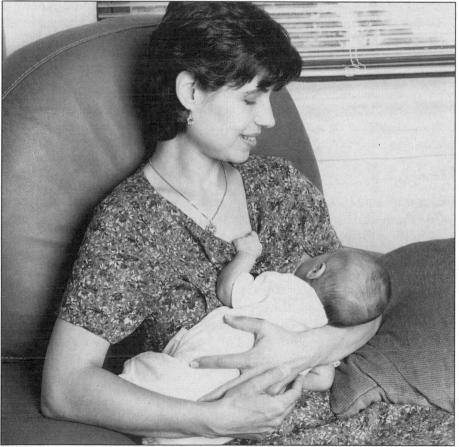

Robin Holland

A loving moment shared by a nursing mother and her baby.

Childhood Illnesses Prevented or Minimized by Breastfeeding

In the strongest, most well documented statement it has ever issued about the value of breastfeeding, the American Academy of Pediatrics states:

"Research in the United States, Canada, Europe and other *developed* [emphasis in original] countries, among predominantly middle-class populations, provides strong evidence that human milk feeding decreases the incidence and/or severity of diarrhea, lower respiratory infection, otitis media, bacteremia, bacterial meningitis, botulism, urinary tract infection, and necrotizing enterocolitis. . . .

"[A] number of studies . . . show a possible protective effect of human milk feeding against sudden infant death syndrome, insulin-dependent diabetes mellitus, Crohn's disease, ulcerative colitis, lymphoma, allergic diseases, and other chronic digestive diseases. Breastfeeding has also been related to possible enhancement of cognitive development."

"Breastfeeding and the Use of Human Milk"
American Academy of Pediatrics, Work Group on Breastfeeding
Pediatrics, volume 100, no. 6, December 1997

Health

Breast milk confers many other important health benefits. In underdeveloped countries, the survival rate for the breastfed baby may be six times greater than for his bottle-fed cousin. And even among the children of middle- or upper-class parents in highly developed countries, breastfed babies are healthier and have better chances for survival.

In technologically developed countries like ours, where sanitary conditions are generally good, the gap in health between the breastfed and the bottle-fed baby is narrowed considerably. In addition, modern medical techniques can now vanquish many of the illnesses that used to be fatal to infants. Still, it's better to prevent disease than to cure it. And there's a great deal of evidence that breast milk does indeed have preventive, protective powers, even in the most technically advanced countries.

Breastfed babies make fewer visits to doctors' offices and hospitals than bottle-fed babies do, especially for diarrhea and other gastrointestinal disorders, rashes, and respiratory infections. They are less likely to suffer from diaper rash, a common problem in infancy, apparently because breastfed babies' higher level of fecal acidity helps to protect them against the yeast infections that can lead to diaper rash.

Breastfed babies also seem to be protected in varying degrees from a number of other illnesses (see the box on page 10). When they do get sick, their illnesses are likely to be less severe and their recovery faster. Breastfeeding also seems to enhance babies' vision through the presence of the nutrient DHA (more about this later in this chapter, and in Chapters 3 and 7); it also seems to further their healthy neurological development later in childhood.

Breastfeeding's advantages are most striking during the first six months of life, very evident during the first two years, and still apparent later in life. In fact, as the American Academy of Pediatrics points out, breastfeeding may even help to prevent various illnesses in adulthood. For example, having been breastfed as a baby lowers a woman's risk for breast cancer, both before and after menopause. There is also evidence to suggest that breastfeeding may increase your child's bone mineral density, and that it also protects against such lower respiratory diseases as bronchitis, pneumonia, and asthma during middle childhood.

The greatest health differences between breastfed and formula-fed babies show up when the babies compared are fed exclusively by either method. The differences narrow in proportion to the amount of formula or other foods given in addition to breast milk.

Digestibility

Babies can digest human milk more easily than the milk of any other animal, probably because human milk contains an enzyme to aid in its own digestion. Breast milk forms softer curds in the infant's stomach than cow's milk (the basis for most formulas) and is more quickly assimilated. While it contains less protein than does cow's milk, virtually all the protein in breast milk is used by the baby. By contrast, about half the protein in cow's milk is wasted, passing through the baby's body and making extra work for the baby's excretory system. Similarly, iron and zinc are absorbed better by breastfed babies.

Breastfed babies are less apt to get diarrhea, and they do not become constipated, since breast milk cannot solidify in the intestinal tract to form hard stools. While your breastfed baby may soil all her diapers in the early days or go several days without a bowel movement later on, neither of these situations necessarily indicates intestinal upset (see Chapter 6).

Some premature infants and other babies with sensitive digestive systems thrive best on breast milk. If their own mothers cannot or do not provide it, they may be able to get it from a milk bank. (For information about milk banks, see the Resource Appendix.)

Human Milk for Human Babies

In country after country, language after language, the most common way that young children call their mothers is with the two syllables "ma-ma." This universal word gave rise to the Latin word for breast, *mamma*. And in 1758, the importance of a mother's ability to nurture her babies from her breasts was scientifically acknowledged for perhaps the first time, when the Swedish scientist Carolus Linnaeus coined the name *mammalia* for the class of animals designed to breastfeed their young. No doubt he chose this particular female trait because he considered it so significant. As indeed it is.

The milk of every species of mammal is different in its composition from every other milk. We can logically assume from this that each animal produces in its milk those elements most important for the survival of its young. Human milk contains at least one hundred ingredients that are not in cow's milk, and while artificial formulas try to imitate mother's milk, they can never duplicate it exactly. No manufacturer has ever officially claimed that a formula product is just as good as or better than breast milk, and none is likely to make such an audacious claim.

For one thing, breast milk changes in composition from day to day, and even from feeding to feeding. For another, each mother's milk is custom-designed for her own baby: Women develop specific antibodies against bacteria and viruses in their own lungs and intestines, which also appear in their milk. Thus, they manufacture the mix of antibodies that is best for their own babies.

The perfect match between a baby and its mother's milk is dramatically evident in the case of premature infants: The milk of a woman who has delivered prematurely is higher in protein and in fat than that produced by the mother of a full-term baby and is, therefore, better suited to the special growth needs of her preterm baby.

In addition, we're constantly discovering new ingredients in mother's milk. One recently discovered component in breast milk is a fatty acid known as DHA (docosahexaenoic acid), which appears to be vital for newborns' brain and eye development. As of this writing, in the United States DHA is not added to formula, which means that the *only* way babies can get it is through their mothers' breast milk. Another newly discovered constituent in human milk is mucin, an acid-based protein that prevents intestinal illness in nursing animals.

Through trial and error, formula manufacturers have learned that many ingredients are essential for babies' nutrition. A few years ago when a manufacturer lowered the salt content in its formula, the resulting compound ended up with so little chloride that babies who drank it became se-

How Breastfeeding Protects Against Disease

In some countries around the world, especially in parts of Africa, South America, and the Middle East, mothers put breast milk in their babies' eyes or on the sites of circumcisions to prevent or treat infections. We have not seen scientific evidence for the value of these particular folk treatments, but there is a great deal of evidence supporting breastfeeding's disease-protection benefits. These probably occur in several ways, including the following:

• Mother's milk transmits immunoglobulin A proteins (IgA), which are antibodies against pathogens (disease-causing organisms) to which the mother has been exposed. These IgA proteins are unique in that they line the baby's respiratory and intestinal surfaces, forming a protective coating to prevent many bacterial and viral agents from invading the baby's body and causing disease. Thus your breastfed baby is afforded time during the vulnerable first few months, until his own immune system matures. In their role as your baby's guardian, various versions of this unique protein fight specific organisms.

• Breast milk also contains other protective substances. Eighty percent of the cells in breast milk are *macrophages,* cells that in other parts of the body are known to kill bacteria, fungi, and viruses and to help stop the growth of cancer cells. The mystery is that the macrophages in human milk are inactive. As one prominent microbiologist has said, "We don't know exactly what they do in human milk—but they probably do *something*." (Again, we see why it is impossible to make a formula that duplicates human milk exactly. There is too much that science does not know about why human milk does such a good job helping babies grow.)

• The complex sugars in all human milk are thought to protect a baby against pathogens to which the mother has *not* been exposed, but to which the baby may have been, including some that cause diarrhea and ear infections. They do this by preventing the first step in infection, the binding of a pathogen to the infant's cells.

• Other elements in breast milk also confer protection, as we'll see in Chapter 3, which compares human milk with cow's milk.

• Some benefits of breastfeeding are procedural: The milk in your breast cannot be contaminated by the harmful bacteria that can multiply in animal milk left out of the refrigerator for too long a period of time. It's always served in a clean container. It can't be overdiluted to save money. It can neither be counterfeited nor prepared incorrectly (both of which have occurred from time to time in baby formulas, sometimes with disastrous results).

Some of the Ways Breastfed Babies Differ from Formula-Fed Babies

Although we don't know the implications of the many physiological differences between breastfed and formula-fed babies, the fact that there is a difference seems significant in terms of species-specific development. In other words, the milk of each species is designed to further the optimal development of the young of that species. What, then, are some of the differences between babies fed human milk and babies fed with the milk of other animals?

• Breastfed babies grow differently. Formula-fed babies not only grow longer and fatter, but they also develop bigger and heavier bones during the first year of life, probably due to the larger amounts of calcium in cow's milk. Formula-fed babies may grow faster than nature intended them to; bigger is not necessarily better.

• The bacteria in their intestinal tracts are strikingly different. Those in the tracts of breastfed babies consist largely of *Lactobacillus bifidus,* a beneficial organism that prevents the growth of certain harmful bacteria and that's present in only small numbers in the stools of bottle-fed babies.

• *Lysozyme,* another substance found only in the stools of breastfed infants, also protects against harmful microorganisms.

• The ratio of vitamins in their systems is different.

• Human milk contains more cholesterol than does formula, and animal studies suggest that exposure to cholesterol early in life may help program the individual to metabolize cholesterol more efficiently in adulthood, offering some protection against heart disease. Breastfed infants have higher cholesterol levels at first than do bottle-fed babies, but this difference disappears after weaning. In any case, the higher levels are not unhealthy.

verely ill. An earlier disaster had followed another manufacturer's use of higher temperatures for sterilization, which destroyed vitamin B_6, an element that until then had not been known to be vital. Who knows what other ingredients will be identified in mother's milk for formula-makers to try to imitate?

Teleology, the ultimate purpose or design in nature, is revealed in various ways. For example, newborn babies see best at a distance of between twelve and fifteen inches, precisely the usual distance of a baby's eyes from the face of a nursing mother. And neuroscientists point to the importance of repeated experience, as in gazing intently at a loving face, in aiding babies' brain development. As Aristotle said so many centuries ago, "There is reason behind everything in nature."

Other research has found that seven- to eight-year-old children who had been fed breast milk scored higher on IQ tests than children who had received only formula. All these children had been born prematurely and had been fed through tubes to eliminate the bias of bonding with the mother. This evidence strongly suggests the presence of some substance in human milk that affects mental development.

Even though we don't know the precise reasons for, or the significance of, all the differences between the baby nourished at the breast and the baby fed by bottle, it seems logical to assume that the best first food for your baby is the kind you provide yourself. As Dr. Paul György, the pioneering researcher who discovered vitamin B_6, said more than seventy years ago, "Human milk is for the human infant; cow's milk is for the calf." As two nurses proposed more recently, breast milk substitutes should carry a label stating: "Warning: This product is inferior to human milk."

Less Chance of Allergic Reactions

Although many babies do well on formulas, an occasional infant has an allergic reaction like indigestion or diarrhea. As a breastfeeding mother, you won't have to experiment with different milks and nonmilk formulas.

As a breastfeeding mother, you would never have this concern, since no baby is allergic to breast milk. Some babies do develop allergic reactions like vomiting, diarrhea, skin rash, hives, or sniffles, to something in the mother's diet that's transmitted through the milk. But, as explained in Chapter 7, it's usually possible for the mother to identify and stop eating that particular food for the duration of nursing.

Some research suggests that breastfeeding reduces the likelihood of such allergic reactions as eczema and other skin ailments, asthma, and runny noses. This makes nursing particularly important if you have a family history of allergy. Cow's milk allergy is fairly common, and babies are protected from this as long as they are taking nothing but breast milk and their mothers significantly reduce or eliminate cow's milk products from their own diets.

It seems that the earlier a baby with a predisposition to allergy receives cow's milk, the greater the risk of developing an allergy. For this reason, some authorities recommend that babies with a family history of allergy be exclusively breastfed for at least six months. After this time breastfeeding should continue, and supplemental foods should be carefully chosen to avoid common allergies (to wheat, for example).

Cognitive Development

Researchers recently reported on a study of one thousand children born in 1977 in New Zealand who were followed until age eighteen. The research findings showed that the longer infants are breastfed, the more likely they are to do well in school and on tests of intellectual ability. The children were divided into four categories: not having been breastfed at all, and having been nursed for four months, four to seven months, and eight or more months.

The longer these children had been breastfed, the higher they scored on IQ and other standardized tests. Teachers rated the breastfed children higher in reading and math; and they achieved better grades in high school than did students who as babies had been fed formula. The researchers believe that this cognitive advantage may result from the presence in breast milk of certain fatty acids that promote lasting brain development.

Tooth and Jaw Development

Suckling at the breast is good for your baby's tooth and jaw development. Babies at the breast use more muscles to get food than do those drinking from a bottle. The nursling has to draw much or all of the areola (the darker area around the nipple) into his mouth, move his jaws up and down, and squeeze with his tongue to extract milk. To accomplish this task, your baby has been endowed with jaw muscles relatively three times stronger than yours. As these muscles are strenuously exercised in suckling, their constant activity encourages well-formed jaws and straight, healthy teeth.

One factor accounting for many dental malformations that eventually send children to the orthodontist or the speech therapist is an abnormal feeding pattern known as "tongue thrust." This is very common among bottle-fed babies, but almost nonexistent among the breastfed. To understand why, we have to examine the mechanisms of feeding. As we explain in detail in the box on page 107 in Chapter 6, the breastfed baby works her gums and lower jaw quite vigorously to get the milk, whereas bottle-fed babies don't have to exercise their jaws so energetically, since light sucking alone produces a rapid flow. In fact, the milk often flows so freely that the baby has to learn how to protect himself from an oversupply so that he won't choke. He pushes his tongue forward against the nipple holes to stem the flow to a level that he can easily handle. Many dentists believe that such a forward tongue thrust can result in mouth breathing, lip biting, gum disease, and a generally unattractive appearance.

Another factor contributes to breastfed children's healthy tooth and jaw development. Since they get more of the sucking that babies need, they're less likely to suck their thumbs. Bottle-fed babies have to stop sucking on the nipple as soon as the bottle is empty to avoid taking in air; your baby at the breast can continue in this blissful pastime until you or she decide she's been at the well long enough.

Of course, not all bottle-fed babies develop dental problems, and some breastfed babies do. Still, this is one more realm in which breastfeeding remains superior to bottle-feeding.

Availability

Another advantage your nursling enjoys is the virtually constant availability of milk. Her dinner is always ready, always at the right temperature. She doesn't have to struggle to get milk from a nipple with scanty holes, nor does she have to gulp furiously to keep up with a gush from extra-large ones. No snowstorm, no flood, no car breakdown, no dairy workers' strike can keep her food from her. You don't have to worry about running short when you're out with your baby. As long as mother is near, so is sustenance.

Emotional Gratification

When you nurture your baby at your breast, you cannot be tempted—even on your busiest days—to lay your baby down with a propped bottle. You *have* to draw him close to you for every single feeding. While bottle-feeding mothers can also show their love for their babies by holding and cuddling them at feeding times, in actual practice they tend to do less of this. And while they *can* hold their babies next to their bare skin when they offer the bottle, to simulate the body contact of nursing, they rarely do. Research has proved the value of the sense of touch in many different settings. This basic element of breastfeeding is one of the most gratifying aspects of the experience, to both mother and baby.

Babies also gain a sense of well-being from secure handling, and nursing mothers often seem more confident. Whether the woman who's sure of her maternal abilities is more likely to breastfeed—or whether the experience of being a good provider infuses her with self-confidence—is hard to determine. Nursing mothers do seem more likely to know how to soothe their babies when they're upset, maybe because the very act of putting them to the breast is so comforting that they don't have to search for other means of solace. The breast is more than a pipeline for getting food into your baby. It's warmth; it's reassurance; it's succor.

Much has been written and said about the psychological benefits that babies derive from breastfeeding. Dr. Niles Newton, a psychologist who made extensive studies of lactation in people and in laboratory animals, found many psychological differences between breast and artificial feeding, most of which tip the scales in favor of nursing.

For example, lactating mice demonstrate a greater drive than non-nursing mouse mothers in overcoming obstacles to reach their infants, indicating some mechanism in lactation itself that triggers maternal behavior. It may well be the hormone prolactin, called "the mothering hormone":

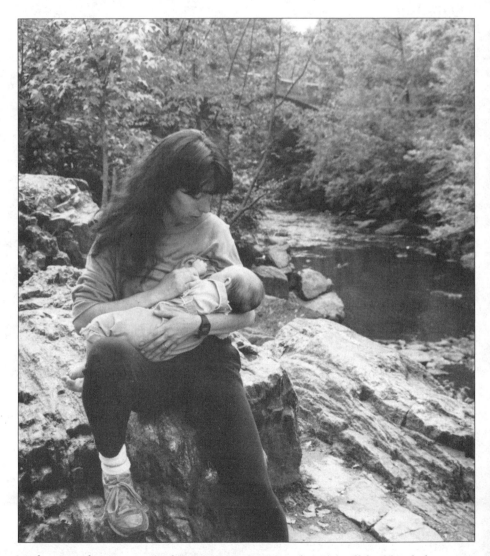

Miles away from store or refrigerator, a nursing mother can still feed her baby.

when injected into a hen, prolactin will make her take care of nearby chicks, even if they aren't her own. Another important hormone in lactation is oxytocin, which Dr. Newton described as "the hormone of love"; it also triggers nurturing behavior. (For more about prolactin and oxytocin, see Chapters 3 and 13.)

Human infants seem to recognize and become attached to their nursing mothers very early, as shown by the fact that when one-week-old babies are presented with breast pads that their own mothers had worn and with pads worn by other nursing women, they seem to prefer their mothers' smell. They turn their heads more often and are more likely to suck toward their mothers' breast pads.

However, we do need to point out the conclusions of researchers who have, over the past sixty years, conducted studies that tried to correlate methods of infant feeding with later personality development. Their findings: As important as early feeding experiences may be to a child's later development, there are so many variables in parent-child relationships that it's impossible to claim definitively that any one factor, including breastfeeding, is, in and of itself, a prescription for healthy adjustment.

Still, psychiatrists and other students of human and animal nature do state categorically that babies gain a sense of security from the warmth and closeness of the mother's body. Also, it seems that the more intimate interaction between the breastfeeding mother and child, the warm skin-to-skin contact, and the more immediate satisfaction of the nursing baby's hunger would make for healthier psychological development.

BENEFITS FOR THE MOTHER

Your primary reason for wanting to breastfeed is probably your awareness that it will be better for your baby. You may not have realized how many benefits nursing offers you, too.

Good for Your Figure

Nursing their babies helps many women to regain their figures more quickly after childbirth, since the process of lactation causes the uterus (which has increased during pregnancy to about twenty times its normal size) to shrink more quickly to its prepregnancy size. During the early days of nursing, you can feel your uterus contracting while your baby suckles. As she nurses, she stimulates your pituitary gland to secrete the hormone oxytocin, which brings about uterine contractions. These contractions hasten your uterus's return to its former size, while helping to expel excess tissue and blood. The uterus of the nonlactating mother, on the other hand, always remains somewhat larger than it was before she became pregnant.

Also, since breastfeeding uses up so many calories, you may be able to lose weight while eating more. A number of research studies have found that nursing mothers, who eat more than women who bottle-feed their babies, lose more weight over the first year after childbirth. This is especially true if they nurse for at least six months. Not only do they shed pounds—they lose more fat from their bodies, especially the hips and thighs, which affects how they look as well as how much they weigh.

Furthermore, despite what many people believe, nursing does *not* break down the connective tissues in your breasts. In Pulitzer Prize–winner Maya Angelou's memoir, *Gather Together in My Name,* she quotes her mother as having said to her: "You don't have stretch marks and because you breastfed, your breasts never got out of shape." Research confirms this folk wisdom: Changes in the breasts that occur, such as a loss of firmness, are the results of pregnancy, weight gain, heredity, and maturity, not lactation.

Convenience

Even today, when formula comes ready-mixed in nursing bottles, breast-feeding is easier than bottle-feeding. No efficiency expert has been able to outdo nature's way of feeding an infant. Your baby's daily batch of food prepares itself in its own permanent containers.

It's so easy just to wake up in the morning, pick up your baby, and put her to your breast. You don't have to scrub and sterilize bottles and nipples. You don't have to pad barefoot into a chilly kitchen to heat up a bottle. You never have to make up an extra bottle at the last minute or throw out formula that your baby doesn't want. Working on the time-honored principle of supply and demand, your mammary glands produce the amount of milk your baby wants. Your actively lactating breast is never empty, so that no matter how often your baby is hungry, your breasts will be able to supply milk to her.

You'll find it easier to go visiting or traveling with your baby, since you won't have to take along bottles, nipples, and formula, nor will you have to worry about refrigeration, dish-washing facilities, or changes in the water supply. When you have to be separated from your baby—if you work outside the home, for example—you can express and store your milk, to be given in a bottle when you're away.

Your Health

Breastfeeding offers you a number of important health benefits also. First, you reap benefits right after your baby's birth; then you gain an advantage from the temporary cessation of your menses; and in later life, you appear to have some protection from both breast and ovarian cancer, and also from osteoporosis.

- *Postpartum:* Breastfeeding your infant within the first hour of birth offers you three health benefits: (1) It helps to prevent postbirth hemorrhaging; (2) it facilitates the expulsion of the placenta; and (3) it speeds up the process of involution by which your uterus returns to its prepregnancy size.

Then, every mother of a newborn needs adequate rest. The many physiological changes of pregnancy, the hard work of labor and delivery, and the demanding care of a new baby all deplete your energy. When you breastfeed, you're forced to relax during your baby's feeding times, since you cannot prop a bottle or turn the baby over to someone else while you run around doing chores. Your baby's feeding times are your enforced rest times.

- *Respite from menstruation:* As an exclusively breastfeeding woman you probably won't menstruate for at least six months after childbirth, and possibly longer if you are feeding your baby with breast milk alone. This is the only time in your reproductive life when you're not losing iron through your menses or through nourishing a baby in your womb. Although you do provide iron in your milk, the amounts taken from your body are much less than you would be losing through your menstrual periods. Thus, this is a chance to build up your stores of iron and to correct any anemic tendencies you may have.

- *Protection from cancer:* Another advantage of not menstruating is a protective effect against ovarian cancer, which, according to recent research, is directly related to a woman's lifetime number of ovulations. Therefore, the fewer times in your life you ovulate, the lower your risk may be for ovarian cancer. Lactating women tend to ovulate later.

Another major health benefit of breastfeeding is its role in lowering the risk of breast cancer, especially among younger women, that is, women who have not yet experienced menopause. Breast cancer is the second leading cancer killer among women (after lung cancer), and breastfeeding is one of the few actions that you can take to lessen your risk for this disease.

The protective effect against breast cancer is particularly striking among women who begin to breastfeed in their teens and then nurse their babies for at least six months. However, women who begin to breastfeed after age twenty and breastfeed from three to six months also have a lower risk of breast cancer than women who do not nurse. The protective effect is strongest among women who nurse for longer durations. There is also some evidence that breastfeeding may protect women from postmenopausal breast cancer, the time of life when most cases occur. In China and in Mexico, studies have found protection extending to postmenopausal women, too. (In China, more than half of women nurse for at least three years.)

• *Protection from osteoporosis:* Osteoporosis is a thinning of the bones that causes "widow's humps" and bone fractures later in life, and this is one more condition for which breastfeeding seems protective. Women who breastfeed tend to have increased bone mineral density later in life, and denser bones are a protective factor against fractures of the hip and other sites, a major health risk for older women. Older women who have ever breastfed have half the risk for bone fractures as women who did not nurse their babies. The longer a woman's lifetime lactation lasts, the lower her risk of fracture.

Economy

Breastfeeding saves you money. In the decade spanning 1980 to 1990 the average wholesale price of formula doubled. Since all three of the major formula producers were charging almost identical prices, the Federal Trade Commission investigated pricing policies and charged these companies with violating antitrust regulations. But even if competition in the marketplace does bring down the price, nursing is still cheaper. In fact, one study concluded that two newborn babies could be breastfed for the cost of feeding only one baby by formula.

If you already eat right, you don't have to change your diet. You just need to eat small amounts of extra food to make up for the calories you expend in producing and giving milk. (See Chapter 7 for recommended eating patterns during pregnancy and lactation.) This will cost you less than you'd have to pay for bottles, nipples, sterilizing equipment, and formula. For the average family, formula takes twice the bite from the family budget as does the mother's extra food.

Another economic benefit stems from the better health of breastfed babies, which means fewer days the parents need to miss from work and fewer doctors' visits.

In view of the cost-saving nature of breastfeeding, the fact that women in low-income groups are less likely to breastfeed than more affluent women is doubly troubling. There is cause for optimism, though, in the increase in breastfeeding during the 1990s among low-income women. Programs of education and assistance—such as WIC (the United States Department of Agriculture's Special Supplemental Nutrition Program for Women, Infants, and Children)—that are planned especially for women of limited means have paid off. One such program is operated by the provincial government in Quebec, Canada, which pays low-income women to nurse their babies, on the basis that "encouraging nursing could ultimately save the publicly financed health care system millions of dollars a year."

Aesthetics

If you have a sensitive nose you'll appreciate the fact that your breastfed baby smells sweeter. Both bowel movements and excess milk spit up after feedings smell mild and inoffensive, unlike the strong, nose-wrinkling odors emitted by the bottle-fed baby.

Birth Control

Breastfeeding acts as a natural—although not totally reliable—means of spacing children. While your baby is receiving nothing but breast milk—no solid foods or formula at all—and is still being nursed during the night, you are less likely to become pregnant than is the non-nursing or partially nursing mother. This is because the fully lactating woman rarely ovulates. This is the basis of LAM, the Lactational Amenorrhea Method of child spacing, which will be explained more fully in Chapter 13.

Nursing a baby is not a guarantee against pregnancy, however. Although you are less likely to conceive while you're nursing, it is possible that you might become pregnant. If you want to plan the size and spacing of your family, you need to use some form of contraception. (See the discussion in Chapter 13 regarding forms of birth control that are suitable for nursing women.)

BENEFITS FOR SOCIETY

At a time when so much of our life has an unsettlingly unnatural aspect—with chemicals in the air we breathe, the clothes we wear, and the foods we eat—more and more of us are striving to recapture some of the natural joys of life on earth. When you breastfeed your baby, you know you're giving him the natural food intended just for him. Its purity is tainted by no synthetic compounds, no preservatives, no artificial ingredients.

If you're concerned about the environment your child will grow up in, you can appreciate the ecological superiority of breastfeeding. Feeding the bottle-fed baby entails the use and disposal of innumerable cans and bottles of formula, the cardboard cartons that package them, and the baby's bottles and nipples, which are also discarded, either after one use or after a few months. Then there's the energy used to transport the milk, and to heat it in the home, and the soap or detergents and water used to wash all that equipment.

WHY SOME WOMEN DECIDE AGAINST BREASTFEEDING

The reasons why women decide not to breastfeed are almost as varied as the arguments in its favor. There are a very, very few instances when a woman is physiologically unable to nurse her baby, as indicated in the box on page 25. Fortunately, such cases are extremely rare. Virtually every healthy woman can breastfeed her baby if she wants to.

Why do some women prefer not to breastfeed? This question has no simple answer. Some of the most common reasons given are listed in the box on page 27. All of these concerns are answered somewhere in this book.

None of these reasons exists in a vacuum. Most were born in history, either society's or the individual's. Many stem from a lack of knowledge; others from a lack of support even today. While it's up to each individual woman to look at her own personal reasons for her choice, we can take a look here at some relevant societal trends. In the next chapter we'll answer some of the questions that are most often on women's minds, and throughout this book we'll deal with these issues.

A HISTORY LESSON: HOW OUR SOCIETY HAS INFLUENCED WOMEN

Rigid Beliefs About Child Rearing

At the beginning of the twentieth century, psychologists, psychiatrists, and physicians were convinced that babies developed best if they were raised according to certain hard-and-fast rules. Mothers were ordered not to feed— or even pick up—their babies more often than every four hours, no matter how piercing or pathetic the infants' wails. Bottle-feeding was far better adapted to these practices. Breastfeeding requires flexibility, not rigidity;

When Breastfeeding May Not Be an Option

Breastfeeding may be either inadvisable or impossible in the following circumstances:

• When the mother has had surgery or trauma to the breasts that has severed the ducts. (In some cases the ducts have been known to reconnect, however, and therefore some women give nursing a try while closely monitoring their babies' weight and hydration status.)

• When the mother is so ill that she can't be with her baby and is too sick to pump her breasts.

• When the mother is infected with human immunodeficiency virus (HIV) that can be passed to the baby through breast milk. HIV has been linked to the disease known as AIDS (acquired immune deficiency syndrome). Although some research suggests that the risk of a child's contracting at least one type of human immunodeficiency virus (HIV-1) by breastfeeding is low even if the mother was infected with it prenatally, most public health advocates in developed countries advise against an HIV-infected mother's breastfeeding when a safe alternative is available.

• When the mother has insufficient glandular tissue, a very rare condition that affects fewer than 2 percent of women and usually can be detected in a prenatal breast examination (an important reason why your obstetrician should examine your breasts before you give birth). In this kind of situation, the baby can still be put to the breast, if he is receiving appropriate supplements to ensure proper nutrition for growth and development.

• In those rare circumstances when the baby has some condition or illness that makes it impossible to nurse. In such cases the mother's expressed breast milk may be given to the baby, if the baby is being closely monitored for proper growth and development.

understanding of a baby's needs, not the ability to tell time; and an intuitive response, not an adherence to a cultural fad. Also, because the child-care experts insisted that only they knew what was best for children, mothers believed them—and lost confidence in their own capabilities. And lack of confidence itself can sabotage breastfeeding.

Thus for about fifty years—from the 1920s till the 1970s—the United States served as the laboratory for the largest and most dangerous uncontrolled "scientific experiment" in history, perpetrated on subjects who, because they were infants, could not give their informed consent. The feeding method that had sustained our species for millions of years was discredited and abandoned, with no evidence to justify this wholesale rejection.

Changing Status of Women

At the same time mothers were being intimidated in the nursery, they were, in the "Roaring Twenties," asserting themselves on the street. Demonstrating to achieve the right to vote, bobbing their hair, and daring to carve out their own careers, women were eager to free themselves from their traditional roles in the house. The baby bottle became an instant symbol of emancipation.

Furthermore, as the quality of formulas improved during the 1930s, the act of giving a bottle achieved a certain status of its own. Women who wanted to be modern wanted to bottle-feed. Unfortunately, this urge to keep up, to be "modern," has wooed many poor women in both developed and underdeveloped countries around the world away from the breast, often with disastrous results. When money is scarce, mothers dilute the milk and babies starve; when refrigeration and sanitation are inadequate, the milk becomes contaminated and babies sicken. The World Health Organization, governments of many nations, and numerous private health organizations have mounted major campaigns around the world to encourage women to go back to safe, healthy breastfeeding.

Sexualization of Breasts

During the flapper era of the 1920s in the United States, tight binders hid and flattened women's breasts. Then, by the 1940s, pin-up photos were gracing barracks walls, exhibiting the new ideal of feminine beauty—a pretty young woman with large breasts. These organs, molded into fashionably pointed (and highly unnatural) shapes by the brassieres of the day, became purely decorative in nature, valued for their sexiness and forgotten for their function. This cultural attitude contrasts with that in most societies around the world, which do not view the mammary gland as erotic or sexual.

Embarrassed by the sexual nature of their breasts, many women shyly shrank away from touching them or using them in nonsexual ways. Many men jealously looked upon their wives' breasts as their own property and resented the idea of those breasts being seen by anyone else, even their infant children.

More recently, as more women have gone braless and as nudity has become more prevalent in the media, many women have become more com-

Reasons Women Give for Not Wanting to Breastfeed

- They think there's no difference between breast milk and formula as far as their baby's well-being is concerned.

- They're embarrassed about the idea.

- They're modest and neither want to nurse publicly nor have to run into another room whenever people are around.

- They think body secretions of any kind are "icky."

- They don't want to be tied down.

- They have to go back to work and don't want to start something they can't finish. (See suggestions in Chapter 12.)

- They want the babies' fathers to share more equally in the baby's care. (For ways this can be done, see Chapter 14.)

- They're afraid of ruining their figures.

- Their husbands or partners don't want them to.

- They think they don't have the right kind of breasts.

- They think they're too nervous.

- They're afraid they won't know whether their baby is getting enough to eat.

- They're afraid that they will have to restrict or radically change their diet.

- They think that breastfeeding plunges women back into traditional roles, negating many societal advances over the past several decades toward equality of the sexes.

- The whole business just seems too complicated.

- Occasionally, there is a reason that goes unspoken, but that often influences women against breastfeeding. For a woman who has suffered sexual abuse sometime in her life, among its many painful vestiges are feelings of shame and embarrassment around bodily sensations. Unless she understands where these feelings are coming from, she may be so uncomfortable with her body that she shrinks from breastfeeding.

fortable with the notion of touching and baring their breasts, at least to the extent required for nursing. As we'll see in Chapter 11, it's possible to nurse so discreetly that observers can't even tell what you're doing, which sets to rest a concern of many women and men.

TODAY'S SOCIETY
AND BREASTFEEDING

First, the Bad News

It's ironic that a society that equates motherhood with apple pie seems to choke over linking motherhood with mother's milk, as seen in the following ridiculous events:

• As we'll see in Chapter 11, women are still being arrested for breastfeeding in public—even when they are sitting in their own cars.

• The word *breast* has been held obscene as recently as early 1996, when the Internet server America Online (AOL) banned the word from its chat groups, thus making any discussion of breastfeeding or breast health impossible, unless subscribers used other (more colorful?) synonyms. (Fortunately, AOL changed its stance on this, after much protest by users.)

• The December 1997 issue of a leading national magazine for young women showed a breastfeeding mother and baby on its cover. But while its editor in chief said the photo moved her with its tenderness and its family feeling, she put a different cover photo on the version of the magazine that went to subscribers. Why? She wrote, "I know some people are uncomfortable with breast-feeding. I did not want to force that on anyone who is a subscriber."

• A 1996 article in another major women's magazine discussed cosmetic breast surgery with no mention of the care needed to preserve a woman's ability to nurse.

• Several retail chains refused to sell a 1993 issue of *Life* magazine whose cover showed a woman nursing her baby.

• A prominent pediatrician writing in *The New York Times* in 1996 used the phrase "an affected earth-motherism that flies in the face of common sense" to refer to mothers who nurse their children past the typical ages for weaning in our society.

• Greeting cards offering congratulations on a new baby, television shows, and movies trumpet the baby bottle as the symbol for infant care, routinely assuming that babies will be fed with artificial baby milk.

- Too many physicians, nurses, and hospital personnel are uninformed and unenthusiastic about the value of breastfeeding, and too many hospitals send new mothers home with samples of baby formula.

No wonder so many women are confused or embarrassed by the idea of breastfeeding!

Now the Good News

Today's woman is more comfortable with her body than in times past, is concerned with fitness and health for herself and for her family, and is less embarrassed to be herself. Our ideals of beauty have changed from the heavily made up, elaborately coiffed look of yesterday to the healthy, natural look of today. Thus, the contemporary woman is more likely to want to feed her baby in the healthiest and the most natural way.

In fact, the modern counterparts of those feminists who moved away from breastfeeding—the well-educated, middle- and upper-class women who set trends—are now among its staunchest supporters. They often, in fact, have to call upon the same qualities of strength and assertiveness to achieve their right to nurse as to achieve choice in other areas of their lives. Many women see their choice to breastfeed as a liberating one, one that challenges ingrained practices in the workplace and society in general.

Furthermore, society *has* changed in many ways. As new scientific findings affirmed the value of human milk, the 1990s saw strong statements urging virtually universal breastfeeding for at least the first year of life, and as long thereafter as mutually desired by mother and baby, by such major health organizations as the American Academy of Pediatrics, the United Nations Children's Fund (UNICEF), and the World Health Organization (WHO).

Meanwhile, in the United States many hospitals and pediatric practices have hired lactation consultants to help new mothers, and breastfeeding is once again becoming the preferred way to feed babies. Probably the first half of this century will go down in history as an aberration in its temporary rejection of this age-old natural means of nurture.

Still, even if you know you want to breastfeed, you may have many questions and concerns. Even after your questions are answered, you may decide that breastfeeding is not for you. You don't have to breastfeed to be a good mother. You shouldn't do something you find displeasing to please your partner, your doctor, your mother, your next-door neighbor, or your best friend.

WHAT WILL YOU DO?

A baby raised in a loving home can grow up to be healthy and psychologically secure no matter how she or he receives nourishment. Although nursing is usually a beautiful, happy experience for both mother and child, the woman who nurses grudgingly, tight-lipped, and stiff-armed, because she feels she *should,* may do more harm to her baby by communicating her feelings of resentment and unhappiness than she would if she were a relaxed, loving, bottle-feeding mother.

Ultimately, how you feel about your children is more important than how you feed them. When psychologists from Harvard University followed up seventy-eight people in their thirties whose mothers had been interviewed twenty-five years earlier, they found that neither the fact nor the duration of breastfeeding, like many other specific child-rearing practices, had any discernible effect on the way these people turned out as adults. The only thing that did matter was whether the parents had truly loved their children—and had shown their children that love.

If you are unsure about whether you want to breastfeed, you will want to learn as much as you can about the benefits of breastfeeding. And then you might ask the women in your family and your friends about their experiences with infant care—how they fed their babies, what the experience was like for them, and how they decided between breast and bottle. You might also attend a nursing mothers' support group, like La Leche League, and learn about other women's experiences. Then, weighing all the evidence, you can make up your own mind.

As we said earlier, we urge you to give breastfeeding a try. If you never give it a chance, you may well look back on this time in later years and wonder whether you and your baby missed one of life's greatest gifts—the bond shared by the nursing pair. The regrets we have in life are less often for the things we have done than for those missed opportunities that will never come again. This priceless chance to nurse your baby comes only once in each baby's lifetime. Make the most of it. You may count these nursing days among the most beautiful and fulfilling of your entire life.

Questions You May Have About Breastfeeding

I had so many questions and no one to go to with them. No one in my family ever breastfed, I had just moved to a new town where I didn't know anyone, and my doctor was so busy I was nervous about bothering her.

—ALIX, BOULDER, COLORADO

E veryone has questions about something they haven't done before—and until you've had a baby, you haven't breastfed one. We know you must be wondering about many aspects of this new activity and how it will affect your life, and so we want to address some of your concerns right away, even though most of them will also be answered somewhere else in this book.

Q: Will nursing make my breasts sag?
A: No, it will not. Some women notice little or no change even after bearing and nursing several children; others develop a definite droop after only one. Most women do find that their breasts become less firm and less erect after childbirth, but these changes are caused by pregnancy, not lactation. How much your breasts change will be determined by your genes, how old you are, and by the amount of weight you gain during pregnancy. Many nursing mothers feel that wearing a good, well-fitting nursing bra, even during the night, not only makes them more comfortable, but helps to maintain breast shape.

Your breasts will be larger during lactation, but if you're like most women, your breasts will return to their former size after you wean your baby. Some women feel their breasts are smaller after nursing, some feel they are larger, but most find no change at all. In any case, the die is cast by the time your first child is born; the change occurs as a result of pregnancy, and whether you nurse this child or not will have no permanent effect on the size and shape of your breasts. One small-breasted woman told us with a grin, "My figure never looked so good as when I was nursing—I felt as if I were wearing a WonderBra!" And fuller-bosomed women can also feel and look good during this time, with the help of a supportive bra and flattering clothing.

Q: Will I gain weight if I nurse?
A: No—on the contrary. Breastfeeding will help you return more quickly to your prepregnancy size. Many women have breastfed several children and ended up just as slim as they were before they became pregnant. Proper diet during pregnancy and lactation, combined with moderate exercise, will keep you slender. In fact, there's some evidence that nursing helps women to regain their figures, since the fat stores developed during pregnancy are laid down specifically for lactation. Women who do not nurse may have a harder time working off this fat. Just think of it—you're burning approximately 500 calories a day through lactation, as many calories as you'd expend on a five-mile run.

Q: If I nurse my baby, will I have to stay with her twenty-four hours a day? I can't bear the thought of being so tied down.
A: Parenthood itself, like any major commitment, restricts your freedom. After the first few weeks, when your milk supply has been established, your baby has become an expert nurser, and her feeding times have become fairly regular, you'll be able to work out a schedule allowing you to be away from your baby for various periods of time. Many employed mothers breastfeed despite full-time work schedules. (For suggestions, see Chapter 12.)

The first couple of months after childbirth tend to be confining for most mothers, no matter how they feed. You'll need to rest and you'll want to stay near your baby, both of which will keep you close to home. So even if you plan to go back to work or to resume an active schedule that would make breastfeeding difficult, you can still nurse your baby in the early months and give him the benefits of colostrum and the milk itself.

Some women successfully combine breast- and bottle-feeding on a regular basis after the first four to six weeks. The babies of working women may receive one or more bottles of formula or expressed or pumped breast milk while their mothers are on the job. Some fathers feed their babies bottled milk in the middle of the night or in the early morning while the mother catches up on sleep. And some mothers of twins regularly alternate breast and bottle for each baby.

The course of breastfeeding almost always runs smoother when the mother provides almost all of her baby's nourishment herself, at the breast, and relies on only an occasional bottle. In most cases it's best to wait awhile before

combining the two forms of feeding, until your milk supply is well established—at least six to eight weeks after birth. But combining the two forms of
feeding works well for some women and prevents that tied-down feeling.

Q: How long should I continue to breastfeed?
A: There is no one best time to wean your baby from the breast. The American Academy of Pediatrics recommends breastfeeding for at least the first
year of life—and longer, if both mother and baby want to continue. The
Academy states that exclusive breastfeeding for the first six months provides
ideal nutrition for your baby's growth and development. The World Health
Organization advocates breastfeeding for at least two years. However, you
will make your own decision about when to wean, based on many different
factors in your and your baby's life.

Q: Will weaning hurt?
A: No, gradual weaning should not hurt and should not be traumatic for either you or your baby. For a detailed discussion of weaning, see Chapter 18.

**Q: I have to go back to work when my baby is three months old; is it
still worth starting to breastfeed when I know I'll have to stop so early?**
A: Yes, it's well worth it. During those early weeks you will have given your
baby a good start in life, providing antibodies and immunities in both your
colostrum and your milk. Some breastfeeding is definitely better than no
breastfeeding. Besides, you may find that after you return to work, it will be
easier than you thought it would be to continue to breastfeed. For possible
ways of doing this, see Chapter 12.

Q: I like the idea of nursing, but won't it be embarrassing?
A: It doesn't have to be. You don't have to bare your breasts to feed your
baby; there are ways of nursing discreetly so that no one is even aware of
what you are doing. However, even if people do realize that you're feeding
your baby, what is shameful about this?

Our society's erotic interest in women's breasts has generated a taboo
against showing them in public, thus keeping many women from nursing.
It's a pity that the nursing mother, one of the loveliest subjects in art or nature, should be such a rare sight in our society. If you had been more accustomed to seeing breastfeeding women, you probably would not be so shy
about doing it yourself.

You can deal with these feelings in a number of ways, however. When
you begin to nurse, insist on privacy. In the hospital ask the nurse to draw a
screen around your bed; at home find a quiet nook where no one is likely to
disturb you. Chances are that after you have nursed your baby a few times,
you'll be so gratified by the experience that you won't find it embarrassing.

Furthermore, by being savvy about the clothes you wear, you can nurse in such public places as airplanes, department stores, or park benches without anyone being aware of what you're doing. Advice on nursing modestly in front of friends or even delivery people who suddenly appear at the door is given in Chapter 11.

Q: I hear so many stories about women who really wanted to nurse their babies but had to switch to the bottle because they didn't have enough milk or they couldn't nurse for some other reason. How can I be sure this won't happen to me?
A: Every healthy woman who has ever had a baby has had milk come into her breasts, and nearly all women can breastfeed when they receive encouragement, information, and support. The first two to three weeks are the most crucial: It's important to build your support network and reach out for help. For suggestions on doing this, see Chapter 4. With this help, you can develop the attitude that you can overcome any problems that arise. With this viewpoint, you're virtually assured of a gratifying nursing experience.

Q: My mother didn't have enough milk to nurse me. Will I take after her?
A: Probably your mom didn't get enough encouragement or information. The ability to breastfeed is not inherited, nor is it instinctual. Women need to learn how to breastfeed. Almost all cases of insufficient milk supply are due to mismanagement of one sort or another and to lack of encouragement from doctors, hospitals, family, and friends. Your mother may not have had enough milk because at the time you were born, the value of breastfeeding was not appreciated. Today, with a renewed realization that this is the best way to feed an infant, we have relearned the old ways of building a mother's milk supply (explained in Chapters 7 and 10) and are constantly coming up with new ways to help mothers and babies.

Q: How can I tell whether I have enough milk for my baby?
A: If you have enough information and encouragement, and if you nurse your baby frequently, you are almost assured of having enough milk. There are a number of markers to tell whether your baby is getting enough—most importantly, your baby's elimination patterns. These and other signs are clearly described in Chapter 6.

Q: I'm almost perfectly flat-chested. How could my breasts possibly hold enough milk to nourish a baby?
A: Women are often surprised to learn that the size of their breasts has no relation at all to their ability to produce milk. Many small-bosomed women breastfeed very successfully, and some have even donated extra milk for the benefit of sick or premature babies!

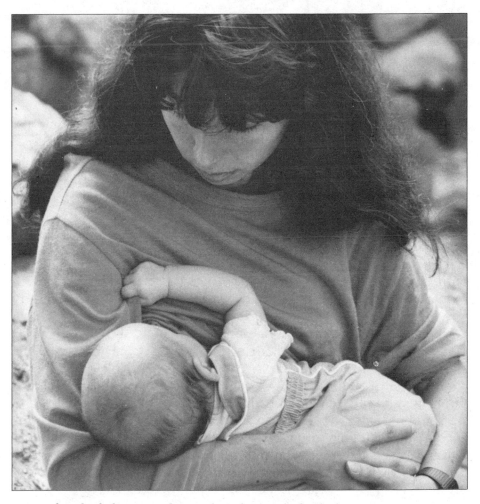

No one but this baby can see her mother's breasts, and onlookers may not even realize that she is nursing.

The size of your breasts depends on the amount of fatty tissue in your mammary glands. But the amount of milk you produce is determined by a process that is completely independent of the fatty tissue, as you'll see in Chapter 3. Your bra size is completely irrelevant to your ability to nurse your baby.

Q: Does breastfeeding hurt?

A: No, it should not. Some women do feel some tenderness, usually in the very beginning as the baby starts to latch onto the breasts. This initial discomfort usually goes away fairly quickly as the nursing mother becomes more expert in helping her baby feed. However, if you experience pain that lasts throughout a feeding and persists after the feeding is over, call your doctor or lactation consultant immediately to diagnose and resolve the problem, which is usually one of nursing technique. Chapter 6 describes the right way to put the baby to the breast, and also offers simple suggestions to alleviate discomfort.

Q: What happens when my baby gets teeth?
A: Probably nothing. The baby who's nursing properly cannot bite the breast. Some teething babies may try to bite down toward the end of a feeding, after their initial hunger has been satisfied. As little as they are, these infants can be gently taught, and can learn, not to do this. See Chapter 10 for suggestions for teaching a baby that biting is a no-no.

Q: Can I breastfeed if I have inverted nipples?
A: Most nipples that seem inverted (pushed in) work themselves out during pregnancy so that they're able to function normally after the baby is born. Sometimes exercises during pregnancy will help to bring out such nipples. Other cases may be helped by wearing special breast cups. It's very rare that nipples don't respond to these measures, which we describe in Chapter 4. But even in these cases, your baby will probably be able to nurse. Fortunately for the human race, right from birth we are born with strong survival skills.

Q: How can I tell if my milk is rich enough for my baby?
A: Your breast milk may look thin and watery, but if you are in reasonably good health and eating adequately, your milk will have enough of all the essential elements that your baby needs. Human milk normally has a bluish tint to it. See Chapter 7 for suggestions on how you should eat and take care of yourself.

Q: Suppose my milk doesn't agree with my baby?
A: Breast milk agrees with every baby. No baby is allergic to it. Some babies do react to certain foods that you eat, and if you find that your baby is rejecting the breast or developing colicky symptoms, examine your diet for possible offenders, as explained in Chapters 7 and 10.

Q: I've always been the "nervous type" and I hear you have to be calm to breastfeed. Am I doomed to failure?
A: Definitely not! A calm, relaxed mother may have an easier time breastfeeding than does a tense, nervous one. But over the centuries, millions of women have nursed during wars, natural disasters, and other highly stressful events. During times of emotional upset, the flow of milk may be de-

creased because the let-down or milk-ejection reflex is inhibited, but the quality of the milk is unchanged. If you find it hard to relax when you start to nurse, you can help yourself by following some of the suggestions in Chapter 10.

For many women the act of breastfeeding is a relaxer itself. This is probably due to the action of the hormone *prolactin,* which is released by the process of lactation, as explained in Chapter 3. Laboratory studies have shown that female rats fight less, maintain their body temperature better, and respond less to stressful situations when they're lactating. This moderation of the nursing mother's responses probably serves to protect babies from extreme changes in maternal behavior caused by outside stress. So you may be among the many "nervous types" who discover a new calmness through nursing.

Q: I want to breastfeed, but my husband doesn't like the idea. Is it worth making an issue about this?
A: Your husband may need both information and reassurance. You may want to point out some of the advantages nursing holds for him—like relieving him of the responsibility for those middle-of-the-night feedings. You can also reassure him that he can still play a major role in his baby's care; new babies need much more than food, as he'll see if he reads Chapter 14, which is addressed to fathers.

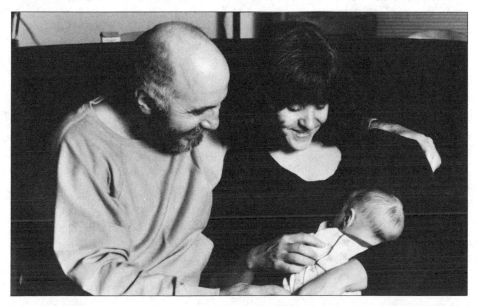

Many men become strong supporters of breastfeeding when they learn how it benefits the entire family.

Many a husband initially opposed to his wife's breastfeeding goes on to become her staunchest supporter. The help and reassurance of a supportive partner are enormously valuable, so it pays for you to make extra efforts to find out what his concerns are and to answer them as well as you can.

Q: Ever since I decided to breastfeed, everyone has been trying to talk me out of it. How can I deal with all this opposition?

A: Opposition to breastfeeding is less common these days than it was a few years ago, but you may still sometimes hear put-downs like "You wouldn't make a good cow" or "Why can't you be like everyone else and do the natural thing—give the baby a bottle?" or "What are you trying to prove?" Or people may blame your baby's every crying spell on your milk (or what they diagnose as your lack of it) or your doctor may suggest that you stop breastfeeding if you run into a minor problem.

When these situations arise, try to think why people say these things, and then respond accordingly. When people have good intentions but poor information about the normal course of breastfeeding, you can enlighten them. When a trace of jealousy affects a grandmother (who sees you care for your baby so competently without her help) or a friend (who did not have a good nursing experience herself), you can help build up *their* morale. And when a doctor seems to be misinterpreting your questions, thinking that you're asking for permission to stop nursing, while you're actually asking for support and information, you can be clearer in your communication.

In any case, once you make your decision to breastfeed, stick with it. You may not be able to change other people's minds, but you don't have to let them change yours.

Q: How will my older children react to my breastfeeding the baby?

A: Most youngsters are fascinated. They'll respond to your own attitude. If you let them know that you're doing the right thing, they'll accept this as the way things are. But if you feel guilty and afraid of making them jealous, they'll sense your vulnerability and will capitalize on it.

One study found that the older siblings of babies who were being bottle-fed misbehaved more at feeding time than did the siblings of babies being breastfed. Apparently, then, breastfeeding doesn't seem to add to the older children's stress. For more about emphasizing the positive with the older brothers and sisters of a nursing baby, see Chapter 11.

Q: When my baby is born, I'll be a single mother. Will it be too hard for me to take on the responsibilities of breastfeeding?

A: You certainly will have your hands full, but if you are like many other

Fighting Sabotage

When I (Sally Olds) was nursing my first baby, the baby nurse I had hired seemed to be jealous of my ability to feed my baby, and in subtle, and not so subtle, ways tried to sabotage the course of breastfeeding. Fortunately, my mother saw the nurse heating skim milk in a saucepan to give to the baby and told the nurse in no uncertain terms not to give the baby anything unless I asked her to. Soon after that, we told the nurse to go!

single mothers, you may well find that breastfeeding actually makes your life easier—and more gratifying. In fact, some single nursing mothers find that they especially appreciate the activity of nursing itself, partly because it ensures close physical contact with another human being and partly because of the relaxing properties of the high levels of prolactin in their system.

It's particularly important to take as good care of yourself as you can and to make special efforts to find people who can become part of your support network. This is one time in your life when you don't want to become too isolated. You may find help from an organization of other single mothers, or from a local breastfeeding or parenting group. Call upon your family and friends—upon anyone who can offer encouragement, as well as practical help. And try not to let your day-to-day practical concerns overshadow the pleasures you can get from this time in your life. It makes its demands on you, but it also proffers rich rewards.

Q: I hate milk. Do I have to drink a quart a day to make milk?
A: You don't even have to drink a cup a day. Although milk is an excellent source of protein, minerals (especially calcium), and vitamins, it's not the only source. You can either substitute other foods or take a vitamin and mineral supplement. (See Chapter 7 for suggestions on diet during lactation.) Recent research has found, however, that pregnant and nursing women do *not* need calcium supplements. The nursing mother is especially efficient at absorbing calcium—one more piece of evidence that nature intends women to nurse their babies!

Q: Do I have to eat special foods while I'm nursing?
A: Probably not, but that depends on what you've been eating up till now. If you've been eating a variety of healthful foods, you don't have to change your eating habits—except to take in about 500 extra calories a day to make up for the ones you use in making and giving milk. If your diet has been de-

ficient, however, this is a good time to make a change. Suggestions for a well-balanced diet are given in Chapter 7.

Some babies don't react to any foods their mothers eat, but others do. You may occasionally find that certain foods in your diet may upset your baby's stomach; common offenders are cow's milk and gas-producing foods in the cabbage family, like broccoli and cauliflower. Or your baby may seem especially wakeful after you've been drinking cup after caffeine-loaded cup of coffee or soda. You can then cut back on the foods in question while you're nursing.

Be sensible—and moderate. One mother called her pediatrician to say that her baby was fussy. "Do you think it might be due to the fact that I ate chocolate last night?" she asked. When the doctor asked her what she had eaten, she replied, "Half a cake." It's surprising she wasn't on the phone to her own doctor.

Q: Can I have a glass of wine or beer while I'm breastfeeding?
A: Yes. There's no evidence that moderate amounts of alcohol—a glass of beer or wine or one cocktail occasionally—will have any ill effects on your nursing baby. Heavy drinking, however, can be harmful: It can affect your ability to care for your baby, it can make your nursing baby drowsy by depressing his nervous system, and it may diminish your let-down or milk-ejection reflex. For more information about alcohol, see Chapter 9.

Q: Can I breastfeed if my baby is born by a cesarean delivery?
A: Yes. Your milk will come in just as quickly after a surgical birth as it does after a vaginal delivery if you breastfeed frequently. If you have not had general anesthesia, you will be able to nurse immediately, just as if you had had a vaginal delivery. If you did have general anesthesia, you will be able to nurse as soon as you are awake and alert enough to hold your baby. You will probably need extra rest, since you have just had surgery, and at first you will want to protect your incision with a pillow when you hold your baby. But these minor adjustments are only temporary. More information about postcesarean breastfeeding is in Chapters 5 and 6.

Q: Can I breastfeed while I'm menstruating? I've heard that milk given at this time isn't good for the baby.
A: Not true! You may find you have less milk when you menstruate, but the simple solution to that is to nurse more frequently. In any case, only the quantity of your milk will be affected—not the quality. Your milk is good, even though some babies are fussy and may refuse their mothers' milk during the menses, possibly because the flavor may be different.

As a matter of fact, you may not menstruate at all while you're nursing. But if you do, there's no reason not to nurse during your period.

Q: Will my baby's suckling at my breasts arouse me sexually? Or will breastfeeding make my breasts seem less erotic during sex?
A: Every woman is different. Most women do not experience sexual sensations from breastfeeding, but some do. Both responses are normal. Some women find that breastfeeding enhances their sense of themselves as sexual beings, whereas others feel that it seems to relegate their sexuality to the "back burner."

The most important thing to remember is that you can enjoy nursing if you do become erotically aroused by breastfeeding—or if such feelings are the farthest thing from your mind. Female sexuality is a complex issue that involves many aspects of your history and self-image. To explore some of these aspects, you will want to read Chapter 13, which discusses the relationship between breastfeeding and female sexuality.

Q: Does breastfeeding prevent pregnancy?
A: It may under certain circumstances. You have only a very slight chance of becoming pregnant if *all* of the following conditions are met: your baby is under six months of age, your menstrual periods have not returned, you are breastfeeding frequently (no less than every four hours during the day and every six hours at night), and your baby is receiving no food or drink other than what you give her from your breast. These criteria are the basis for the Lactational Amenorrhea Method (LAM), which we discuss in more detail in Chapter 13, along with various other methods of birth control.

Generally, if your nursing baby is receiving no supplemental bottles or solid food and is being nursed regularly during the night as well as the day, the hormonal balance in your body, with its low levels of estrogen, will prevent ovulation and therefore pregnancy for three to six months or even longer. Your first menstrual period after childbirth may be sterile; however, this period is a signal that you have either begun to ovulate or are about to do so.

Most women who breastfeed exclusively and often do not ovulate for at least the first two months after delivery. Most women, then, can use these first months to think about the kind of birth control they'll start to use by the third or fourth month after the baby's birth. In some cases LAM is effective even beyond six months.

But—and this is a big but—some women have become pregnant while fully lactating and before their menses have resumed. If you want to be absolutely, positively sure not to become pregnant, you will want to use contraception as soon as you resume sexual intercourse. You have to look closely at your own situation and make your contraceptive decisions accordingly. For more information about birth control choices, see Chapter 13.

Q: If I do become pregnant, can I continue to nurse my first baby?
A: You *can* continue to breastfeed, but most women do not. It's probable that your milk supply will diminish somewhat after the first few months of your pregnancy. Some women nurse one child right through pregnancy and then nurse both the first and the second (known as "tandem nursing"); others choose not to. Lactation and pregnancy both demand energy from the mother; the two of them together may take too much of a toll. Also, you need to be sure that the infant gets the colostrum he needs and an adequate supply of milk, which may be difficult if you're also nursing a toddler. Most women around the world wean a nursling as soon as they learn that they're pregnant. It is up to you to decide what is best in your circumstance.

Q: Can I breastfeed a premature baby who has to stay in the hospital for several weeks?
A: Yes, and giving your milk to your baby is one of the very best things you can do for her. The milk of women who have delivered prematurely has higher percentages of protein and fat, and a lower percentage of lactose (milk sugar) than does the milk of women who have had full-term babies. Because this milk's higher caloric density meets the special growth needs of preterm infants, it's better for them to get their own mothers' milk than to receive formula or even human milk from a milk bank. Therefore, many women feel it's well worth the extra effort to maintain their supply of milk until the baby comes home.

    Although you may not be able to actually feed your preterm or very small baby at your breast, you can express your milk and take it to the hospital until she is big enough and strong enough to suckle at your breast. More about this in Chapters 16 and 18.

Q: Can I still breastfeed after breast surgery?
A: You may be able to, depending on the kind of surgery you had. In recent years more surgeons have tried to perform breast operations in ways that would permit future breastfeeding. If you had implants inserted to make your breasts larger and if the incision did not cut the nerves around the areola (the dark area surrounding the nipple), you can probably breastfeed, at least partially. If you had surgery to make your breasts smaller and if the nipple/areola complex is still attached to the breast tissue beneath it, most likely you will be able to breastfeed. In any case, you will want to discuss

your surgical history with your obstetrician during your prenatal examination. You will also want to consult the surgeon who operated on your breasts. For more on this topic, see Chapter 16.

Q: I've heard that environmental contaminants like the insecticides DDT, dioxin, and dieldrin, the PCBs (polychlorinated biphenyls), and other chemicals are in breast milk. How harmful are they to babies?
A: *There is absolutely no medical evidence that breastfed babies suffer any ill effects from such chemicals*—except for a few rare cases of heavy occupational or accidental contamination. Scientists who have studied the levels of such pollutants in milk have stated repeatedly that the advantages of breastfeeding far outweigh the risk from these chemicals. No baby has been known to fall sick or become injured because of contaminants in human milk.

Human milk does contain some pollutants, as does the milk of every mammalian species that has been investigated. While some human milk does contain some chemicals at levels higher than that allowed in milk for commercial sale, this commercially acceptable rate is an extremely conservative one. For suggestions on protecting yourself and your baby from pollutants, see Chapter 7.

Q: Shouldn't breastfeeding come naturally? Why has it become so complicated that whole library shelves are stocked with books about it, a whole new profession (lactation consultant) has developed, and a bunch of organizations focus on it?
A: Human beings do very little by instinct alone. Practically everything we do has to be learned. If you had seen women nurse, and if your mother, your aunts, your older sisters, and your neighbors had breastfed, you would have learned from them, as women in traditional societies still do. But most of us did not grow up in a culture where breastfeeding is the norm. In fact, since the late 1960s and early 70s had the lowest rate of breastfeeding in American history, many new grandmothers don't have the know-how to pass on to their daughters. So new mothers need to find other ways to learn how to nurse their babies.

With this book we aim to offer the information you need to have a happy, fulfilling breastfeeding experience. You can learn more, of course. You can call a lactation consultant right after your baby is born. You can "talk shop" with other nursing mothers, either individually or in breastfeeding support groups. And one day you'll be so expert that you'll able to help other new mothers.

*T*he Miracle of Lactation

My baby is growing up strong and healthy and I am secure in my belief that I am doing the best thing for him.

—*Bonnie, Odessa, Texas*

*I*f you're curious about the technology of breastfeeding, this chapter is for you. Some of the material here may tell you more than you want to know at this point, so you may want to skim through this chapter and read only those parts that answer your questions, then look back later as questions arise. If you do read the whole chapter, we're sure you'll agree that *lactation,* the process by which a mother feeds her newborn baby with the milk produced by her own body, is truly a miracle of biologic design.

Among other information in this chapter, it answers such questions as:

- How do your breasts make milk and get it to your baby?

- How can lactation sometimes postpone menstruation and pregnancy?

- How does human milk differ from cow's milk?

Other sections will help you to understand how breastfeeding works and what is happening in your body.

THE DEVELOPMENT OF YOUR BREASTS

You probably remember when you first noticed your breasts beginning to bud, and the day when you shyly bought your first bra. In fact, your breasts began to develop long before that momentous day.

Your mammary glands, as the breasts are medically termed, began to develop when you were a six-week-old embryo in your own mother's womb. By the time you were born, the main milk ducts in your breasts were already formed.

Right after birth, your breasts may even have swollen and excreted a small amount of milk, known as "witch's milk." This very common phenomenon among both boy and girl infants, which subsides after a few days, is caused by the stimulation of the infant's mammary glands by the same hormones produced by the placenta to prepare the mother's breasts for lactation.

Your breasts are powerful and important parts of your body's glandular system. The parts of the human body that develop secretions are called *glands*. The endocrine glands (*endo* means within) secrete *hormones*, powerful chemical substances that pass directly into the bloodstream and then travel to other parts of the body. These hormones influence such basic processes as growth, sexual development, and even the formation of personality. The exocrine glands (*exo* means outside) secrete substances into ducts that carry them elsewhere in the body.

The breasts are *exocrine* glands, which are stimulated, both in their development and in their production of milk, by the hormones of the *endocrine* glands. Your mammary glands were inactive from shortly after birth until shortly before the onset of puberty, when hormones began to flood your body.

Changes in Your Breasts at Puberty

Your body then took its first step toward changing from that of a girl to that of a woman when your pituitary gland, the "master gland" of the endocrine system, sent a message to your female sex glands, the ovaries, directing them to make *estrogen* in sharply increased amounts.

Estrogen is the principal female hormone, the substance responsible for the growth of female-patterned body hair, for the sexual maturation of the genital organs, and for the development of feminine contours, including the swelling of the breasts that led you to the lingerie department for the first time. The pituitary gland also stimulated the manufacture of other female hormones, most notably *progesterone,* a hormone that actively prepares the body for pregnancy.

A combination of growth hormones and female sex hormones spurred the development of your breasts throughout your adolescence, until you reached your full body growth sometime in your late teens or early twenties.

Changes in Your Breasts During Your Menstrual Cycle

Although your breasts will not begin to produce milk until after the birth of your baby and the delivery of the placenta, they have been preparing for this time for many years. From the time you reach the *menarche* (your first menstrual period) until you arrive at menopause, a rhythmic cycle regulates your body.

Every month your system produces a series of hormones that prepare your body to bear children, thickening the lining of your uterus and increasing the blood supply to it. In the months you do not conceive, these preparations are washed away at the time of your menses. Ever optimistic, however, your body begins the entire cycle anew the next month.

The female sex hormones, estrogen and progesterone, produce changes in your breasts every month, ever hopeful that this will be the month that sperm and egg will find each other to create a new being. Just before you menstruate, your breasts may enlarge and may also feel tender. This is because the high levels of estrogen in your body make the blood vessels and glands in the breasts increase in size somewhat during this premenstrual phase, in preparation for a possible pregnancy. While estrogen stimulates growth, it inhibits the production of milk. This is why your breasts will not begin to produce milk until after you have a baby.

With the beginning of each menstrual period, your breasts quickly return to their previous state. If, however, you become pregnant, the heightened levels of sex hormones in your body produce many changes in your breasts.

Changes in Your Breasts During Pregnancy

When you first go to have your pregnancy confirmed, your doctor will perform a pelvic examination and will closely examine your breasts to look for signs that you have indeed conceived. Some of these signs that appear by the fifth or sixth week of pregnancy include a persistent fullness and tenderness of your breasts similar to premenstrual sensations, the sudden prominence of the glands of Montgomery (little bumps located on the areola), and the enlargement and darkening of both your nipples and your areolae.

The complete duct system in your breasts develops only now, when you are pregnant, stimulated in large part by the hormones from your placenta. The duct system is completed sometime during the middle trimester of your pregnancy. Thus milk is available for your baby even if you should deliver prematurely.

By the time your baby is born, glandular tissue has replaced much of the fatty tissue in your breasts. The development of this glandular tissue is responsible for the enlargement of the breasts during pregnancy and lactation. By the time of your baby's birth, your breasts will be larger by about a pound and a half each. They will remain at about this size during the early months of lactation and then will probably revert to their previous size— once you revert to your prepregnancy weight.

The placenta, that organ that transmits nourishment and oxygen from your system to your unborn baby's, also has another function. It serves as a chemical factory: In early pregnancy it takes over from your ovaries the job of producing large amounts of hormones.

Somewhere around the fifth month of your pregnancy, the placenta begins to produce a new hormone, *human placental lactogen.* This hormone stimulates the development of the alveoli, the little sacs where the milk is made. Once these are formed, your breasts begin to produce "early milk," or *colostrum,* a sticky colorless or slightly yellowish liquid that may occasionally drip from your nipples during the latter part of your pregnancy. (More about this "liquid gold" later.)

During pregnancy your body experiences rising levels of *prolactin,* a hormone that's very important for lactation. Your pituitary gland has been producing prolactin all your life, but when you are not pregnant or nursing, its release is usually blocked by a hormone known as *prolactin-release inhibiting factor (PIF).* During pregnancy prolactin levels are high, but its action is inhibited by the high levels of estrogen in your system.

Changes in Your Breasts After Childbirth

Once your baby has been born and the placenta has been delivered, the estrogen and progesterone levels in your body drop sharply. No longer inhibited by estrogens, your prolactin level rises dramatically, enabling the full-scale production of milk within twenty-four to forty-eight hours after childbirth. Your baby's suckling stimulates your pituitary glands to inhibit the secretion of PIF and to permit the production and release of high levels of prolactin.

Besides producing milk, prolactin also seems to have psychological effects. As we stated earlier, it has been dubbed "the mothering hormone" since laboratory experiments have shown that injecting it into a virgin animal induces motherly behavior.

The changed hormonal balance in your body sets in motion a chain of events necessary for lactation to occur. Extra blood is pumped into the small blood vessels of the alveoli, causing these vessels to enlarge and become visible beneath the skin, and making the breasts firmer and fuller. The manufacture of milk and the vascular expansion are responsible for the engorgement experienced by many—but not all—women. This engorgement (swelling caused by the pressure of the newly produced milk) and the temporary discomfort associated with it is almost always relieved by the baby's early and frequent nursing. (This is discussed in more detail in Chapter 6.)

Immediately after birth, the cells in the center of the alveoli undergo dissolution and are extruded into the first milk as colostrum. This high-protein, low-fat, and low-lactose substance has so many protective elements that it constitutes your baby's first immunization at this most vulnerable stage of life. Colostrum, then, is the first milk. At approximately three days after birth to the end of the first week, it gradually turns into the much more plentiful transitional milk. By about ten days to two weeks postpartum the mature milk has replaced the transitional milk.

The sooner and more frequently you put your baby to your breast, the sooner your transitional milk will replace the colostrum. If you have nursed a baby before, your milk will come in earlier, since your breasts have previously been conditioned for breastfeeding. Women who have nursed a baby previously seem to have a greater number of mammary gland receptors for prolactin. Therefore, they seem to produce more milk in the beginning, explaining why later-born infants begin gaining weight a little faster than firstborns.

When a New Mother Doesn't Breastfeed

The woman who does not breastfeed is apt to experience a great deal of discomfort from engorgement, which in her case may last from twenty-four to thirty-six hours. She may develop fever, headache, and throbbing pains in her breasts and under her arms. A firm bra, a mild pain reliever like aspirin, and the application of cold packs usually help to relieve discomfort until her breasts stop producing milk. In the absence of a suckling baby, this should happen within a few days. While medication used to be administered to a non-nursing mother to dry up her milk, this is no longer done. The strongest factor in drying up the milk is the lack of stimulation to the breasts. If a baby does not nurse and the milk is not otherwise removed from the breasts manually or with a pump, the alveoli get the message that they are not needed and they stop producing milk.

THE ANATOMY OF YOUR BREASTS

No matter what the size and shape of your breasts, you can have a gratifying breastfeeding experience. Whether your breasts are broad or narrow, high or sloping, small or large, you can happily nurse your baby. Just as women differ in height, general body build, and facial characteristics, they vary considerably with regard to the size and shape of their breasts. Furthermore, most women have one breast that's larger than the other. None of these characteristics are important for feeding a baby.

This is because the milk-producing glands are just one of the four types of tissue that make up the breasts. These four types are the *glands* that secrete milk, the *ducts* that carry it, the *connective tissue* that supports and attaches the breasts to the muscles of the chest, and the *fatty tissue* that encases and protects these other structures.

The size of your breasts is determined by the amount of fatty tissue they contain, and since the only purpose of this tissue is to encase and protect the more functional elements, it has no bearing at all on your ability to produce and give milk. You can be an excellent breastfeeder, no matter what the size or shape of your breasts.

The Nipple

Let's look at the breasts with a baby's-eye view. The nipple is the handle by which the infant grabs hold of the breast and also the spout through which she receives her milk.

The size of the nipple is usually as unimportant for nursing as is the size of the breast itself. Nipples come in different shapes. They are cylindrical in some women and conical in others.

The nipples of some women look flat or folded in and do not become erect when cold or when stimulated. Most often, however, by the end of pregnancy such "pseudo-inverted" nipples protrude normally and come out fully when the baby starts to suckle. In very rare cases, a woman has truly inverted nipples, which do not protrude enough for the baby's mouth to grasp them and which do not protrude with the baby's suckling. Fortunately, this condition is almost always correctable during pregnancy by the measures described in Chapter 4.

You have probably noticed that your nipples become erect when they're cold, or when you become sexually excited. The erect nipple becomes two to three times longer than in its softer state. The same thing will happen when your baby nurses.

Each of your nipples has fifteen to twenty tiny openings through which milk is excreted. As the nursing baby stimulates the many nerve endings in the nipple, this causes uterine contractions that help return the uterus to its prepregnancy size.

The Areola

Surrounding the nipple is a darker-colored circle called the *areola*. In most women the areola is between one and two inches in diameter, but it can be considerably larger. The areola and nipple are darker than the rest of the breast, ranging from a light pink in very fair-skinned women to a very dark brown in others.

The areolar pigmentation deepens in pregnancy and remains darker during lactation, after which the color fades somewhat; it never reverts, however, to the lighter shade it was before pregnancy. (This is one way doctors sometimes determine whether a woman has ever borne a child.) The

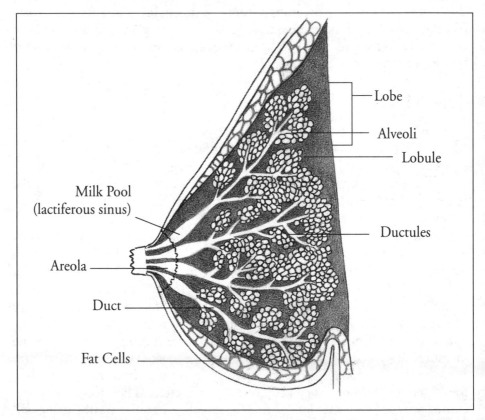

A cross-section of the breast showing the alveoli (milk-producing glands) and the duct system (milk-delivery apparatus).

darker color of the areola may be some sort of visual signal to newborns, since they must close their mouth upon the areola, not upon the nipple alone, if they are to obtain milk.

You may have noticed little bumps on your areola. These are called *Montgomery's glands*. They become enlarged and quite noticeable during pregnancy and lactation, because they secrete a substance that cleanses, lubricates, and protects the nipple during nursing. The antibacterial properties in this substance also help to prevent infection in both mother and baby. After lactation, these glands recede to their former unobtrusive state.

How Your Body Makes Milk

Directly beneath and behind your areola is a group of *milk pools* (known scientifically as *lactiferous sinuses*). These pools are widened parts of the milk-carrying canals *(lactiferous ducts)*, which transport the milk from the place in the breast where it is made to the nipples, where your baby can obtain it. (See the illustration, opposite.)

Each of your breasts has from fifteen to twenty ducts, each of which ends at the tip of the nipple. These ducts branch off into smaller canals within the breast toward the chest wall; these canals are called *ductules*. At the end of each ductule is a grapelike cluster of tiny rounded sacs called *alveoli*. The milk is made in these alveoli. Each cluster of alveoli is referred to as a *lobule* (a small rounded complex); a cluster of lobules is called a *lobe*. The lobes, each of which is a miniature gland, are situated at the base of the breast next to the chest wall. There are from fifteen to twenty lobes in each breast, each lobe connected to one duct, each duct emptying into one nipple opening, or milk pore.

Both the ducts and alveoli are covered with smooth-muscle cells. Under the influence of the hormone *oxytocin* (more later about this important hormone), these smooth-muscle cells squeeze the milk out from the alveoli into the duct system. Then the cells in the alveoli burst and extrude fat cells to form the *hind milk* (the fatty milk released at the end of a feeding session).

The Supporting Structure

In some cultures, women deliberately pull at their breasts to make them longer, so that it will be easier to nurse a baby strapped to their backs. Since this is probably not your aim, you'll want to give your breasts as much support as possible.

Nature provides some support—through the muscles attached to the ribs, the collarbone, and the bones of the upper arm near the shoulder. You can help Mother Nature along by wearing a good, supportive bra, even during sleep, during the latter part of your pregnancy and during lactation.

Although wearing a bra or going without one has no effect at all upon the breastfeeding function, the force of gravity will tend to pull down the heavier breasts of the pregnant or nursing woman. A supportive bra helps to prevent undue stretching of the suspensory ligaments of the upper part of the breast. Some doctors feel that a woman whose breasts are wide at the base will retain her figure, whether or not she wears a bra.

THE LET-DOWN REFLEX—HOW YOUR BABY GETS YOUR MILK

When your *let-down reflex* is operating well, you are overjoyed, not "let down" in the sense of feeling disappointed. Also known as the *milk-ejection reflex (MER)* and, in England, the "draught" (pronounced "draft"), the let-down reflex lets down your milk from your breast to your baby. The let-down reflex is automatic, and in almost all cases it does operate well, as it has for millions of years for almost all women.

In the early stage of lactation, it takes anywhere from several seconds to several minutes of your baby's suckling to produce a let-down reflex. After lactation is well established, you may find that hearing your baby cry or even just thinking about your baby will bring it on.

How can you tell when your let-down reflex is working to get your milk to your baby? The box on page 54 lists the usual signals, from the mother's point of view. To judge whether your baby is getting milk, which is a clear indication that your let-down reflex is working, see "Is My Baby Getting Enough Milk?" on page 118 in Chapter 6.

As your baby suckles, she stimulates the nerve endings in your nipples, which then send signals to your pituitary gland, directing it to produce more of the hormone prolactin. The prolactin stimulates the alveoli to produce milk. As long as your breasts are suckled or otherwise stimulated (as with a breast pump or with manual manipulation), they will continue to make milk.

Your baby's suckling also causes your pituitary to release *oxytocin,* another very important hormone for lactation. Oxytocin travels through your bloodstream to your breast, where it causes the smooth-muscle cells surrounding the alveoli to contract. As they contract, they squeeze the milk from the alveoli into the ducts. The walls of the ducts also contract, sending the milk out to the milk pools beneath the areolae.

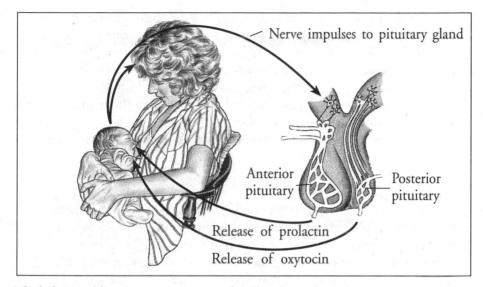

The baby's suckling initiates nerve impulses that direct the endocrine system to produce the hormones prolactin (which makes the milk) and oxytocin (which causes contractions that send the milk down the duct system into the milk pools).

While prolactin makes the milk, oxytocin makes it available to your baby. Animal research suggests that oxytocin also plays a part in stimulating the release of prolactin. In addition, oxytocin released into the brain promotes calming and positive social behaviors. Oxytocin has been called "the quintessential mammalian hormone," "the satisfactional hormone," and the "hormone of love." Besides its role in fostering bonds between parents and offspring, it also causes the uterus to contract during childbirth, orgasm, and lactation.

The Renaissance artist Jacopo Tintoretto portrayed a beautiful representation of the let-down reflex in his work *The Origin of the Milky Way.* The painting tells the story of Hercules, Zeus's son by a mortal woman, whom Zeus put to the breast of the sleeping goddess Hera to make him immortal. After the infant had stopped drinking of Hera's milk, the milk continued to flow from the goddess's breasts. Some went up into the sky, forming the galaxy, and the rest dropped on the ground, forming a garden of lilies.

The British scientist S. J. Folley points out that this picture illustrates two important attributes of the milk-ejection reflex: first, that the stimulus of suckling creates an increased pressure of the milk inside the breasts, causing it to spurt from the nipples, and second, that even though only one breast may be suckled, milk will flow from both.

Although the let-down reflex operates like clockwork in almost all women, occasionally some women need a little help to "oil the mechanism." Problems with let-down can usually be resolved quite easily. The let-down reflex has a strong psychological basis. The pituitary gland, which controls the release of oxytocin, is itself controlled by the *hypothalamus*. This walnut-sized organ in the brain is often referred to as the "seat of emotion," since it receives messages about the individual's psychological state and, acting on these messages, sends its own orders to the glands, translating emotions into physiological reactions. The emotions, therefore, exert a powerful influence on such hormone-regulated functions as the menstrual cycle, childbirth, and lactation.

When you have the confidence that you will have milk for your baby, even major stresses like war or natural disasters will not dam up the flow. But when you live in a society like ours, in which women often worry about their ability to provide milk, the slightest of emotions can interfere with your milk production. Pain, embarrassment, fear, fatigue, illness, or distraction can inhibit the let-down reflex and hold your milk back from your baby. If your nipples hurt you, your let-down may not work right. If you are distressed by the disparaging remarks of relatives and friends, your let-down may let you down. If you overtire yourself, don't eat properly, don't respect your own needs for privacy and for relaxation, your let-down reflex may be affected.

This is why it's important to prepare yourself for breastfeeding, both emotionally and intellectually. Chances are that even if you did nothing and

Signs of an Active Let-Down Reflex

Some of the most common signs that your let-down reflex is functioning are:

- A tingling sensation in your breasts
- A feeling of warmth and/or fullness in your breasts
- Dripping of milk before your baby starts to nurse
- Release of milk from the nipple other than the one your baby is suckling
- Cramps caused by the contractions of your uterus
- The relief of nipple or breast discomfort as your baby nurses.

Some women with very powerful let-downs do not experience many of these sensations, and some feel a brief period of pain in the early days when their milk lets down. Another way to check your let-down reflex is to look at your baby for signs of active swallowing (listed in the box on page 109 in Chapter 6); if she's swallowing, you're getting milk to her!

knew nothing, you would probably still be blessed with good milk production and an active milk-ejection reflex. But the more you know and the better you can manage the course of breastfeeding, the better your experience is likely to be.

MENSTRUATION, OVULATION, AND PREGNANCY

Women who do not breastfeed usually begin to menstruate and ovulate within one to three months after childbirth, while nursing mothers may not resume their cycles for more than a year. Your baby's suckling at your breast maintains high levels of prolactin in your system for at least the first few months of exclusive breastfeeding. These quantities of prolactin tend to suppress the action of your ovaries, preventing them from producing the hormones that trigger *ovulation,* the periodical release of *ova* (eggs).

Most women do not ovulate or menstruate at all while their babies are receiving no food other than breast milk and are suckling frequently, day and night, especially in the first few months after birth. If you are not releasing fertilizable eggs, you cannot become pregnant.

Nursing mothers who give their babies no water, no solid foods, and no milk other than their own breast milk in the first six months, who continue breastfeeding frequently thereafter, and who have not yet resumed menstruating have only a small likelihood of ovulating during this time. LAM, the Lactational Amenorrhea Method of birth control, is based on this premise.

However, as soon as your baby takes any supplementary bottles or solid foods, the baby's suckling becomes less vigorous and the prolactin level in your system drops. When your baby does not nurse for long stretches of time (during the night, or during the day for working mothers), your prolactin levels also drop. When there is not enough prolactin in your body to inhibit your ovaries from functioning normally, you will again resume your regular ovulatory and menstrual cycles. And you will be fertile.

There's a great deal of variability among women. One woman may have one "sterile" menstrual period before ovulation begins; that is, she may begin to menstruate but not yet be able to conceive. Another is fertile with her first menstrual period after childbirth. Some women don't begin to ovulate and menstruate for several months after their babies are completely weaned from the breast. Others ovulate even while they're fully lactating and before their menses resume.

So while you are *less likely* to conceive when your baby is totally breast-fed, you *might* become pregnant. Since it's impossible to tell when any particular woman will begin to ovulate, if you want to be sure to space your children you will want to use some kind of contraception. (Birth control for nursing mothers is discussed in Chapter 13.)

HUMAN MILK, THE ULTIMATE HEALTH FOOD

Colostrum, the Early Milk

"One of the dumbest things I was told in the hospital," one mother told us, "was that I shouldn't bother nursing for the first few days after my baby was born, since I wouldn't have any milk anyway."

Yes, this advice was truly unfortunate, since this mother's baby could have begun receiving the many benefits of colostrum right from birth instead of having to wait for this good food.

As we said earlier, probably from as early as the beginning of the second trimester of your pregnancy, your breasts have been producing *colostrum*, a wonderfully protective fluid that will give your child a head start toward a healthy life. For the better part of the first week after giving birth your breasts will be providing colostrum for your baby.

This clear or golden-colored fluid is an ideal first food for your baby for several reasons. While it's similar to true milk, it's easier to digest and richer in disease-fighting antibodies.

Over the past three decades, a great number of additional components have been identified in human colostrum, thirteen of which are unique to breast milk. The composition of colostrum is different from milk in a number of ways. Colostrum contains more protein, minerals, salt, vitamin A, nitrogen, and complex carbohydrates (mostly oligosaccharides). It contains nearly three times the amount of protein as mature milk; it has several amino acids and antibody-containing proteins that are not found in mature milk.

Colostrum has higher levels of immunoglobulin A proteins (IgA), which ward off disease. Secretory IgA, the most prevalent antibody in colostrum, coats the baby's intestinal and respiratory tracts, acting as a barrier to prevent the invasion of harmful organisms. Colostrum also contains higher numbers of white blood cells than milk does. And it's lower in calories since it has lower levels of fat and sugar.

The fat that colostrum does have is, however, higher in cholesterol than the fat in mature milk, which in turn has higher levels of cholesterol than formula. This seems to confer an advantage on breastfed babies, who have higher cholesterol levels than formula-fed children during the first year of life. These higher cholesterol levels may reflect a natural programming that helps breast-fed babies handle cholesterol later in life, and may explain why babies who have been breastfed are apt to have lower cholesterol levels as adults.

The main function of colostrum seems to be to protect the newborn against infection, but it may also provide important nutrients. It is especially beneficial for sick and premature infants. Another valuable function it performs is a laxative one of cleaning out the *meconium* from the baby's bowels. This greenish-black waste matter formed in the baby's intestinal tract before birth decreases the likelihood of jaundice in the baby by carrying a substance called *bilirubin* out of the baby's body. (More detailed information about jaundice is given in Chapter 6.)

Colostrum is very important to most animals, because it provides many essential immunities in the early weeks. Antibodies from colostrum have been found in the feces of breastfed babies, showing that the babies received these antibodies through their mothers' milk and that they are not destroyed by the digestive enzymes. These antibodies are not present in the intestines of babies who receive only formula. It seems probable that the breastfed baby's superior resistance to disease is due in part to these early antibodies, and in part to the oligosaccharides in human milk, the presence of which is highly correlated with resistance to disease.

Therefore, providing infants with this valuable fluid is a prime argument for feeding newborns as soon and as frequently as possible. It's also a good reason for beginning to breastfeed even if you feel you can do it for only a short time.

The Mature Milk

The mature milk itself is another magical elixir. Your baby's fare is custom-made by you especially for her at each stage of her development. Breastfeeding provides everything your baby needs—appetizer, main course, and dessert all wrapped up into one delicious food.

First, as we said, comes the colostrum. Then, from about four or five days to two weeks after birth, the breasts produce what's known as *transitional milk*. And finally, from about two weeks on, they produce a more *mature milk*. What is this true milk like?

The milk of every mammal has the same basic structure, but there are striking differences in chemical composition and proportion among the milks of various species. It seems reasonable to suppose that the milk of each species is especially suited to the needs of its young.

A Comparison of Cow's Milk and Human Milk

	COW'S MILK	HUMAN MILK
Color	Creamy white, due to high level of fats.	Bluish cast reflects lower fat content. Toward the end of a feeding, when fat content is higher, it looks creamy.
Vitamins	More D and K. Virtually no vitamin C.	More A and E, which may protect against anemia. Mother who eats well produces enough vitamin C for her baby. Babies need supplemental vitamin D if they or their nursing mothers don't get enough exposure to sun and if their nursing mothers are strict vegetarians. Vitamin K should be administered to newborns to aid in blood clotting.
Iron	Very little.	About the same amount of iron. However, the iron in human milk is better absorbed by the breastfed baby. Half of the iron in human milk is absorbed by the baby, compared to only 10 percent in cow's milk and only 4 percent in iron-fortified formula. Breast milk meets a baby's iron requirements for at least the first six months of life.

	COW'S MILK	HUMAN MILK
Other Minerals	Four times the amount of *calcium,* seven times the *phosphorus,* and twice the *sulfur* as human milk. The bottle-fed baby excretes a large portion of these minerals as excess.	*Zinc* is more available in breast milk, preventing one skin disorder that's never seen in breastfed babies. Two to three times the amount of *selenium* as in formulas. This mineral helps form a protective enzyme and is critical to developing and protecting a growing child's lungs.
Protein	More than twice as much as in human milk, and in a form utilized less efficiently by the baby. About half the protein in cow's milk is passed in the stool. Present recommendations for infant protein needs are based on cow's milk and therefore may be set too high. Casein is the predominant protein in cow's milk and is responsible for the harder (and smellier) stools of formula-fed babies.	Virtually all the protein in breast milk is used by the baby. Also, human milk has different kinds of proteins: Whey proteins (such as alpha-lactalbumin, lactoferrin, and secretory IgA) are abundant. Also present are *L. bifidus* and an antistaphylococcal factor. The whey protein portion of human milk contains most of its protective substances. Other small proteins present in human milk and absent from formula are growth factors that promote a baby's growth and development.
Sugar	Half that in human milk.	Lactose, the predominant sugar in human milk, (1) provides an important source of energy; (2) is essential for brain cell functions and enhances the development of the

(continued on the following page)

(continued from page 59)

	COW'S MILK	HUMAN MILK
		central nervous system; (3) is responsible for the beneficial acidity of the breastfed baby's intestinal tract (which, along with the presence of the *L. bifidus* factor, makes it harder for harmful bacteria to flourish); and (4) being less sweet than other sugars, may help in appetite control and the development of taste. Furthermore, the complex sugars in human milk seem to protect breastfed babies from a number of disease-causing bacteria and fungi.
Fats	Usually polyunsaturated vegetable fats are put into formulas to replace saturated fats in cow's milk. Do not contain DHA and AA, fatty acids essential for brain and eye development.	High in essential saturated fats (which are largely converted to cholesterol in the body). Breastfed babies have higher cholesterol levels during the first year of life, which may be the way nature programs them to help them handle cholesterol later in life. Human milk provides the long-chain fatty acids DHA (docosahexaenoic acid) and AA (arachidonic acid), which are not only essential for brain and eye development but which are thought to raise IQ scores in childhood.

	COW'S MILK	HUMAN MILK
		Babies digest human milk fat more efficiently than cow's milk fat because of the presence of the enzyme lipase.
Enzymes	Appropriate for calves.	Contains *lipase,* an enzyme that helps babies digest the fat of human milk more efficiently.
Growth Modulators	Appropriate for calves.	Constituents in human milk that help various cells develop and differentiate, these factors may have other roles, too. *Taurine,* an amino acid, aids in digestion and is also thought to be important in brain and nervous system development.
Hormones	Appropriate for calves.	Human milk contains *oxytocin* (may help foster a loving mother-baby bond), *melatonin* (helps regulate the baby's biological clock, letting the baby know when to eat), *gonadotropin-releasing hormone* (influences sexual development), *thyroid hormones* (may prevent certain disorders), *prostaglandins* (help to regulate body functions), *endorphins* (painkillers), and other hormones.

The whale, for example, gives milk that's rich in fats and calories—elements important for survival in cold water. Cow's milk is high in protein, calcium, and phosphate, ingredients that are important for the rapid growth of young calves. While human babies usually require about six months to double their birth weight, calves do this in a month and a half. It stands to reason that the higher protein and mineral levels in cow's milk (which are four times greater than those in human milk) foster this rapid growth, whereas the lower levels in human milk are more suited to the human growth timetable.

Even though we're constantly learning more about the unique structure of human milk, we'll probably never be able to identify every single one of its more than one hundred different components. Over the last forty years, hundreds of scientific papers have been published on the biochemical properties of human milk, and ongoing research continues to find new substances in human milk. The box on page 58 ("A Comparison between Cow's Milk and Human Milk") compares these two types of milk.

Like the milk of other species, human milk is mostly water—88 percent. Its nutrient portion—the other 12 percent—is made up mostly of fat, carbohydrate in the form of lactose (milk sugar), undigestible complex carbohydrates (mostly oligosaccharides), and protein. While this ratio is fairly constant, there is some variability from woman to woman and in the same woman at different times. Some of this variation stems from what you eat. The vitamins and minerals you take in will be reflected in your milk, as will the kind of fats you eat. As you'll see in Chapter 7, it's important for you to eat a variety of different kinds of foods.

Milk composition varies during a single feeding session. The milk secreted at the beginning of a feeding, the *fore milk*, is leaner than the *hind milk* secreted toward the end of the feeding, which may be 50 percent higher in fat. This high-fat content of the hind milk may give your baby a feeling of fullness, letting him know that it's time to stop eating. Milk composition also seems to vary from one feeding to another, although research is somewhat conflicting on this. Some studies have shown breast milk to be richest in fat in the morning and leaner as the day goes on, while others have shown it to be fattiest in the afternoon, leanest in the morning.

The protein content of milk also varies, with slight differences sometimes recorded even between the left and right breasts. Substantial change takes place over the course of nursing, as the very high protein level in the colostrum drops sharply in the first week and then continues to drop gradually throughout lactation. After about eight to ten months babies generally need other sources of protein.

The Uniqueness of Human Milk

It's most probable that, even with all our scientific know-how, no one will ever be able to isolate, identify, and copy all the constituents of human milk—the best food for the human baby.

Manufacturers of formula products do try. Aware of the differences between human milk and raw cow's milk, they use the latest scientific knowledge as a guideline for the preparation of nutritionally sound baby formulas. They use tables of recommended minimum daily requirements—and all their ingenuity.

Most formulas, for example, replace the butterfat in cow's milk with some combination of oleo, soy oil, corn oil, coconut oil, palm oil, olive oil, or peanut oil. They experiment with various types of sugars, add substances to help the baby's body synthesize fatty acids, and in other ways try to copy breast milk.

From time to time, however, scientists discover new compounds in breast milk, requiring new modifications of cow's milk. However, they will never be able to duplicate the species-specific ingredients in human milk.

One of the most exciting discoveries of recent years has been the finding that the composition of the milk secreted by women who have given birth prematurely is different from that of women who have borne a full-term baby. Nature's design is so elegant that each mother of a preterm baby produces milk that has the specific constituents needed by her own baby. This preterm milk is higher in protein, fats, and the salts sodium, nitrogen, and chloride. Thus it's better constituted to meet the needs of the preterm baby; however, the tiniest preterm babies may need additional supplementation.

As in so many cases, human milk is a sterling example of the inability of human invention to equal the creativity of nature.

Before Your Baby Comes

Now I have this incredibly healthy baby and I can be very proud knowing that I directly contributed to this by staying healthy during my pregnancy.

—CAROLE, HARRISBURG, PENNSYLVANIA

Even before you feel your baby's first stirrings inside your womb, you can prepare for your happy breastfeeding experience. You're already doing your baby and yourself a favor by reading this book and getting answers to some of your many questions.

During the months before your baby's birth, you'll have many decisions to make. In this chapter we'll answer questions like: What kind of medical and birth practitioners will you want? Where will you want to have your baby? What kind of delivery will you want?

Other questions will be answered in later chapters. For example, we offer suggestions on diet during pregnancy and after childbirth in Chapter 7. And in Chapter 12 we talk about issues that concern the breastfeeding working mother, such as how soon you'll be going back to work, what kind of maternity leave you'll ask for, and what kind of child care you'll arrange for.

CHOOSING YOUR HEALTH CARE PROVIDERS

Because the kind of medical and nursing care you and your baby receive before, during, and after the birth has such far-reaching impact on your health, as well as your baby's, you want to be sure that the people you consult are knowledgeable and skilled. And because how you feel about the experiences of pregnancy, childbirth, and your family relationship has such a major influence on the emotional well-being of everyone in your family, you want to feel comfortable and happy with your helpers.

These days, you have many options, and you should be able to find caregivers who match your needs and your preferences. The kind of practitioner you choose will depend on many factors—the community you live in, your philosophy about childbearing and medical care in general, your physical condition, financial considerations, the kind of health plan you have, and possibly the personality of the particular practitioners you meet. You may want an older, well-established parent-figure type, or you might be happier with a partner type close to your own age. You may prefer a woman or a man. The location of the practitioner and the medical facility she or he is affiliated with may be important as well.

The text that follows briefly describes the different kinds of health care providers you may be calling on. For help in choosing a specific practitioner, see "Finding a Practitioner Whom You Trust" later in this chapter. Also consult the Resource Appendix.

To clarify your thinking and help you decide, you can talk to friends, as well as representatives of childbirth education organizations. You can also consult books about pregnancy that describe the specialties described in the following section in greater detail.

TYPES OF HEALTH CARE PROVIDERS

Obstetrician-Gynecologist (OB/GYN): Most women in America have their babies with the help of a physician who specializes in treating women and in delivering babies. Such a doctor will see you periodically throughout your pregnancy, will monitor the progress of your baby while it's still in the uterus, will deliver your baby, will examine you after childbirth, and then will see you throughout your life for routine checkups and care of your reproductive organs and your breasts. Women whose medical histories or present circumstances put them in the "high-risk" category are especially likely to seek the services of an obstetrician.

Family Physician: This up-to-date version of the general practitioner who takes care of everyone in the family is a far cry from the old-fashioned GP who used to make house calls in a horse and buggy. Family practice has been a recognized medical specialty since 1969, and family physicians can now receive certification after passing rigorous examinations enabling them to be the doctor of first contact. Family physicians can provide a continuity of medical care born from long years of treating family members. Many family doctors undergo special training to deliver babies, after which they continue to care for the new baby, as well as for the rest of the family.

Midwife: The tradition of women who are not trained as physicians but who assist women giving birth is an old and respected one. Today, such practitioners generally care for women with low-risk pregnancies and uncomplicated births. They usually devote a great deal of time to their patients and offer emotional, as well as physical, support. They help both before and after childbirth, lend helping hands when needed, and offer experience-based advice. Most will assist at home births.

Midwives range considerably in terms of training and accreditation. Before engaging one, learn her qualifications, talk to other women who have used her services, and discuss with her in what circumstances she would call in a physician who could respond quickly in case of a medical emergency. (To find a midwife, see the Resource Appendix.)

Certified Nurse-Midwife (CNM): A CNM is a registered nurse who has completed a course in midwifery training and passed a certification examination given by the American College of Nurse Midwives Certification Council (ACC). Certified nurse-midwives generally work in conjunction with physicians in private practice, in maternity or birth centers, and in some hospitals.

Other midwives, who are not nurses, are known as "direct-entry midwives" or "lay midwives." Some are licensed and legally permitted to practice in some states. Some have served as apprentices to experienced midwives and/or studied at private or college-affiliated midwifery schools. *Certified Professional Midwives* (CPMs) become certified after successfully completing a written examination and skills assessment, like the one administered by the North American Registry of Midwives (NARM). Other midwives practice independently (legal status varies by state) with neither certification nor license.

Pediatrician: These physicians are specially trained and certified to take care of children from birth through adolescence, although some pediatricians continue to see their patients into young adulthood. Since they usually see at least one parent, and often both, when they see a child, they come to know the entire family and often serve as the doctor of first resort for everyone.

If you plan to consult a pediatrician for your child, it's a good idea to choose one at least three months before your due date. While this doctor will not care for the developing fetus, she or he will be able to examine your baby immediately after birth. If you deliver prematurely or if any complications arise with your baby's health, you'll feel more confident placing your baby's care in the hands of someone you have already met rather than having to deal with a complete stranger.

Lactation Consultant (L.C.): This relatively new kind of health professional specializes in promoting, protecting, and supporting breastfeeding, largely by hands-on, person-to-person contact with a nursing mother and baby. Such consultants can give telephone or in-person counseling for breastfeeding problems, either in private practice or in affiliation with a pediatrician, a hospital, or a maternity center. L.C.'s come from many different backgrounds; some started out as nurses, midwives, or physical therapists, while others come from completely different fields, including lay breastfeeding support organizations.

They function independently to evaluate a breastfeeding problem, come up with a treatment plan, and then report to the client and her physician. Look for an L.C. who has passed an examination given by the International Board of Lactation Consultant Examiners (IBLCE) and can use the letters *IBCLC* (International Board Certified Lactation Consultant) after her name. For more information about IBLCE, see the Resource Appendix.

Volunteer Breastfeeding Consultant: The women who lead local groups of La Leche League International are experienced nursing mothers who have undergone training to become accredited leaders. They hold monthly meetings for pregnant and nursing women; the first meeting is free, and after that women who want to continue attending meetings are asked to become League members. The leaders provide answers to breastfeeding questions, either over the phone or in person, and also refer women to professional sources of information. In some communities, other groups help nursing mothers in this way.

It is helpful to attend meetings during your pregnancy to get a preview of what to expect after your baby arrives, to establish a relationship with people knowledgeable about breastfeeding, and to meet other nursing mothers. To find the closest La Leche League group, look in your local telephone directory, or contact the League's headquarters, listed in the Resource Appendix.

Doula: Anthropologist Dana Raphael coined the term *doula* for a person (almost always a woman) who "mothers the mother." As compared to a "baby nurse" who is hired solely to care for a newborn, a doula focuses on the mother. She provides emotional and practical support before, during, or after delivery—or at all three times. Her involvement may center around infant care, breastfeeding, and other postpartum needs like cooking, laundry, and caring for older siblings. Research has found that the support of a doula results in shorter labors, less use of childbirth medication, fewer forceps and cesarean deliveries, and more positive breastfeeding outcomes.

In traditional societies, and also in our own, a new mother's doula is often her own mother or another woman in the community. In addition, the profession of doula has been launched. Professional doulas receive special training, register with agencies, and go into families' homes for pay. Two agencies that refer doulas are listed in the Resource Appendix. Although this service can be costly, if you have no one else who can help you and if your budget will allow it, it is often well worth the expense.

Baby Nurse: Some new mothers hire someone whose principal duty is to care for the new baby. The baby nurse is often a licensed practical nurse (L.P.N.) or a personal care aide (P.C.A.) rather than a registered nurse (R.N.); or she may be a woman who has had no further training beyond her experience in raising her own children. Typically a baby nurse diapers, bathes, and comforts the baby, and cares for the umbilical cord site. She also launders the baby's clothes and bed linens. In the case of a breastfed baby, she takes the baby to the mother for feedings. Often, the nurse will also prepare simple meals for the family and do light housework.

This service is also costly. If your pregnancy and delivery have been uncomplicated and you feel good, and if you are breastfeeding, you would probably be better served by a doula, or someone who comes in to do household chores, so that you can be your baby's principal caregiver. However, if you are not feeling well and you have no family members who can help you, and you can afford it, you may want to hire a baby nurse for the first week or two of your child's life. You should interview baby nurses with particular emphasis on their positive attitudes toward breastfeeding.

In addition to personal recommendations from other women, you can find a baby nurse (or a housekeeper) through local employment agencies that specialize in home health care. They are listed in the Yellow Pages under Home Health Services or under Nurses.

Finding Possible Candidates

It sometimes requires some effort to find the right person or people for you—someone who is skilled, who shares your philosophy about childbearing and child care, and who is both knowledgeable and enthusiastic about breastfeeding. Although many doctors are very helpful to the breastfeeding family, recent surveys of physicians' knowledge, attitudes, training, and experience have found dismaying gaps in breastfeeding knowledge in all three of the specialties most involved with nursing mothers and babies (obstetricians, pediatricians, and family practitioners). In one study, while more than 90 percent of the doctors expressed enthusiasm about the value of breastfeeding, almost one out of three practicing physicians was not able to give the correct advice to mothers who felt they did not have enough milk. Hence, you need to look carefully for the doctors and other practitioners you'll want to help you with your pregnancy, childbirth, and child care. To find the most helpful people, you can:

- Ask friends who have recently had babies.

- Ask your family doctor or gynecologist for a recommendation.

- Call a local hospital or birthing center and ask for a recommendation to one or more people on their staff.

- Call your local medical society and ask for referrals.

- Call representatives of the organizations listed in the Resource Appendix. Look in your local telephone directory first; if you don't find a listing, contact the national offices.

Finding a Practitioner Whom You Trust

Once you have the names of one or more practitioners in the categories you're looking for, you'll want to make your selection based on a number of criteria. Basically you'll want to know the following:

- *Is the practitioner competent?* After you locate an accredited hospital or maternity center whose maternity policies are at least close to those in the Baby-Friendly Hospital Initiative described later in this chapter, you can ask whether a particular practitioner is affiliated with the institution and has staff privileges (the ability to admit and treat patients).

 You can contact one of the organizations listed in the Resource Appendix to find out whether a practitioner is a member. And you can consult your library's copy of *The Directory of Medical Specialties* for information about a doctor's credentials. Or you can ask the practitioner or his/her office staff about the practitioner's degrees, accreditation, and certification.

- *Can you schedule a consultation?* Call the practitioner's office and ask to make an appointment for a consultation. Ask what the fee is, as compared to a complete examination. If the practitioner does not offer consultations, go in for an examination and spend time talking to him or her. Ask your partner to go with you, since this decision will affect him and his child, too.

 In your preliminary consultation, you can find out how a prospective birth attendant feels about issues like those covered by the questions in the box on page 70 and any other childbirth- and child-care-oriented issues that

Questions to Ask
Your Birth Attendant

- How do you feel about anesthesia during labor and delivery? (See the discussion of childbirth medication in Chapter 9, which can help you talk to your attendant about this.)

- In what circumstances would you use forceps to deliver a baby?

- How frequently do you perform an episiotomy on the mother?

- What circumstances would call for induction of labor?

- Do you routinely give enemas to women giving birth?

- Do you routinely shave women's pubic hair?

- What conditions do you feel warrant a cesarean delivery?

- How soon after birth do you recommend that a mother breastfeed?

- When do you recommend rooming-in for mother and baby?

- Do you recommend circumcising newborn boys?

- At what age do you think babies should begin to eat solid foods?

- If I go into labor at a time when you are not available, what backup coverage do you have?

- What provisions do you have for childbirth emergencies?

For pediatricians and family practitioners you can also ask:

- How many breastfed babies are in your practice?

- About how long do the mothers in your practice breastfeed?

are important to you. Before you go, prepare a list of the questions you want to ask—with the most important ones first so you'll be sure to ask them. If you go in with a fair, nonbelligerent attitude, you should get a friendly and open-minded reception.

If, however, the practitioner seems impatient or annoyed with your questions, wants to impose his/her views on you, or tries to soothe you with a "doctor-knows-best" attitude, you will have learned something valuable right at the beginning, and you may want to continue your search for a more compatible caregiver.

If you emerge from your consultation feeling confident that you made the right choice, your shopping is over. If you're not completely convinced, you don't have to say anything yet. Meet the other people on your list and then make up your mind.

• *Is the practitioner knowledgeable and enthusiastic about breastfeeding?* Ask the practitioner what percentage of his/her patients nurse their babies (the higher the percentage and the longer they nurse, the more helpful the practitioner is likely to be), which hospital she or he is affiliated with, and how available she or he is to answer questions outside of regular office visits. A practitioner who has the letters *IBCLC* after his or her name has been certified by the International Board of Lactation Consultant Examiners (IBLCE). At the very least, you know that this person has passed a standard qualifying examination as a knowledgeable lactation consultant. Many pediatricians these days have on their office staffs certified lactation consultants, whom you can consult by phone or in the office. An increasing number of pediatricians are becoming certified as lactation consultants themselves.

• *Actions may speak louder than words.* What does the practitioner do? If, for example, you have already consulted an obstetrician, ask yourself these questions: Did s/he examine your breasts at your first prenatal visit; assure you that there is no reason why you cannot breastfeed, or else pick up problems that need to be taken care of; point out the benefits breastfeeding confers on both mother and baby; and answer your questions patiently and knowledgeably?

• *Especially for doulas and midwives.* You can ask your prospective candidate whether she provides prenatal and/or postpartum visits to your home, and what she will do in these visits; how many births she has attended; what her training has been; what references she can provide; what kind of backup arrangements she has in case of emergency; and how she defines her role during labor, birth, and the postpartum period.

• *Fees.* Ask the practitioner directly, or talk to the office receptionist. Also ask whether a sliding scale, a barter arrangement, or an extended payment plan is available.

You may find that you're not 100 percent happy with any of the practitioners you meet. Few matchings are perfect—most of us don't love everything about our spouses or our children, either. But if the good outweighs the bad by a comfortable margin, you're probably headed for an acceptable situation. Supportive health care providers are immensely helpful, but you can have a good nursing experience without them. You can find your own support among your family, your friends, local support groups, and written materials. You can take the best that your practitioner has to offer—and help him or her learn through your experience—and both of you will gain.

As you read this, you may be well along in your pregnancy—and unhappy with your practitioner. Or your baby may be born already and you feel that your doctor is not as helpful as you had expected. Changing birth attendants or doctors is not a decision to be undertaken lightly, but it is possible, and sometimes advisable. Your first obligation is to your own and your family's mental and physical health, not to your practitioner's feelings. Besides, health care professionals are made of pretty durable stuff; they recognize that they can't be all things to all people and that sometimes a switch is better for everyone concerned. The possibility of such a change is an important reason for not prepaying your entire obstetric fee.

• *Who is the expert here?* You are. No matter how knowledgeable and experienced a professional person is, you are ultimately the expert on your own life. This is your pregnancy, your labor, your birth experience, and your baby. While the practitioner may be an expert in his or her field, you are an expert on your body and your child. You need to have enough faith in yourself and in your good judgment to know when to follow advice and when not to. Yes, of course, you will follow your doctor's advice in medical matters and your lactation consultant's in breastfeeding matters—but when they express their beliefs about parenting (like what constitutes "spoiling" a baby, or at what age you should wean your child from the breast), you need to remember that such opinions are only opinions, nothing more. No one has all the answers on what is right for you and your baby, but everyone has advice for new mothers! So you need to treat all advice, including this book, as a smorgasbord from which you take what seems to make sense and leave the rest.

Your Health Insurance

Often we have little or no say over which insurance plan will cover our medical care. We take what we can get from our employer or our spouse's employer—and feel lucky to be insured at all, in these days of soaring medical costs. However, if you are in a position to choose your health insurance provider, you will want to choose the plan that offers the most benefits to you as a breastfeeding mother.

These days, more and more patients are being asked to choose a "managed care" plan. Such a plan usually stipulates that you get your services only from the providers included in the plan network (or else pay extra for your care) and that you are assigned to a primary care physician who makes all referrals to specialists.

If you are exploring different plans, you will want to ask the following questions:

• Do you cover the services of a lactation consultant (L.C.)?

• If so, how many visits are allowed under the plan?

• Do you pay all the costs for the L.C.'s services? If not, what percentage do you pay?

• If lactation consultants are not covered under the basic plan, do you have another type of policy that I can upgrade to?

• If I have a breastfeeding problem, do you offer a free follow-up visit on the second or third day after birth with a physician or a lactation consultant?

Even if you do not have a choice of plans, it is worth raising these questions. If consumer demand is great enough, your employer or other organization that contracts for your health plan can sometimes negotiate a special rate for special services.

A powerful argument for including lactation consultants in a health plan is its cost-effectiveness. According to the cost analysis prepared by Miriam H. Labbok, M.D., director of the World Health Organization Collaborating Center on Breastfeeding, if insurance companies spent money to provide lactation consultants, fewer babies would get sick because they would be breastfed. If infants nursed for twelve weeks, the insurance companies would save 57 cents for every dollar currently spent for care of the illnesses that would not occur among these babies. Nationwide, over the next ten years, public and private insurers and HMOs would save about $2 billion.

If your health insurance does not cover the services of lactation consultants, some L.C. agencies will give you the opportunity to self-insure. Wellcare, Inc., in New York City, for example, ordinarily charges $165 for the first home visit and $120 for follow-up home visits, and $150 for the first office visit and $100 for follow-ups. But if a woman signs up before she gives birth, she can pay a flat rate of $550 that covers one prenatal breastfeeding class, an initial visit in hospital or home, and as many follow-up visits as are necessary. If she signs up after delivery, the flat rate is $650. This, then, is one possible option, one that might be well worth the money *if* you have received glowing recommendations for a particular L.C. or agency, and especially if you do not have other knowledgeable resource people to help you.

CHOOSING WHERE
YOU'LL GIVE BIRTH

At about the same time that you choose your birth attendant, you'll be deciding where you want to have your baby. The practitioner of your choice may not have staff privileges at the institution of your choice, so you may have to compromise on either the "who" or the "where." On the facility, there are three basic options:

Hospital

While many hospitals are big and impersonal, with rigid rules that often seem designed for the smooth functioning of the institution rather than the individual, others are run with the comfort and well-being of the patient more in mind.

Furthermore, as more has been learned about the optimal conditions for successful breastfeeding, more hospitals have implemented at least some of the policies of the "Baby-Friendly Hospital Initiative," launched in 1991. According to this program, every facility providing maternity services and care for newborn infants should follow ten steps to support the breastfeeding mother and baby. Although these steps represent the ideal, as of this writing the United States has only fourteen certified Baby-Friendly Hospitals. So the odds are that your hospital won't be practicing all ten steps listed in the box on page 75.

However, the policies in the initiative have been gaining ground. For one thing, as hospitals have needed to compete more for fewer maternity cases, they have become more responsive to the desires of patients. Many now have rooming-in policies, permit fathers or other labor coaches to remain with the mother during labor and birth (including cesarean births), and offer such other aspects of family-centered maternity care as birthing rooms and family rooms that let siblings be present during childbirth. (Some even have queen-size beds that allow fathers to spend the night.) Another policy that benefits nursing mothers and babies is *not* distributing discharge packs of infant formula (or coupons for them) to nursing mothers. Research has shown that mothers breastfeed for a longer time when they have rooming-in and when they do not receive formula when they leave the hospital.

Hospitals *can* change and be more humane, in response to demands from patients and medical and nursing professionals. If you have a choice of

The Ten Steps to Successful Breastfeeding in a Baby-Friendly Hospital

A baby-friendly hospital should:

1. Have a written breastfeeding policy and routinely communicate it to all health care staff. (The policy should assume that breastfeeding is the standard method of feeding.)

2. Train all health care staff in skills necessary to put the policy into practice.

3. Inform all pregnant women about the benefits and management of breast-feeding. (Ideally, the hospital should offer prenatal classes for couples.)

4. Help mothers begin to nurse within about an hour of birth.

5. Show mothers how to nurse, and how to maintain lactation even if they should be separated from their infants.

6. Give newborns no food or drink (including water) other than breast milk, unless there is a medical reason.

7. Establish rooming-in: Allow mothers and babies to remain together, twenty-four hours a day. A major advantage of rooming-in is that, by being with her baby, the new mother can learn to recognize signals of hunger (like rooting, sucking on his fist, or making small sounds) before the baby starts to cry vigorously. He is likely to nurse better if he can be fed *before* he gets very hungry and frustrated.

8. Encourage breastfeeding on cue; that is, whenever the baby seems to want to nurse, as shown by rooting, sucking on his fist, or crying.

9. Give no pacifiers to nursing babies.

10. Help to establish breastfeeding support groups and refer mothers to them when they leave the hospital.

hospitals in your community, ask about their regulations and policies, and go with the one that offers more family-centered services. The more often patients ask for these services, the more hospitals will offer them.

The big plus of a hospital birth is that, should any complications occur, you will have an array of modern technology and professionals. If your pregnancy is considered high-risk, you'll certainly want to give birth in the hospital. According to a federal law enacted in 1998, neither your hospital nor your insurance company can demand that you leave the hospital sooner than forty-eight hours after a vaginal delivery and ninety-six hours after a cesarean birth. If, as usually happens, your vaginal birth proceeds smoothly and your baby is healthy—and if you have helpful resources at home—you may elect to go home within eight to twenty-four hours.

Even if your hospital does not have ideal family-centered policies, you can still have a good birth experience. You can ask your doctor to leave these written instructions: to help you nurse your baby within one hour of birth; to have your baby brought to you whenever she seems hungry, including the middle of the night (if you do not have rooming-in); not to give her any bottles of water or formula; and any other procedures that will help launch a successful course of breastfeeding.

And you need to remember one very important thing: Even if your hospital stay does not go the way you'd like it to, remember that you'll be there for only a short time and that many women have overcome less than ideal hospital practices to go home and embark upon long and happy breastfeeding experiences.

As one mother told us after reading an earlier edition of this book: "When I was crying in the hospital because I was getting such conflicting ad-

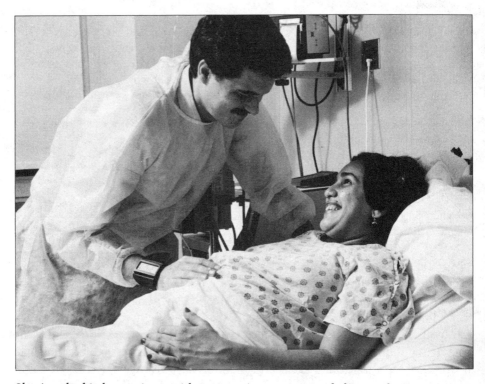

Sharing the birth experience with a supportive partner can help to make it more comfortable and more exciting.

Packing Your Bag

About six weeks before your due date pack a small bag containing the items to take with you to the hospital or birth center. Among those you may want to include:

- *A nursing bra.* Buy one or two in your eighth month of pregnancy. For suggestions on how to choose a nursing bra, see Chapter 8. Some hospitals supply halter-type tops. Although your own bras are more attractive, the hospital launders its supplies but not your personal items. The choice of beauty or convenience is up to you.

- *A nursing nightgown.* This will have hidden side slits on the bodice. You'll look prettier than you would in those one-size-fits-all less-than-flattering hospital gowns and you'll have it to wear at home.

- *A few pairs of underpants.* Whatever you wore while you were pregnant—bikini or maternity panties—will still fit since it takes a while to regain the waistline you once knew. The hospital will provide sanitary napkins, but you'll feel more comfortable wearing your own undergarments.

- *Telephone numbers.* These should include your childbirth educator, your obstetric care provider and your pediatrician or family doctor (so you can call your doctor in the office, for example, instead of trying to catch him or her in the hospital), your lactation consultant, and a local La Leche League leader, so you can reach them easily if you have questions. And of course, the friends and family members you'll most want to talk to.

- *Your favorite books about pregnancy and breastfeeding.* Questions will arise and it's good to have something to refer to.

vice, I read what you said about trying to nurse in less than an ideal situation, and I felt so much better. I had almost gone to bottle-feeding, but I stayed with the breastfeeding, and once I got home everything worked out fine."

Maternity Center/Birthing Center

These freestanding centers offer a happy compromise between the comfort of home and the security of a well-equipped medical facility. They're usually staffed principally by nurse-midwives, with one or more physicians and nurse assistants. They are designed for low-risk, uncomplicated births, and offer prenatal care, birth in a homelike setting, and discharge the same day. Should complications arise, patients are transferred to a hospital. The most vital bits of information to find out about a birthing center are its staffing and its provision of emergency backup services (contract with an ambulance service, agreement with a nearby reputable hospital, and on-premises emergency equipment).

Home Birth

Some women choose to have their babies at home. They prefer to be in familiar surroundings, with family and friends and any older children they already have, and to treat the birth as a normal family event. These births are often staffed by certified nurse-midwives or lay midwives (also known as direct-entry midwives), but are sometimes attended by physicians who believe in the benefits of home births and assist in them. If the pregnancy is low-risk and the birth uncomplicated, this can work fine.

If you are thinking about a home birth, you should have no reason to think that your baby's birth will be at all complicated. You should not have heart disease or diabetes, there should be no family history of genetic disorders, you should not be expecting a multiple birth, the fetus should not be in the breech position, and your pregnancy should have gone to full term.

Because it's often impossible to predict a sudden emergency during childbirth, however, it's vital to have backup plans in case of emergency so you and your baby can get to a hospital quickly. Your home should be no more than ten minutes away from the hospital and previous arrangements should have been made with physician and hospital in case their services are needed. It's especially important to check out the qualifications of your birth attendant if you're planning to have your baby at home.

PRENATAL CLASSES

No matter whom you choose as a practitioner and where you decide to bring your baby into the world, both you and your partner will benefit from enrolling in a prenatal education course. If you're a single parent or if your husband cannot or chooses not to attend, another supportive person (like a mother, sister, or friend) can go with you to learn how to coach you during labor and delivery. Ideally, you should begin attending classes during your second trimester, since if you wait for the last trimester, you might, if your baby comes early, miss some of the most important sessions.

Besides teaching techniques to help you during the birth, these classes help you plan your delivery, familiarize you with hospital procedures, and teach you how to get started with breastfeeding. Some hospitals also give courses to prepare children for the birth of a new sibling, to prepare grand-parents for the birth of their grandchildren, and to educate couples expect-ing a second cesarean birth.

As a bonus, it's fun to attend classes with other pregnant women, and you may well meet someone with whom you'll develop a friendship that will continue many years after the births of your babies. To accommodate the needs of prospective parents who cannot schedule eight consecutive weekly classes, some childbirth educators have developed weekend "cram" classes. To find out what's available in your community, you can call the obstetric department of a local hospital or contact ASPO/Lamaze or the Interna-tional Childbirth Education Association (see the Resource Appendix).

PREPARING YOUR BREASTS

You don't have to do anything to prepare your breasts for nursing. Mother Nature does it for you. Most women around the world do nothing at all to their breasts before their babies are born, yet they breastfeed with hardly any problems. Although a number of routines are often recommended in our country, some actually hinder successful nursing and most don't make much difference one way or the other.

One pregnancy manual from the 1940s advised women to throw open the windows every morning and stand topless before them, while giving themselves a good brisk nipple scrub with a nail brush. Ouch! This and other measures that have sometimes been recommended in the past are *very* harmful. They irritate the nipples and predispose them to cracking and pain. Among the biggest no-no's:

• Do not rub your nipples with a nail brush to toughen them. For innocu-ous ways to make your nipples less sensitive, you *may* want to do some of the measures suggested in the box on page 81, but for most women they are not necessary.

• Do not apply alcohol, witch hazel, or tincture of benzoin to harden the nipples. These drying agents irritate the nipples and predispose them to cracking and pain.

• In fact, during the last two or three months of pregnancy and while you're nursing, you don't need soap on your nipples—and you're best off to avoid using it on them. When you're soaping up in the bath or shower, just skip your nipples. The glands on and around them will be secreting substances to keep them clean, so there's no need for soap, which can dry them out.

• Do not engage in prenatal hand-expression of colostrum. At one time this was thought to open the milk ducts and prevent engorgement, but there's no evidence that it makes any difference. Also, since no one yet knows whether there's a fixed amount of colostrum in the breasts or whether it replaces itself, there's a chance that you might waste this "liquid gold" through hand-expression.

• Do not massage your breasts. This has sometimes been recommended to bring the colostrum from the alveoli to the milk pools under the areolae, to stretch and prevent clogging of the milk ducts, to improve circulation and help prevent engorgement of the breasts after birth, and to help women get used to handling their breasts. However, there's no evidence that it's helpful, and this too might stimulate uterine contractions, so it's better not to engage in vigorous breast massage.

Inverted Nipples

Inverted nipples constitute the one condition for which prenatal preparation may be of value. These are nipples that retract into the breast tissue instead of becoming erect and protruding when they're cold or stimulated.

To test for inverted nipples, hold your breast at the edge of the areola between your thumb and forefinger and press in firmly but gently about an inch behind the base of your nipple. If the nipple seems to disappear within the flesh of the breast, it is inverted.

Usually nipples like this protrude normally by the end of pregnancy, and in almost all cases they come out fully when the baby starts to nurse. Slightly inverted nipples do not affect breastfeeding. Occasionally, however, they remain severely inverted and pose a real problem to the baby who cannot grasp the breast with her mouth. Fortunately, such a condition is almost always correctable, either through simple exercises you can do in less than a minute when you're getting dressed in the morning and undressed at night, or by wearing special breast shells. Both these techniques can be begun in the last trimester of pregnancy, and both are easy and painless. Although breastfeeding experts disagree on the value of these measures, many women have found them helpful.

Exercise: The basis for the "Hoffman technique" is the belief that this exercise will break any adhesions at the base of the nipple that keep it inverted. The exercise involves placing the thumbs of both hands, opposing each other, at the base of the nipple and gently but firmly pulling the thumbs away from each other. Do this both up and down and sideways. These exercises can be done twice a day at first, and, if they are continued, can eventually be performed up to five times a day in late pregnancy and early lactation.

Nonharmful Ways to Toughen Nipples

Although breastfeeding professionals do not consider any of the following measures necessary, some women feel that they help their nipples to become hardier. And there's no evidence that they do any harm.

• For a few minutes every day (or longer, depending on your schedule and the level of privacy in your life), expose your nipples to the air by leaving your breasts uncovered.

• You might allow your nipples to rub against your clothing occasionally, either by going without a bra, by cutting a little hole in your bra around the nipple area, or by wearing a nursing bra with the flaps down.

• Gentle manual and/or oral stimulation of your breasts can continue to be part of your lovemaking. You don't need to treat your breasts like fragile porcelain.

Breast Shells: Another common treatment for inverted nipples is the wearing of special plastic breast shells* during pregnancy. These shells, also known as shields or milk cups, exert a constant, gentle, and painless pressure that gradually draws out a flat or inverted nipple. (These are quite different from the rubbery nipple shields that are sometimes advised for sore nipples, but which should *not* be used.)

These shells come in two parts, fit easily into a bra, and are easy to wash with soap and water. If you use them, start to wear them in the last trimester of your pregnancy, beginning with an hour a day and gradually increasing the length of time, according to your comfort. If they fill up with colostrum, empty them frequently and wash them every day, since warm moisture is an ideal setting for the growth of infection-causing microorganisms.

If your nipples are still inverted after birth, wear the shells for about half an hour before feedings, again being sure to empty them often. Do not feed the milk they trap to your baby.

You won't need to wear these shells forever—only until your nipples protrude enough for nursing to occur. Your baby's suckling will help to make this happen, and your nipples may protrude well enough in your baby's mouth, even though they may still look flat and inverted when you are not nursing. Since your baby will become more expert at grasping the breast, you'll probably be able to do away with the shells after the early

---

*These shells/shields/cups are made by several manufacturers. You may be able to find them through your childbirth education organization or through catalogs specializing in items for pregnant women and new mothers.

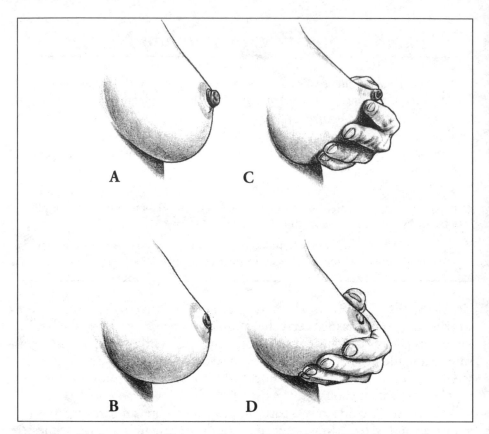

The breast (A) has a normally protruding nipple. The breast (B) is flat. To tell whether it is inverted, hold it at the edge of the areola between your thumb and forefinger. Press back firmly but gently, while at the same time pulling your fingers away from each other. This will either make it protrude as in (C) or invert as in (D).

stages of nursing. Once breastfeeding is well established, you can start to "wean" yourself from the shells by going without them for a couple of hours before one of the midday nursings, not one for which your baby is apt to be frantically hungry. If the baby seems to have trouble nursing, go back to them for a while longer.

WHO WILL "MOTHER" YOU?

In many countries around the world, mothering the new mother is taken for granted. There are plenty of women nearby to help her recover from childbirth and care for her baby. In fact, anthropologists now theorize that in prehistoric days the only reason that families survived was the availability of older women relatives, who could help new mothers and take over their work while they were busy nursing their babies.

In the United States today, however, such help is often not available. A harried mother in Boston confided to us, "When I push my baby in his carriage, I keep wishing that I'm the one being pushed and rocked and taken care of."

The key word for most Western women today is *independence*. You may live far away from the relatives and friends who would ordinarily help you. Or you may feel that you need to prove your adulthood, your womanhood, or your maternal competence by doing everything yourself. This puts a tremendous amount of pressure on you at a time when you need all the help you can get. So look out for yourself, and before your baby is born, look for the person or persons who will be *your* special helpers.

What Kind of Help Will You Need?

You'll need several kinds of helpers. First, although you'll be excited about your baby's arrival, you'll also be tired. The biggest surprise for many new mothers is the constant fatigue they feel for the first few weeks. Aside from your body's reaction to the delivery itself (it's called "labor" for a reason!), the lack of a full night's sleep, night after night, makes you long for someone who can help you with household chores, at least for the first week or two. Meanwhile, you'll have dozens of questions: Why is the baby fussing? How can I organize the diaper-changing area? Is my baby getting enough nourishment? And so forth.

When you identify the person or persons you feel most comfortable with, see if you can ask for the particular kinds of help you think you'll need most.

• If your partner can take time off from work for the first week or two after your baby's birth, or if your mother or mother-in-law can stay with you (and if you get along well), this might be a lifesaver.

• You might hire someone or take up a friend's offer of help and have him or her come over for a couple of hours a day to help with household chores while you take care of the baby, to take care of the baby while you catch up on sleep, or to help you care for your baby by making suggestions on calming him when he's crying or holding her for nursing.

• You may need nothing more than knowing you can phone at any time of the day or night with your questions about child care or breastfeeding. Depending on who the person is, you can work out some means of reciprocating this help, either now or in the future.

Who Will Your Special Helpers Be?

You may be lucky enough to have a mother or mother-in-law like the Long Island grandmother who told us, "Among the most rewarding experiences of my life has been the opportunity to breastfeed my six children—and now, as grandmother to five, to watch them flourish and grow as I help my daughters to continue the 'best-feeding' tradition."

Becoming a mother often opens new connections between you and your own mother or your mother-in-law. You will understand them as you never could before you had children of your own! But if neither of your baby's grandmothers is supportive or knowledgeable about breastfeeding, if they live far away, or if for some other reason they would not be your best helpers, you can reach out to develop a larger support network.

Over the next few months, part of your mothering experience will include "talking shop" with other new mothers, expanding many of your relationships in new baby-oriented ways, and developing new ties. You might, for example, find a great source of support in your sister, your father, your husband or life partner, a friend or neighbor, your midwife, your doctor, a lactation consultant, a member of a breastfeeding support group like La Leche League, your childbirth educator, a professional doula, and/or someone you hire to help out with marketing and household chores.

A great deal of help and emotional support can come from another new mother, or a more experienced mother, whom you may meet at your doctor's office, at the hospital, in a prenatal class or workshop for new parents (given in many communities by family service agencies or other social welfare organizations), or in a baby-sitting co-op. If you're planning to go back to work, try to find another working mother.

Raise your questions about breastfeeding and parenthood with the people who might be able to help you. Find out which ones you'll be able to count on for support and how much each is able and willing to give. You'll also find out whom to stay away from for a while—anyone who is negative, discouraging, or uninformed about the importance of and the techniques involved in breastfeeding. Some friends and relatives may want to help you but may know so little about breastfeeding that they may be too ready to urge you to switch to formula. So acknowledge their good intentions but don't take their bad advice! Take advantage of their interest in helping by asking them to bring you casseroles, so they'll focus on feeding you instead of telling you how to feed your baby.

You'll need the most help in the first few weeks after your baby is born, the time period that's most crucial for the success of breastfeeding. If you can't find anyone to count on, you may have to be your own doula, with the help of books to give you basic information and your telephone to contact resources. Whatever your situation, though, when questions come up, don't just stew over them privately. Seek help. If you try hard enough, you'll be able to come up with answers.

Now you're ready to meet someone you will love for the rest of your life. And you're about to embark upon one of the most exciting—and challenging—adventures of your entire life. It will be full of everything: questions, worries, and anxieties, yes—but also thrills and joy, and gratification like nothing else. Sound like a rollercoaster? Hold on—and enjoy the ride!

Your Baby Is Here

I couldn't believe how tiny she was. She weighed over seven pounds, but still those teeny shirts that had seemed too small for a doll were way too big on her. I couldn't get over how I could have so much love for such a tiny being.

—HEDY, SHAKER HEIGHTS, OHIO

Finally you set eyes upon that squalling, squirming mite of humanity whose arrival you have so eagerly awaited all these months. You marvel at the wonder of tiny fingers and toes. You are amazed to realize that this small person actually grew in your body. You draw the little body close to you, to cuddle and love.

And then, if you are a first-time mother, the questions rush through your mind. How will you be able to care for such a dependent little creature? How will you know what to do? And when and how to do it? It may buoy up your confidence to stop for a minute and consider that women have been having first babies since the beginning of humankind and have somehow coped well enough so that each succeeding generation has survived to bear its own progeny.

Like every other new mother, you have questions about every aspect of child care—how to diaper, burp, bathe, and dress your infant. Or you may already have other children but are now breastfeeding for the first time, or wanting to refresh yourself on the many aspects of feeding your baby. In this chapter we talk about the first few days after birth, when you and your baby take your first steps toward bonding as a nursing duo.

If your experience is like most other women's, breastfeeding will get better and better for both you and your baby. A month from now, you and your baby will most likely have settled into an easy, comfortable breast-feeding relationship. Now, over these first two weeks, you and your baby need to learn about each other and about breastfeeding. Human beings are not born knowing how to breastfeed; both mother and baby need to *learn* how to do it.

Actually, other animals do, too. Not too long ago, when keepers at the San Diego Zoo were troubled because its gorilla was not nursing her infant, they asked some local nursing women to go and take seats in front of the gorilla's cage so that she could learn from their example!

If you know what to expect and what to do, you'll be better prepared for these first few weeks. You can make the beginning of breastfeeding easier if you arm yourself with information, if you start out right, and if you know when you need help and where to go for it. Meanwhile, you may need to be patient to give the two of you time to develop your relationship. You may have a love-at-first-sight relationship, with nothing but good experiences right from the start. Or you may have a longer courtship, taking a few weeks to establish a smooth and mutually satisfying bond.

THE IDEAL BEGINNING

In the best of all possible worlds, every baby would be born healthy, after the full gestation period. Every mother would have an easy, fast, unmedicated birthing. Both mother and baby would be alert and feeling good. Right after birth the mother would put her baby to the breast. The baby would latch on and nurse eagerly. Mother and baby would then spend their time together in the same room, where the mother would rest, nursing her baby every time he wanted to feed. She would have supportive health care professionals to go to with her questions, as well as helpful friends and relatives.

In the real world, this scenario *sometimes* unfolds exactly as it's written here. Too often, however, one or more of the elements just described are not present. Some babies are born prematurely; some mothers have long, difficult deliveries or cesarean sections for which they need some form of anesthesia; some hospitals do not permit immediate breastfeeding, feeding "on cue," or rooming-in; some babies are not eager nursers. And still mothers and babies can and do go on to have wonderful breastfeeding experiences. Let's look at how much you can do to achieve the ideal scenario—and what you can do when you need to follow a different script.

Recommendations for Successful Breastfeeding from the American Academy of Pediatrics

1. Put your baby to your breast within an hour of birth.

2. Keep your baby in your own room during the day and night.

3. Breastfeed "on cue," as soon as your baby shows signs of hunger, such as increased alertness or activity, smacking her lips, making sucking motions, or rooting (moving her head around in search of the breast). Do not wait until your baby begins to cry, which is a late sign of hunger.

4. Nurse your newborn about eight to twelve times in every twenty-four-hour period, until the baby seems full, usually ten to fifteen minutes on each breast. By the fourth to the sixth day after birth your baby should be nursed at least six to eight times in every twenty-four-hour period. If he does not "request" this many feedings, wake him at four-hour intervals to be sure he gets his daily allotment of meals.

5. Do not give your baby any formula, water, or glucose water unless medically indicated.

6. If you must be separated from your baby and cannot breastfeed directly, express your milk to be given to your baby.

7. During the first twenty-four to forty-eight hours after delivery, have a lactation expert monitor breastfeeding to be sure everything is going well. Receive a follow-up evaluation forty-eight to seventy-two hours after hospital discharge.

8. Give your baby nothing but breast milk for the first six months of life. After this time you may add iron-enriched solid food.

9. Breastfeed your baby for the first year of life or longer.

BREASTFEEDING IN A HOSPITAL OR BIRTHING CENTER

The growth of modern hospitals as places for babies to be born coincided with the popularity of feeding babies with artificial baby milk. So it's not surprising that many hospital routines were developed to fit the patterns of bottle-fed babies—and the convenience of hospital staff. Some of these routines have included separating mother and baby, feeding infants on strict four-hour schedules, and limiting the length of feeding sessions.

In recent years, however, as we pointed out in the previous chapter, many hospital administrators have recognized that breastfed babies thrive best according to very different practices. Now what do we find? An unexpected bonus is that many of the changes fought for by nursing mothers have been better for the physical and emotional health of bottle-fed babies, too.

The box on page 88 lists the most recent research-based recommendations from the American Academy of Pediatrics for providing ideal nutrition to babies through a happy breastfeeding experience. Although the Academy recommends that, ideally, breastfeeding continue through a baby's first year, if for any reason you cannot nurse for this long, you can be assured that for whatever length of time you do breastfeed, you will be giving your baby the best start in life.

Healthy Mother, Healthy Baby

If you got good prenatal care, took care of yourself and your unborn child throughout your pregnancy, and enrolled in a prenatal class that armed you with information, you did the best things you could toward improving your chances for bearing a healthy, full-term baby. Preparing yourself for childbirth improved your chances for a drug-free delivery and a wide-awake baby who is more likely to be an eager nurser right from the start.

If, however, unforeseen circumstances occur and your baby's birth turns out differently from the way you planned it—if your baby comes early, if you need medication for labor and delivery, if you need to have your baby by cesarean surgery, or if for some other reason your birthing experience does not live up to your expectations for it—don't berate yourself. Instead, focus on what you can do *now* for your baby and yourself. We'll talk specifically about postcesarean breastfeeding later in this chapter, and in Chapter 16 we'll talk about nursing premature babies.

THE FIRST NURSING

If you were awake during your delivery in a facility that supports prepared childbirth, you will most likely be encouraged to hold and nurse your baby moments after he emerges from your body. This is ideal, since your baby is likely to be more wide awake now than he will be several hours later.

Many a mother has been thrilled to see her newborn infant inch himself up from her belly, where he was placed immediately after birth (often even before the placenta has been expelled), and reach the breast, to which he attaches himself, with no help at all. Many other babies need help in finding the breast. You can help your baby latch on (see the section "Latching On" later in this chapter), and if you need help, the attending nurse should be able to help you.

The new policy statement on breastfeeding issued in 1997 by the American Academy of Pediatrics advocates breastfeeding during the first hour after delivery. Perhaps this statement will change the practice that has been followed by those hospitals that take power away from the mother by not permitting her to breastfeed for several hours. Doctors have justified this delay by their concern that the baby might not be able to swallow properly and might get into serious trouble by taking food into the windpipe. For this reason they have told the mother to postpone breastfeeding until after the baby has had a bottle or two of water.

None of this is necessary—neither the delay nor the water. Colostrum is easily absorbed and nonirritating. Besides, breastfed babies get enough fluid in their milk; they do not need any water, not even in hot weather.

Immediate breastfeeding is *not* a good idea if you are very drowsy from heavy medication or if your baby is very premature, tiny, ill, or fragile for some other reason. If you cannot nurse right away, either because of hospital regulations, your condition, or your baby's, don't worry. Immediate is best, but most women who have not been able to nurse right away have gone on to have satisfying, gratifying breastfeeding experiences.

Breastfeeding Within One Hour of Childbirth

Immediate breastfeeding is one of those issues that you probably discussed with your doctor and hospital staff before you gave birth, letting everyone involved know that you wanted to do it. If not, as soon as you go into the hospital or birthing center, ask your doctor to leave orders accordingly.

As in so many cases, the most natural thing is the best thing. For you, the most natural time to offer your breast to your baby will be as soon after birth as possible. The exact time for this will vary, depending on how you are feeling, how your baby is doing, and where you give birth.

Why You'll Want to Breastfeed Right Away

Recent research has confirmed the value of doing what most mothers intuitively want to do—nurse their babies as soon as they're born. Even though the mature milk has not yet come into your breasts, they have, from the last weeks of pregnancy, had a rich supply of colostrum, that fluid that provides such a good start to an infant's life (see Chapter 3).

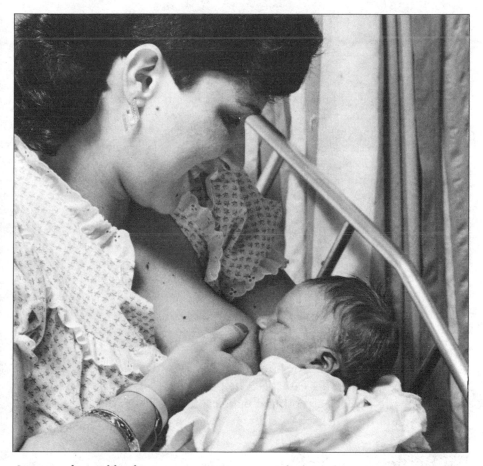

Some newborns, like this one, are eager nursers right from the start; others need a little time to get going.

Also, while your baby is getting the benefits of colostrum, she is also helping to "prime the pump," to establish her future food supply. Your milk will become more plentiful if you begin to nurse early and then nurse frequently. Women who do this usually get their milk on the second day after birth, while those who begin to nurse later and keep to four-hour schedules don't get theirs till the third day, or later. The best way to produce an abundance of milk is to allow a hungry infant to suck vigorously and frequently soon after birth. The more she sucks, the more milk you will produce.

Also, babies fed within one hour of birth pass their first stool earlier, expel meconium earlier, and have lower levels of *bilirubin* (a waste product formed by the breaking down of red blood cells; high levels in the blood cause jaundice, which we'll talk about in Chapter 6).

A Gift That You Don't Want

Many hospitals present every new mother—even those who are breastfeeding—with a free six-pack of formula, or coupons for free formula, when she leaves the hospital with her baby. This is usually the result of aggressive promotion practices of the formula manufacturers. Hospitals that have discontinued this practice find that breastfeeding rates rise accordingly. In fact, the guidelines for the Baby-Friendly Hospital Initiative and the regulations from some state departments of health specifically mandate that formula should be given out *only* upon special request by a doctor or mother.

If your hospital offers you free formula, tell them you don't want it. Show your confidence in your body's ability to produce the milk that your baby needs. If you do decide to use formula for an occasional supplemental bottle later on, it's better to buy it then, after your own milk is established, than to have it sitting on your pantry shelf during these vulnerable first days at home when you might encounter a problem and be tempted to feed formula to your baby, thus making breastfeeding more difficult.

Since stimulation of the breasts causes the uterus to contract, your baby's immediate suckling can speed delivery of the placenta. The contractions of the uterus also shut off the maternal blood vessels that formerly fed your baby and, thus, help to discourage excessive bleeding.

No Bottles, No Pacifiers

Your healthy newborn should not be receiving any bottles or pacifiers. While some infants are adaptable enough to go back and forth between bottle and breast with hardly a break in rhythm, about one baby in four becomes temporarily confused when asked to alternate between suckling at the breast and sucking on a rubber nipple or pacifier. And you don't know ahead of time which category your baby will fall into.

As we pointed out in Chapter 1, the two forms of feeding require different mouth and tongue movements. Furthermore, since milk flows more rapidly from the rubber nipple, babies fed bottles early in their lives sometimes get used to this and are less willing to expend the effort required for nursing. Although this "nipple confusion" is probably temporary, it can lead to sucking problems, so it's best to avoid giving your baby a bottle or pacifier until breastfeeding is well established, which may take six to eight weeks.

CESAREAN BIRTH

"I was so disappointed to need a cesarean," one mother told us. "I'd been looking forward to the experience of childbirth, and learned only at the last minute that I wasn't going to have it the way I'd expected to. I felt my body had let me down—it had failed to do its job. So I found breastfeeding very healing and reassuring. It was proof that my body could function properly, after all."

If your baby was born by cesarean surgery (also called c-section), your breastfeeding experience can be just as happy and complete as if you had delivered vaginally. Your breasts filled up with milk just as soon, and you may be able to nurse right after delivery. But if you need to rest and recover from the surgery for a few hours or even a day, this will not interfere with the course of nursing. Keep in mind that the sooner you begin, the better you're likely to feel and the faster you'll recover from your surgery.

Be sure to tell your own doctor ahead of time, as well as the hospital anesthesiologist, that you plan to breastfeed your baby, and that you want medication and treatment compatible with your baby's well-being, as well as

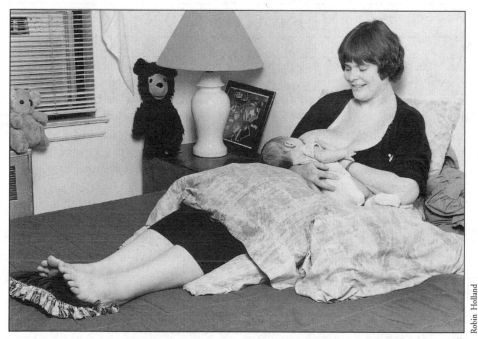

Robin Holland

Mothers who have delivered their babies by cesarean birth appreciate lots of pillows to support the mother's back, knees, and feet, and to bring the baby up to breast level. If your hospital cannot supply enough pillows, have someone bring them from home.

your own. (See Chapter 9 for a discussion of childbirth anesthesia.) After the surgery, it's okay to get relief from any pain through medication that may be administered by injection or pills. Normally, very little of this medication comes through your milk. And even if it does affect your baby temporarily, the American Academy of Pediatrics has stated that the benefits of breastfeeding outweigh the possible mild lethargy your baby might experience after you have received pain medication. You don't have to suffer to breastfeed!

You'll probably stay in the hospital a couple of days longer than women who deliver vaginally. And you'll need more rest, both in the hospital and at home. Because of your abdominal incision, you'll want to make special efforts to find comfortable positions for breastfeeding. Ask the hospital nurses for help, and experiment with different positions until you find the one that you like best. You'll need to position your baby so she isn't lying across or kicking the site of your incision. The most popular postcesarean nursing positions are (1) sitting up, with pillows on your lap to bring your baby up to breast level, (2) the clutch position, and (3) lying down. (See the section on positioning in Chapter 6.)

MOTHER-BABY CONTACT

All other things being equal, mothers and babies usually do best when they're close to each other. This is easy to achieve at a birthing center or at home, and in those hospitals that have rooming-in. This policy lets you keep your baby in your own room rather than in the newborn nursery, either around the clock or during daytime hours only. It's comforting for both mother and baby, and it provides a get-acquainted opportunity for both you and your partner to get to know your baby and learn her natural eating and sleeping rhythms.

Being together makes the beginning of breastfeeding that much easier, since you can nurse your baby when she's hungry and awake, without having to depend on her being brought to you on a set schedule or when it's convenient for the nurse in the newborn nursery. Also, you can feed her when she shows the first signs of wanting to nurse, before she becomes so hungry that she gets frustrated and has trouble latching on. Only through living with your baby can you adjust your milk supply to her needs.

All other things are not always equal, of course. If you're exhausted from a hard labor and delivery, you may not yet feel up to having your baby with you all day long. If your baby needs special care, he may have to be in another room. If you and your baby are not roommates for the first few days of his life, ask to have him brought to you as soon as possible after he awakens. You will, of course, be "rooming in" as soon as you get home.

Don't worry, though, if you can't be with your baby for the first two or three days after birth. You'll have plenty of time to make up for it afterward. Many mothers and babies who have had limited contact at first have still gone on to forge strong breastfeeding relationships.

What about the parent-child "bonding" that is said to take place immediately after birth? In the mid-1970s, a team of pediatric researchers maintained that the first few hours after birth were critical for a deep attachment and that if mother and baby were separated during this time, bonding would not occur and the emotional ramifications could last for years.

However, subsequent research failed to confirm this, and current psychological theory maintains that while early mother-baby contact is desirable, it is *not* essential. Mother and baby can develop a strong relationship

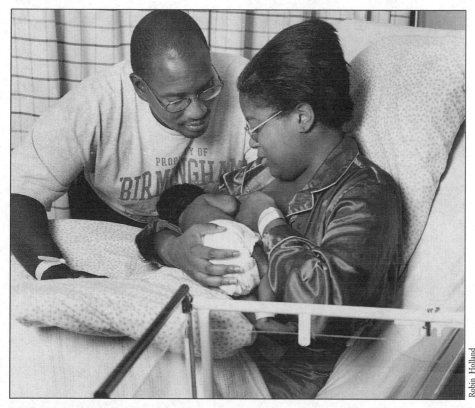

Robin Holland

With rooming-in, mother and baby—and Dad too—can get acquainted sooner, and mother can learn baby's cues signaling his readiness to nurse.

without it. So if you and your baby are not together right after the birth, don't let your natural disappointment at missing this special, intimate time turn into unnecessary worry and guilt over your baby's future development. Human beings are remarkably resilient, and babies can overcome much more traumatic early experiences than brief separations from their mothers to grow up to be healthy and well adjusted.

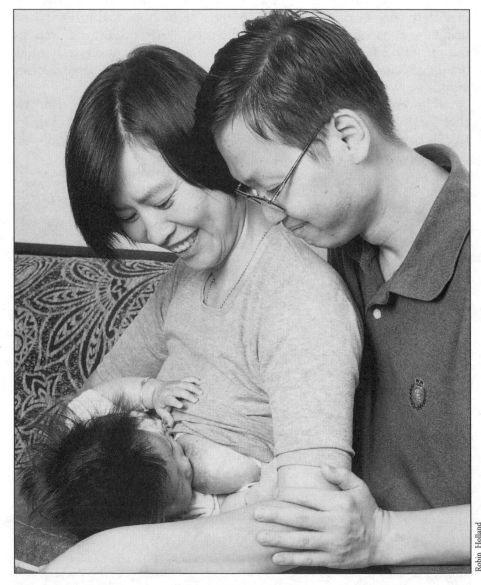

The father is an important member of the nursing family right from the start.

Speak Up in the Hospital

• Ask your doctor to leave written orders for hospital personnel at the time of your baby's delivery, specifying that your baby is not to receive any bottles of formula or water. (You may want to put a note on your baby's bassinet that says "NO, THANK YOU—NO PACIFIERS, NO BOTTLES.")

• If you have not already made arrangements to have your baby room in with you, ask for this when you enter the hospital. Ideally, you will be able to room with another breastfeeding mother. In any case, you may be able to have rooming-in in a semiprivate room with one or more other mothers and their babies, even if the other babies are bottle-fed. (See page 75, number 7 in the Baby-Friendly Hospital Initiative, for the advantages of rooming-in.)

• If your baby cannot be in your room, ask your doctor to leave orders for her to be brought to you whenever she cries or seems hungry, at least every three hours around the clock.

• Communicate your wishes personally to the nursery staff when you first go into the hospital. Remind your baby's doctor and any nurses who come to you that you are breastfeeding.

• Remind your doctor and nurses that you want to feed your baby during the night, as well as during the day. Your breasts need the stimulation, and your baby needs your milk. If you are modest about breastfeeding in front of your roommate or visitors, pull the curtain around your bed. If necessary, ask for help.

• If you need help positioning your baby at the breast, ask the nurse or hospital lactation specialist to help you.

• If your breasts are filling up uncomfortably between feedings (which is not likely to happen during the first couple of days after birth), ask a nurse to bring your baby to you to nurse (if your baby is not rooming with you). If you and your baby cannot be together, the nurse should be able to help you hand-express some of your milk. Or ask for an electric breast pump that you can use to relieve the fullness until feeding time, or to express milk to be given to your baby (see Chapter 17).

• If the hospital nurse asks you to wash your nipples with sterile water before each feeding, you can go ahead and do it. It's not necessary, but it doesn't have any ill effects. But if you're told to wash with a drying agent, do *not* do it just to be a "good" patient. You can always say your doctor told you not to.

• If you're uncomfortable for any reason at all, tell your doctor and nurse.

• If you have any questions at all, ask them. The only dumb question is the one you *don't* ask.

HOSPITAL HELP

If your doctor, midwife, and/or nurses are knowledgeable and supportive of breastfeeding, don't hesitate to take your questions to them. They have probably heard most of them before and will be able to advise and reassure you. Ask whether you can call on them with questions after you go home with your baby; they may be able to give continuing help. If your doctor or nurses act as if they don't want to be bothered, or if they want to help but give misleading or conflicting advice, you'll have to get help from other sources. Go back to the section "Who Will 'Mother' You?" in Chapter 4.

You can do a great deal to help yourself in the hospital. Most important, you need to be both informed and assertive. You are only one patient among many. Hospital personnel, who have other concerns on their minds, may not be as closely attuned to your wishes as you would like. Don't be shy about asking or reminding them about aspects of care that are important for you and your baby. If you're polite and pleasant, no one is likely to take offense. Some of the points you may want to bring up are listed in the box on page 97.

Suppose you meet with resistance in every quarter. Or you're in a non-supportive hospital with outdated regulations (such as four-hour feeding schedules and feeding nursing babies bottles of water). If you have a full-term, healthy baby and someone to help you at home, it may be possible—and advisable—for you to leave the hospital within eight to twenty-four hours of giving birth.

Even if you have to stay the full time (usually only two days for a vaginal delivery, four days for a cesarean) in a less than ideal setting, take heart. You'll be within these walls only a few days. Many other women have borne babies in much more restrictive circumstances and have gone on to nurse them long and happily. You can, too.

NEWBORN HEALTH MEASURES

Immediately after birth your baby should receive vitamin K, which is essential for improving his immature blood-clotting ability and for preventing a rare bleeding disease of the newborn. While the intestines will produce vitamin K within a few days of birth, infants are born without this necessary vitamin, which is present at insufficiently low levels in breast milk. Thus all babies need to have vitamin K administered, and most receive it as a matter of routine.

If your baby is born in a hospital or birthing center, both vitamin K and eyedrops will be administered as a preventive health measure. If she is born at home, your birth attendant should take care of these important procedures.

All fifty state health departments mandate that your baby must be tested a few days after birth for the presence of a few rare birth disorders that can now be easily identified and treated. These screening tests are performed on a tiny sample of blood obtained from your baby's heel.

If your baby is born in a hospital, you'll be informed about the procedures. You can bring your baby back for them within a week of birth. If you have your baby elsewhere, you can find out how to have this screening performed by calling your local department of health. If you leave the hospital within twenty-four hours of your baby's birth, you need to talk to your doctor to make arrangements for any testing that could not be done earlier. Your doctor may be able to perform these simple procedures in her office.

Your doctor may prescribe two other supplements. If your baby is born in winter when sunlight exposure may not provide enough of this vitamin, a vitamin D supplement may be called for. This is especially important if your baby has dark skin and therefore does not readily absorb vitamin D from sunlight. Also, if you wear clothing that covers your entire body in public, you will not receive enough vitamin D and therefore will not be passing it along in your milk. (See Chapter 18 for vitamin recommendations for infants.)

Your Baby's First Doctor's Appointment

Of course, your baby will be examined by a doctor immediately after birth as the first in a long series of well-baby visits to be sure that she or he is developing normally. The next medical assessment, according to the new breastfeeding policy statement of the American Academy of Pediatrics, should take place during the first twenty-four to forty-eight hours after delivery, when a doctor or other lactation expert should evaluate how your baby is doing at latching on and suckling. A follow-up visit should then take place forty-eight to seventy-two hours after you and your baby have left the hospital or birthing center.

Now you will go on to continue to nurture your baby in the best way possible —at your breast. What you as a mother have looked forward to for so long has really begun. We talk about the first days of breastfeeding, the beginning of the unique relationship between a nursing mother and her infant, in Chapter 6.

Breastfeeding Begins

Every time I feed my baby and she looks up at me and smiles or laughs, I break into tears. That look says everything to me that I need to know.

—DEIRDRE, EUREKA, CALIFORNIA

This is the moment you have been anticipating so eagerly—the beginning of nursing. It's exciting and wonderful—and probably a little scary, too. It may comfort you to remember that your normal full-term infant was born with enough reserves to keep him healthy even if he goes without eating much for the first day or two. Aside from the healthy colostrum he receives, the first few feeding sessions are more for education—yours and your baby's—than for nourishment. In fact, some people call these early nursings "practice feeds."

During the first couple of days, while your milk supply is becoming established, you learn how to nurse and your baby learns how to suckle. Of course, it's easier for both parties if your baby is an eager pupil. But if not—if she keeps yawning or snoozing or can't get the nipple in her mouth or keeps letting go of it—ask a lactation specialist to observe your feeding sessions.

BRINGING YOUR BABY TO THE BREAST

Whether your baby first comes to you right after birth or several hours later, he may not at first show a great interest in nursing. Many babies do not nurse well at all for their first few days. One study of six hundred newborns found that 40 percent of them had to be actively helped to suck. They have to learn what it's all about. Some infants start out by licking their mothers' nipples, which is a fine get-acquainted maneuver and also serves the practical function of making the nipples erect. Eventually, with the help you give them, their inborn reflexes assert themselves and they begin to nurse.

If your baby is sleepy the first time or two, offer your breast and try to rouse her by using the techniques listed in the box on page 111. Even if none of these techniques work at first, don't worry about it. She may suck in her sleep or she may enjoy the experience so much that she decides it's worth waking up for. Even if she sleeps through her first meal or two, she'll wake up when she's ready.

Most new mothers feel awkward the first few times they put their babies to the breast. You have to learn an entire new set of movements and sensations. No matter how much you've read or how many other nursing babies you've seen, it's very different when you're actually doing it yourself —just like riding a bicycle. So be patient at the beginning and be reassured that before long you and your baby will both become experts. And again, like riding a bicycle, once you learn it's easy—and you never forget.

Positioning Your Baby at the Breast

There are several different positions that are comfortable and efficient for nursing your baby. As you experiment with various ones, you'll soon develop your own favorites. When you find two or three comfortable positions, alternate them. This will serve to stimulate different milk ducts and thus prevent the ducts from getting clogged. It will also help to prevent sore nipples by spreading out the pressure on different parts of your breast. (If you already have sore nipples, see Chapter 15 for treatment suggestions.)

What Makes a Good Position for Breastfeeding? You'll know a position is good because:

• You are supported in such a way that you are comfortable and can hold the position for some time without feeling cramped or stiff.

• You are not hunched over, trying to bring the breast to your baby; instead, you bring your baby to the breast.

• Your baby's body and face are facing your body; neither her head nor her body is turned sideways.

• Your baby's mouth is directly facing the nipple. She is close enough to take much or all of the areola into her mouth while nursing.

• Your nipples do not hurt. *If feeding hurts, something is wrong!* It is now well known that most cases of women with sore nipples and babies who fail to gain weight can be traced to poor positioning at the breast or poor suckling technique on the baby's part. By readjusting nursing positions, both these problems are often cleared up quickly and dramatically.

See the detailed descriptions below, and the illustrations on the following pages.

Lying Down: For the first few days after your baby's birth and for night feedings afterward, you may find it most restful to lie down to nurse. To nurse lying down, lie on your side with one or two pillows behind your back for support and one or two under your head.

You may find it helpful to place a flat pillow (made of folded cloth diapers, a receiving blanket, or a towel) under your baby's head as he lies facing you; this will put his mouth at breast level and make it easier for him to reach the nipple. Your bottom arm can be up and out of the way of his head or under his head, cradling him.

If you had a cesarean birth, ask your nurse to help get you comfortable. Being a good patient means doing whatever you can to feel good yourself and taking the best care you can of your baby; it does not mean "not bothering the nurses." Keep your legs bent, with a pillow between your knees. Ask the nurse to place something firm, such as a folded blanket, at the bottom of your bed to push your feet against.

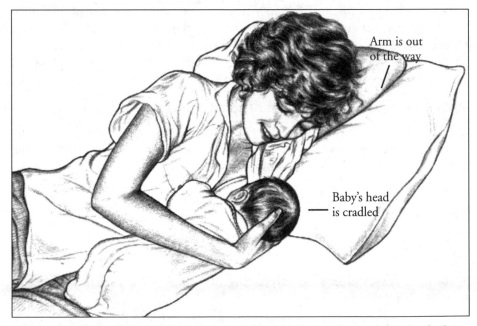

Arm is out of the way

Baby's head is cradled

Nursing while lying down. The baby's entire body is facing the mother, who finds it comfortable to rest her head on her arm. This mom likes a pillow under her head, although it is not necessary. In any case, the baby's head should not be on the pillow.

There is more than one way to shift position from nursing on one side to the other. One is to nurse your baby on one side, then pull your baby over onto your stomach and roll both you and baby over to your other side, using the guard rail on the side of the bed to help. Ask the nurse to show you how. Another way of changing, which some women (especially small-breasted women) find comfortable, involves nursing on the bottom breast, then tucking that breast under your bottom arm, leaning over your baby, and nursing with the top breast. At the next feeding you switch sides.

Sitting Up: Sit up in bed, or in a comfortable chair or couch, with your back and head supported by one or more big pillows. Put your baby on a pillow on your lap, with your arms resting on the pillow. This will make it easier to bring her mouth to nipple level, so you won't have to strain your arm, shoulder, neck, or back muscles.

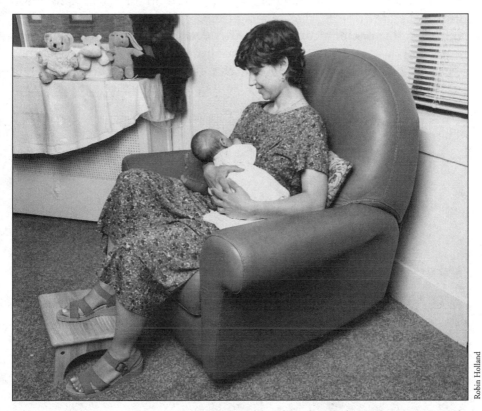

Robin Holland

Nursing in a sitting position is most comfortable when the mother's arm is supported by an armrest, her foot is supported by a stool or other footrest, and the baby's tummy faces the mother's body. This mother is using the cradle hold.

Raise one or both of your knees to bring her closer to your body. If you are in a chair, it may help to rest your foot on a chair rung, a footstool, or a large book like an unabridged dictionary (in these busy postpartum days, that's probably all you'll find time to use the dictionary for).

If your breasts are large, you may be more comfortable if you rest the nursing breast on a rolled-up washcloth or diaper; this will lift up the breast to let your baby latch on more easily, and will take the strain off your hands and arms.

The Cradle Hold: Your baby should be lying on her side so that she does not have to turn her head to reach the nipple. Her face, abdomen, and knees should all be facing your body. Throughout each nursing session, your baby's head should be facing your nipple; if her head is turned to the side, she will not be able to swallow. The rest of her body should be facing your body.

Your baby's pelvis should be up against your abdomen. Her lower arm is under your arm and around your waist, tucked out of her way. Your arm on the side of the breast she's nursing from supports her head as it rests in the crook of your elbow. Your arm is extended as far down your baby's back as possible, with your hand holding her buttocks or lower thigh, keeping her as close to your body as you can. Her knees are held across your other breast, not hanging down. She is horizontal, not diagonal.

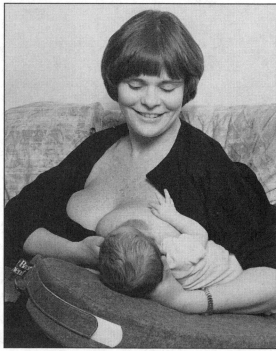

Robin Holland

The "clutch" (or "football") hold is especially good for nursing twins, babies born by cesarean delivery, and babies who need special help with suckling technique. The mother's hand supports the back of the baby's neck, and the baby's feet are close to the mother's body, facing back.

The Cross-over Hold: In this position, you don't hold your baby's head in the crook of your elbow. Instead, the arm opposite the breast he's nursing from goes under his back, and his neck rests on your hand.

The Clutch Hold: This has long been known as the "football hold" but has been renamed. In this position you tuck your baby under your arm as you would a favorite expensive handbag. Her head rests on a firm pillow on your lap; her feet are behind your back. Your hand is at the back of your baby's neck, not pressing the back of her head.

This position is especially good for mothers who had a cesarean delivery, since the baby's legs cannot kick or put pressure on the incision. It's also good for twins, since you can put one on each side and nurse both babies at the same time. And some babies who don't suckle easily in other positions do fine this way.

The Transition Position: This position got its name when described in a medical textbook as the preferred position for preterm babies when they are learning to breastfeed, marking the transition from their previous feeding method. Your baby lies on his side on the pillows on your lap. His abdomen is under the breast you are not feeding from, facing you. His face, chest, and knees are also facing you. When nursing from your right breast, use your left hand to support the base of your baby's head and his shoulders and neck. Use your right hand to support your right breast. Switch hands when you switch breasts.

Latching On

When you and your baby are in position, you're ready to "plug him in," as one five-year-old said of his baby brother. Many babies find the nipple easily, latch onto the breast right away, and take off as if they were born knowing what to do. (Apparently they were.) Others need to learn how.

Briefly, the essentials of latching on are that your baby holds the breast between his upper gum and his tongue (which remains over the lower gum throughout the nursing session) and then sucks on the nipple and much of the areola. Each movement of his lower jaw puts pressure on the milk sinuses under your areola, which sends milk out through the tiny holes in the nipple. The box on page 107 offers a more detailed description of how your baby gets your milk.

To position your baby properly, hold your breast in the "C" hold as follows: Slide your free hand under your breast. Support it underneath with your four fingers and put your thumb on top of your breast. Your hand thus makes the shape of a sideways letter *C.* Your fingers should not touch your

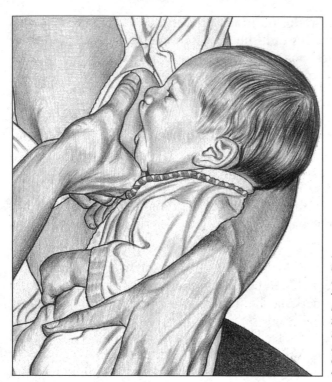

It helps a baby latch on if the mother supports her breast with her free hand —especially if she has large breasts. The baby nurses better when his top lip is open and curled up and his bottom lip is open and curled downward.

areola. If they do, they will be in your baby's way, preventing her from taking it into her mouth properly. Do not use the "cigarette" or "scissors" hold, in which your index finger is on top of the areola, since this sometimes interferes with a baby's grasp of the nipple.

Moving your breast with your hand, tease your baby's mouth open by tickling her lower lip with your nipple. When your baby opens her mouth wide (like a yawn), quickly draw her body even closer to you while centering your breast in her mouth. This will guide your baby's head onto your breast, rather than inserting your breast into her mouth. If she does not open her mouth wide at first, repeat the tickling procedure on the lower lip, and wait until she does open wide before you gently pull her mouth over your breast. It may help for you to open *your* mouth wide, since newborn infants sometimes imitate adults' mouth movements.

Do not try to open your baby's mouth by pressing in on both cheeks. His natural tendency is to turn toward the side being touched; if both are touched at once, he will become confused and move his mouth frantically from side to side. Do not push his head onto the breast. He may become frightened as his nose is pushed into your flesh and be more likely to wail his frustration than to seize the opportunity to nurse.

ANATOMY & PHYSIOLOGY

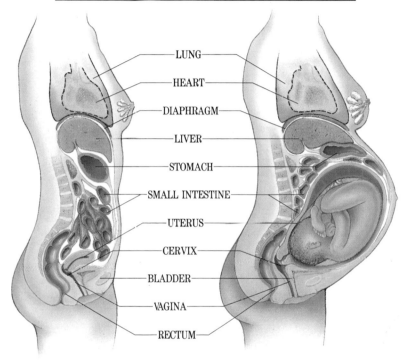

LUNG
HEART
DIAPHRAGM
LIVER
STOMACH
SMALL INTESTINE
UTERUS
CERVIX
BLADDER
VAGINA
RECTUM

NORMAL CHANGES:

Shortness of breath	Skin changes	Backache	Change in balance
Swelling	Heartburn	Constipation	Fatigue
Enlarged breasts	Stretch marks	Loose joints	
Nasal congestion	Hemorrhoids	Frequent urination	

Pamper Your Baby
Keep Them Happy & Dry

POSITIVE POSTURES

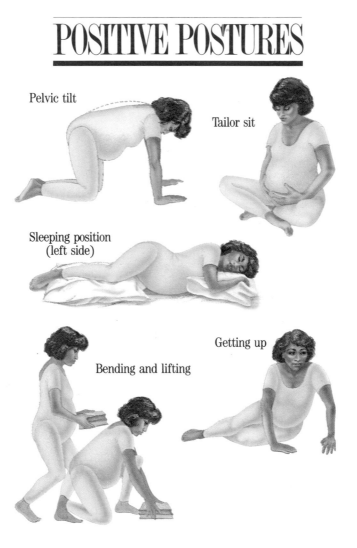

Pelvic tilt

Tailor sit

Sleeping position
(left side)

Getting up

Bending and lifting

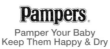

Pampers

Pamper Your Baby
Keep Them Happy & Dry

POSITIONS IN LABOR

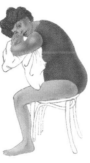

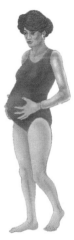

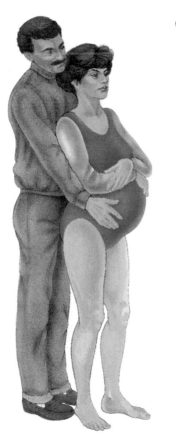

MOTHER:
Change positions
Use gravity
Stay off back
Relax
Urinate often

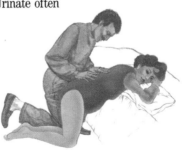

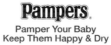

CHILDBIRTH CLASSROOM

LABOR BEGINS

MUCOUS PLUG AND BLOODY SHOW

WHAT IS FALSE LABOR?
Braxton-Hicks contractions
Contractions decrease
Contractions may be lessened
by position change

EFFACEMENT AND DILATATION

MEMBRANE RUPTURE

CONTRACTIONS

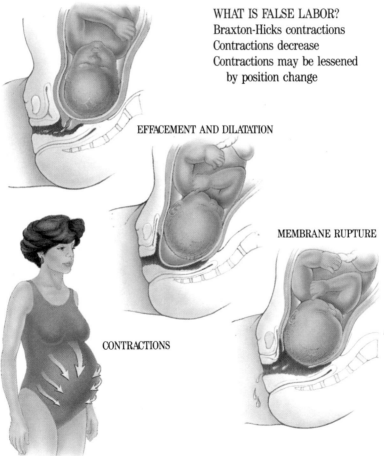

Pampers
Pamper Your Baby
Keep Them Happy & Dry

© Copyright 1994 On Target Media, Inc., Cincinnati, Ohio

ROLE OF THE LABOR PARTNER

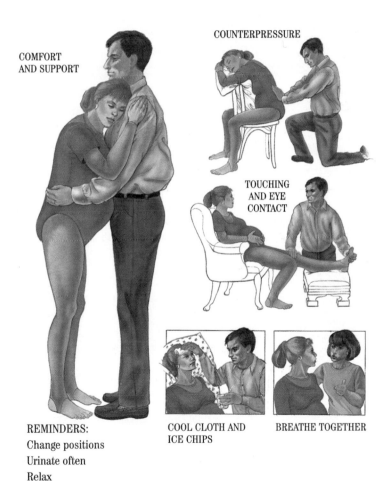

COMFORT
AND SUPPORT

COUNTERPRESSURE

TOUCHING
AND EYE
CONTACT

REMINDERS:
Change positions
Urinate often
Relax

COOL CLOTH AND
ICE CHIPS

BREATHE TOGETHER

Brought to you by

**Pampers.
Parenting
Institute**
EXPERT ADVICE FOR
CARING PARENTS

Visit us at www.pampers.com

11033

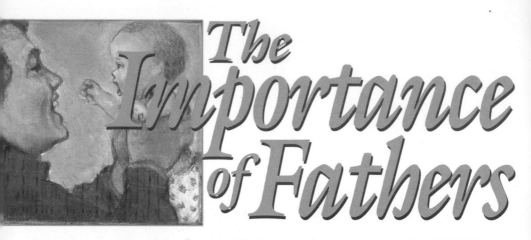

The *Importance* of *Fathers*

Many fathers "play" with their babies even before birth by talking and singing to them or by gently massaging the mother's abdomen.

How do you play with or soothe your baby-to-be?

How does he react?

A father is a very important person in a child's life. Babies who have involved fathers show all sorts of positive benefits. They have a better self-image and do better in school.

Fathers offer babies a kind of interaction that is different from mothers. By four weeks of age a baby reacts differently to the sight of his father. He hunches forward and his face gets a look of eager anticipation — eyebrows up, mouth open, eyes bright. He is ready to play.

Fathers and mothers can also have different styles of parenting. Learning to parent involves learning from successes as well as mistakes. It is important that both mothers and fathers have their own times to take care of their babies.

How involved in the baby's physical care do you want to be?

What caretaking tasks do you want to do?

When will you do these?

Based on *Touchpoints*,
by T. Berry Brazelton, M.D.

Brought to you by

Pampers Parenting Institute

EXPERT ADVICE FOR CARING PARENTS

www.pampers.com

**CHILDBIRTH
CLASSROOM**

EARLY LABOR

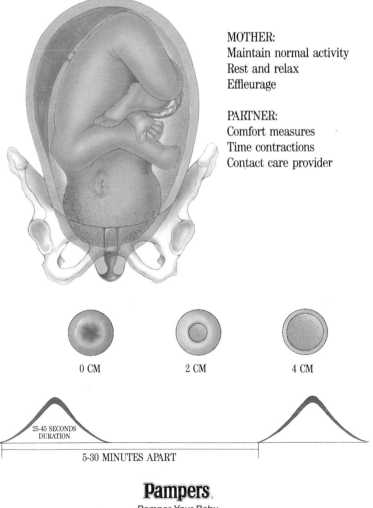

MOTHER:
Maintain normal activity
Rest and relax
Effleurage

PARTNER:
Comfort measures
Time contractions
Contact care provider

0 CM   2 CM   4 CM

25-45 SECONDS
DURATION

5-30 MINUTES APART

Pampers.
Pamper Your Baby
Keep Them Happy & Dry

© Copyright 1994 On Target Media, Inc., Cincinnati, Ohio

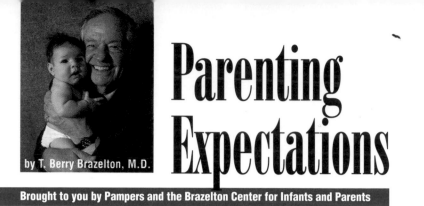

Parenting Expectations

by T. Berry Brazelton, M.D.

Brought to you by Pampers and the Brazelton Center for Infants and Parents

WHAT WILL MY BABY BE LIKE?

Babies help their parents understand them right from the beginning and actually make an enormous contribution to their environment. Through their behavioral reactions to what is happening around them, they shape their parents' responses to them, teaching their parents what gives them comfort, what tastes good, what makes them smile.

When will you learn the most from your baby? When you hold her in a comfortable, cuddled position, and she molds into your body. On your shoulder, she'll snuggle her soft downy head into the crook of your neck. If you lean down to speak in the baby's ear, she'll turn to your voice and look for your face. Finding it, her own face will brighten. A newborn will choose a female voice over a male voice in nearly all cases, and 80 percent of newborns will choose their fathers' voices over other male voices. Why? She has already heard those familiar voices in the womb.

The richness of your baby's various behaviors means there are many ways you can get to know her. When you discover what your baby is especially sensitive to, you will be learning her language — her behavior is her way of "talking" to you.

Your first job, then, in the newborn period is to discover your baby's particular sensitivities. As you try things out, let your baby tell you whether you're right or not. You'll soon learn what she is trying to tell you through her behavior. Listen to it, and trust it.

Excerpted from TOUCHPOINTS, by T. Berry Brazelton, M.D.

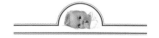

Brought to you by Pampers

Dr. Brazelton is Professor Emeritus at Harvard Medical School, author of numerous books on parenting, and co-founder of the new Brazelton Center for Infants and Parents, sponsored by Pampers.

ACTIVE LABOR

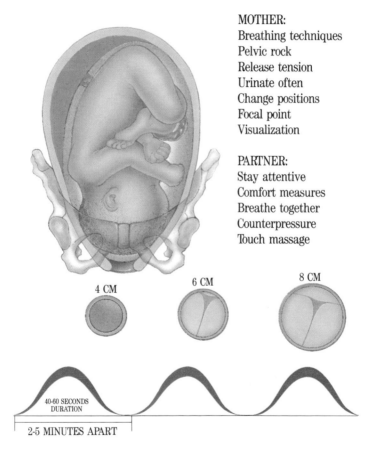

MOTHER:
Breathing techniques
Pelvic rock
Release tension
Urinate often
Change positions
Focal point
Visualization

PARTNER:
Stay attentive
Comfort measures
Breathe together
Counterpressure
Touch massage

4 CM

6 CM

8 CM

40-60 SECONDS
DURATION

2-5 MINUTES APART

TRANSITION

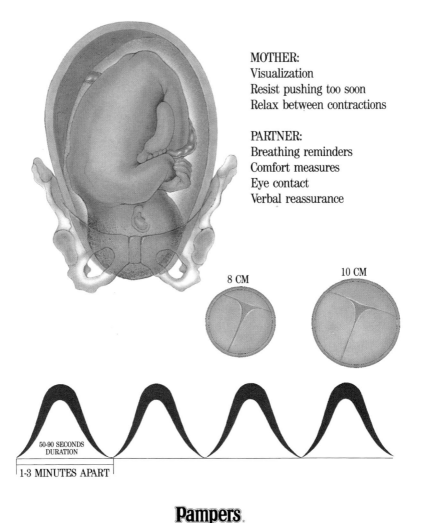

MOTHER:
Visualization
Resist pushing too soon
Relax between contractions

PARTNER:
Breathing reminders
Comfort measures
Eye contact
Verbal reassurance

8 CM

10 CM

50-90 SECONDS
DURATION

1-3 MINUTES APART

Pampers.
Pamper Your Baby
Keep Them Happy & Dry

POSITIONS FOR PUSHING

SIDE-LYING

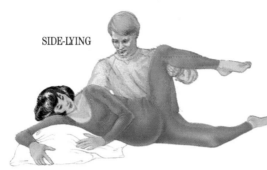

MOTHER:
Breathing techniques
Use gravity
Pushing techniques
Visualize baby's descent

PARTNER:
Breathing reminders
Verbal encouragement
Physical support

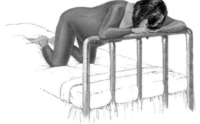

HANDS AND KNEES

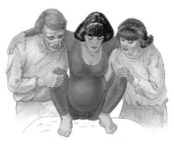

"C" POSITION

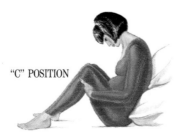

SUPPORTED SQUAT

Pampers.
Pamper Your Baby
Keep Them Happy & Dry

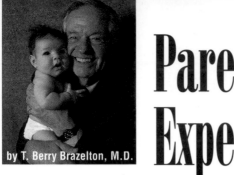
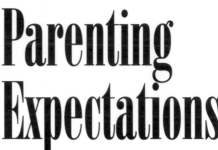

by T. Berry Brazelton, M.D.

Parenting Expectations

Brought to you by Pampers and the Brazelton Center for Infants and Parents

GOING HOME TOGETHER

Going home with a new baby is a very big deal. The first three weeks at home are likely to be challenging. The daily schedule you've been used to will be disrupted; you'll eat your meals wherever you can fit them in between infant feedings; you'll forget what eight hours of sleep were like! New parents may feel overwhelmed and out of touch with the rest of the world during this time.

After an initial period of postpartum withdrawal that most new babies go through after birth, your baby is likely to come to a wide-awake and very active, fussy state at just about the time you are both readjusting to your new schedule at home. Be assured: it's normal and it won't last.

Everything you can do to prepare ahead of time will help. Having a good support system in place before the baby arrives is important. That may mean arranging for a friend or family member to help out with meals and everyday chores for a few days after the birth, or it may even mean hiring an outside caregiver to spend time for a few hours each day in your home.

Prepare to be tired — all new parents are! Don't expect too much of yourselves too soon: this is a recovery period for you and your baby. You are learning about each other, and about coping and working toward the pleasure of making it as a family.

Excerpted from TOUCHPOINTS, by T. Berry Brazelton, M.D.

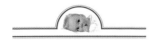

Brought to you by Pampers

Dr. Brazelton is Professor Emeritus at Harvard Medical School, author of numerous books on parenting, and co-founder of the new Brazelton Center for Infants and Parents, sponsored by Pampers.

BIRTH & POSTPARTUM

BIRTH

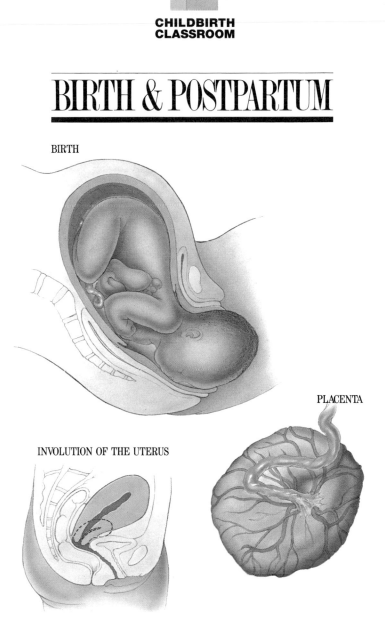

PLACENTA

INVOLUTION OF THE UTERUS

Pampers

Pamper Your Baby
Keep Them Happy & Dry

**CHILDBIRTH
CLASSROOM**

CESAREAN BIRTH

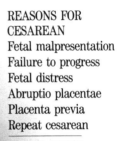

**REASONS FOR
CESAREAN**
Fetal malpresentation
Failure to progress
Fetal distress
Abruptio placentae
Placenta previa
Repeat cesarean

What is VBAC?

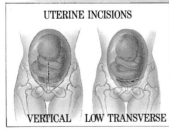

UTERINE INCISIONS

VERTICAL   LOW TRANSVERSE

Pampers
Pamper Your Baby
Keep Them Happy & Dry

CHILDBIRTH CLASSROOM

YOUR AMAZING NEWBORN

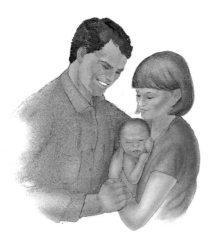

CHARACTERISTICS

Physical
Cyanotic hands/feet
"Crossed" eyes
Umbilical cord stump
Swollen genitals
Fontanelles
Lanugo
Vernix
Milia

Interactive
Can see 8-10″
Hears all sound
Sucking reflex
Grasp reflex
Walking reflex

BREASTFEEDING

Latching on

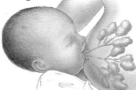

Breaking suction

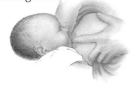

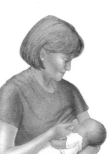

Football hold

Cradle hold

Pampers.
Pamper Your Baby
Keep Them Happy & Dry

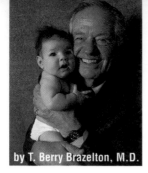

Parenting Expectations

by T. Berry Brazelton, M.D.

Brought to you by Pampers and the Brazelton Center for Infants and Parents

CALMING AND QUIETING

When a baby is over-stimulated by too much activity, her eyes may seem to float, her arms and hands may go limp, her face may frown, or she may avert her gaze. These responses are signs that your baby needs time out to recover and reorganize herself. If parents do too much to try to help her, they just add to the overload. When you've tried everything and nothing works, you may need to step back and just watch her. She will communicate her needs to you through her behavior. Allow her to fuss a bit, and then comfort her. Fussing can be a way to discharge stress and your baby will quiet more readily after five or ten minutes of it.

When your baby is about three weeks old, she is likely to start a fussy period at the end of each day. This is a time in which the baby needs to let out all the overload of stimulation from the day. Try everything you can think of to calm her — feeding, rocking, singing, walking. If nothing works, take a break for a while. She can be over-stimulated by your efforts during such a time and these may prolong her fussing. After seeing to her obvious needs (dry diaper, full tummy) and making certain she is safe, try spending a few minutes in another room. After fussing and then calming, your baby will sleep and eat better and be readier for the next 24 hours.

Your baby's fussing may make you feel like a failure, but it shouldn't. Be assured that you're doing the best job you can and learning more about your baby in the process.

Excerpted from TOUCHPOINTS, by T. Berry Brazelton, M.D.

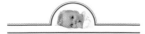

Brought to you by Pampers

Dr. Brazelton is Professor Emeritus at Harvard Medical School, author of numerous books on parenting, and co-founder of the new Brazelton Center for Infants and Parents, sponsored by Pampers.

How Your Baby Gets Your Milk

Through suction created in your baby's mouth, he draws in your nipple, elongating it about three times longer than its length at rest. This lengthened nipple extends far into his mouth, where he holds it between his upper gum and his tongue; his tongue covers his lower gum. The sides of your baby's tongue fold around your nipple, forming a trough; your nipple lies in this trough.

Your baby starts to suckle by curving up the front of his tongue and then closing his mouth around your breast, thus raising his lower jaw. This puts pressure from your baby's gums on the milk sinuses under your areola. The milk being expressed from the milk pools in your breast travels through the large ducts in your nipple. It is carried along by a rollerlike wave along the top of your baby's tongue, which is underneath your elongated nipple. After it exits from the milk pores at the tip of your nipple, it then goes to the back of your baby's mouth. For the first five or ten minutes of nursing, your baby will be suckling vigorously, usually at the rate of one swallow to no more than one or two sucks. After this initial period the rate may slow down, which may signal the need to change him to the second breast.

When properly positioned, your baby's lips will be sealed tightly over your breast, and his jaws will go beyond your nipple to come together on your areola, about an inch and a half in, not on the nipple itself. This is very important for the prevention of sore nipples.

If nipple discomfort occurs, it's most apt to appear when your baby is *first* latching on to your breast. **If your nipples hurt *after* your baby has begun to nurse, he has not latched on properly.** If taking him off your breast and repositioning him does not relieve your discomfort, seek help from a hospital staffer, a lactation consultant, or a La Leche League leader. You should not be grimacing in pain, dreading the next feeding, or seeing cracked or bloody nipples.

If your baby takes only your nipple into her mouth, put your finger into the side of her mouth to break the suction, take her off your breast, and start over again. If you let her mouth the nipple alone, she won't be able to get any milk and you'll get sore nipples. It is important for her to take enough of the areola into her mouth to enable her to "gum" or "jaw" the breast. It is the up-and-down pressure of the infant's jaw that propels the milk into her mouth.

Your baby's chin and likely her nose as well will be touching your breast. If she's facing you squarely, she *will* be able to breathe. Babies' noses are very flat (probably for just this purpose). If your breasts are large or engorged (so full of milk that they are hard), gently press your thumb on your breast to

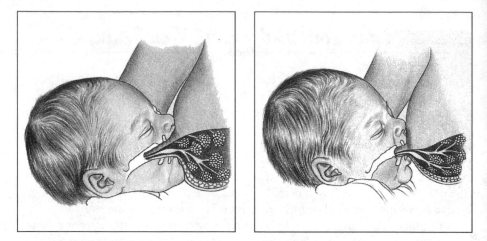

Baby A (on the left) is latched on correctly, with the entire areola in her mouth. The tip of her nose and chin are both touching (but not depressed into) the breast. Baby B (on the right) is sucking only on the nipple, with his chin away from the breast, making it likely that his nose would be depressed into the mother's breast. This would make it hard for him to breathe easily and would also make the mother's nipples sore. This baby should be gently taken off the breast and put back again until he is properly latched on.

keep it away from your baby's nose. Or lift your breast from below to angle your baby's head slightly away from your breast. Or pull your baby's bottom more closely to your body; this will cause the baby's head to tip back slightly.

If your breast is so engorged that your baby cannot get a good grip, express a little bit of milk by hand and then bring her back to the breast. (For suggestions on relieving engorgement, see Chapter 15.) Be sure that she can breathe through her nose, since most babies won't open their mouths to breathe unless they're forced to. (This is why babies are so distressed when they catch a cold.)

If your baby pushes your breast out with her tongue, start over again. Keep doing this until she gets it right. Both you and your baby have to learn how breastfeeding works, and like any other learning process, this takes time and patience. It often takes some weeks for mother and baby to work together efficiently at every feeding. The learning curve will be much faster if you get assistance early on from someone who can help you and your baby work together.

Feeling Your Let-Down Reflex

About the third day after delivery, you may feel a tingling "pins-and-needles" sensation in your breasts within minutes after you begin to nurse.

How to Tell When a Baby Is Actively Suckling

- You can feel a strong suction, especially at the beginning of a feeding.

- You can hear him swallowing and feel him sucking, in a ratio of no more than one or two sucks per swallow. When your milk first lets down, he will swallow milk after every suck. As he begins to slow down, he will swallow after every two sucks. When he is swallowing only after three or more sucks or comes off your breast spontaneously, it's time to switch to the other breast, or to end the feeding.

- You can see her jaws and temples working.

- You can see his cheeks being sucked in as he swallows.

- You do not see dimples by the sides of her mouth, or lips sucked in. If you do see dimples, this means that the baby is not properly latched on. The baby is sucking but not obtaining milk.

- He pauses between sucks, indicating that he got a substantial amount of milk into his mouth.

It may appear within the first minute of nursing, not for several minutes, or not at all. Most women feel this sign of the *let-down reflex*, also known as the *milk-ejection reflex*. Some, however, who produce abundant milk, do not.

The let-down is one sign that your milk is flowing. Other signs include dripping or spurting from the other breast, fullness of the breasts before a feeding and their feeling softer afterward, and signs of your baby's active swallowing. Eventually you'll experience let-down at various times throughout the day, sometimes when you just think about your baby.

You may also feel "after-pains," abdominal pains similar to menstrual cramps. They may be very mild or surprisingly strong. The pains are usually stronger for women who have borne children before. Be happy when you feel them, because they tell you that your uterus is contracting toward its prepregnancy state (another advantage to you as a nursing mother), and that your let-down reflex is operating. If you're really uncomfortable, your doctor may prescribe a mild pain reliever. In any case, these pains are short-lived. Although your uterus will continue to shrink for about six weeks, you'll be aware of its contractions only for the first few days after childbirth.

Taking Your Baby Off the Breast

How do you know when it's time to end a feeding session? The clearest sig-

nal is when your baby has fallen asleep or comes off your breast spontaneously. Another way to tell he has stopped suckling actively is to count the
suck-and-swallow ratio. If you hear only one swallow for every three sucks,
he has clearly slowed down.

If he is still on the first breast, you might detach him as suggested below. Then burp him and put him on the other breast. If he has nursed on
both breasts, you can assume that this meal is over, unless you are trying to
increase your milk production, in which case you may want to put him back
on the first breast.

If you do take him off your breast, insert your finger deeply into the
side of his mouth, between the gums (not just at the edge of his lips), to
break the suction between his mouth and your breast. Do not try to pull him
off the nipple. That will hurt you! He will automatically tighten his mouth;
aside from the immediate pain you'll feel, this can contribute to sore nipples.

One Breast or Two?

There are two schools of thought on this, with reasons for each approach.
We recommend that you offer both breasts at each feeding, especially during the early weeks of nursing, until a dependable milk supply has been established. After that time, some mothers and babies prefer alternating
breasts. Once you have settled into a breastfeeding pattern, you can decide
which feels more comfortable. As long as your baby thrives, you can stick
with your own preference.

Both Breasts: Offer both breasts at each feeding. This will give your baby
more milk at each nursing session; will increase your prolactin production,
which will increase your milk supply; and will help to prevent engorgement.
Don't take your baby away from the first breast while she's actively nursing.
Wait until she stops to rest and her active suckling on that breast has decreased or stopped; then make the change.

If your baby falls asleep on the first breast, changing her diaper or
burping her may wake her up enough to interest her in the second breast. If
not, you may offer her the other breast in about an hour or so. Or you can
express milk from the second breast and save it for a future feeding. (See
Chapter 17 for advice on expressing and storing breast milk.)

Since the first breast is usually drained more completely, alternate first
choice at each feeding, starting on the side that was not suckled or was suckled last at the previous feeding. To keep track of first and second servings,
pin a safety pin to your bra on the side that was offered first; switch the pin
at every feeding. Or you can switch a ring, bracelet, or rubber band from
hand to hand. Soon you won't need these aids. You will be able to tell which

Waking a Sleepy Baby

One or more of the following actions will sometimes rouse a sleepy baby enough to interest him in nursing.

• Speak softly and slowly to your baby, explaining what you're going to do. She won't understand your words, but may respond to your voice.

• If the room isn't too cold, take off all your baby's clothing but the diaper. The feel of the air may do the trick.

• Lay your baby on his back on a hard surface and rock him gently from side to side.

• Sit your baby on your lap and lean her forward slightly—not to an extreme jackknifed position. Then walk your fingers up the back of her spine. Or rub her back between the shoulder blades.

• Gently massage his legs and arms.

• Give her a sponge bath.

• Dab him on the forehead with a sponge dampened with cool water.

• Express a little milk into her mouth.

• Rub your nipple on his lower lip. This will elicit the rooting reflex, one of the many reflexes human beings are born with that help us to survive. In this reflex, a baby responds to a touch on his lip by opening his mouth and making sucking movements. If his head is turned away from your breast, lightly touching his cheek will make him turn his head toward the touch and then open his mouth and suck.

• Do not flick your baby's feet with your fingers. This used to be recommended, but babies do not like it. You don't want to irritate her into wakefulness. (Think about how you feel when you're abruptly awakened by the sound of screeching brakes outside your window!)

side to start nursing from, since the breast suckled last or not at all at the previous feeding will be firmer than the other breast.

If you want to stimulate milk production and increase the amount your baby takes, you might even want to offer both breasts more than once at a single feeding, switching between the two.

One Breast: Offer only one breast at each feeding, and let your baby nurse as long as he wants to. Remember to alternate at each feeding. The advantage of this approach is that your baby will be sure to suckle long enough to get the fattier hind milk, which is produced toward the end of a feeding. Also, although the lactating breast is never emptied completely, suckling only one at a feeding may extract more milk from that one than might be the case if your baby nursed at both breasts.

The disadvantage of this approach is that at the very beginning of nursing the unsuckled breast may become uncomfortably full, resulting in engorgement, but you won't know whether this will occur until you try the one-breast option. If you do get uncomfortably full, you can hand-express or pump out a little milk to relieve your fullness. You probably won't need to keep track of the breast last suckled, but if you do, you can use the same methods described above.

HOW FREQUENTLY SHOULD YOU NURSE YOUR NEW BABY?

In many societies around the world, mothers and their nursing infants are constantly together, and mothers nurse their babies every time the baby fidgets, squirms, or makes a sound. Among the !Kung people, who live in the Kalahari Desert in Botswana, babies nurse several times an hour, day and night. This may involve forty-eight short feedings in one day! Not surprisingly, the babies gain weight well.

In our society women are often cautioned not to feed their babies too frequently as a way of protecting their nipples. (!Kung women would be surprised to hear this, since they don't develop sore nipples even after their forty-eight daily nursings!) But nipples do not become sore from frequent nursing; they become sore from a baby's not latching on properly, not suckling well, or being improperly positioned.

At the beginning—when you're establishing your milk supply and your baby is learning how to nurse—it's better for both of you to nurse frequently. Mothers and babies do best when nursings average between ten and twelve times in a twenty-four-hour period during the first couple of weeks (an average of every two hours). Some infants may nurse more often over twenty-four hours.

One study compared mothers who fed their new babies ten times in a twenty-four-hour period with mothers who nursed only seven times. Even though the total number of minutes of nursing was almost the same, the more frequently nursed babies had a much larger weight gain than the other babies.

Frequent nursings carry another benefit, too. Newborns who are nursed often are less likely to become jaundiced. (See the discussion of jaundice later

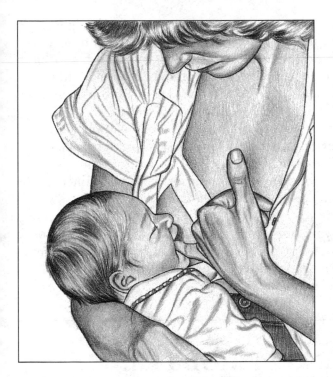

Taking the baby off the breast is easy and painless if you break the suction by inserting your finger deeply in the side of his mouth (not just at the edge of the baby's lips, which does no good).

in this chapter.) In sum, more frequent nursings result in a more bounteous milk supply and greater gains in babies' lengths, weights, and health.

Babies nurse more vigorously at the beginning of a feeding, stimulating the breasts to a greater degree. Since they get most of the milk from a breast in the first four to five minutes of suckling, it's common for them to nurse for five to eight minutes, then doze off for ten or fifteen minutes, wake up, and want to nurse more. (Meanwhile, your breasts have been making more milk.) So while the *average* might be one nursing every two to three hours, this might work out into a regular pattern by which your baby nurses three separate times within an hour, then sleeps for four to five hours, then bunches together another couple of feedings, followed by another sleep.

Fortunately for mothers, this pattern holds true only for the first few weeks of nursing. You don't have to commit yourself to doing nothing but breastfeeding over the next several months!

Prolactin secretion is directly related to frequency of nursing. As we saw in Chapter 3, your baby's stimulation of your nipples causes your prolactin levels to rise, and the higher your prolactin, the more milk you produce. More prolactin is produced at night, with the highest levels between 1:00 and 5:00 A.M., which helps to explain why for at least the first three weeks, most infants are "night owls" who don't know that most human beings (including parents) like to be awake by day and asleep by night. Even after this time, probably for the first six to eight weeks, you may have to feed your baby around the clock. Few things are as exhausting as having to "sleep like a baby" (getting up every couple of hours), but try to think of this as an investment of your time and your energy that will pay off later in a dependable and rich milk supply and a healthy baby.

More important than counting feedings per day or hours between feedings, however, is paying attention to your new baby. When he shows any signs of hunger, like mouthing or rooting, or moving around or looking more alert, you nurse him. You don't wait for him to cry, since by the time he cries for a feeding, he's probably been hungry for a while.

With frequent feedings, your baby is getting good practice in suckling and you're building up your milk supply. She's being comforted and you're not going crazy trying to figure out a way to stop her crying. She's gaining weight and you're gaining confidence. In Chapter 10 we'll talk more about the way feeding "on cue" works *after* the newborn period.

HOW LONG SHOULD EARLY NURSING PERIODS LAST?

Early nursing periods should last as long as your baby is actively suckling. Instead of watching the clock, watch your baby. You can tell when a baby is actively nursing by the signs listed in the box on page 109. When your baby stops suckling, take her off the breast. If she falls asleep at the breast, burp her after one breast and put her to the other.

Doctors used to advise new mothers to nurse their babies for only one minute on each breast at each feeding for the first day of nursing, two minutes on the second day, three minutes on the third, and so on until a maximum of ten minutes per breast per feeding was reached. This advice was given principally to prevent sore nipples. The trouble was that it didn't work. Many women still got sore nipples; the only difference was that they felt the tenderness two or three days later. Again, nipples do not get sore from long feeding sessions.

The big problem with such short nursing periods is that they don't give the let-down reflex a chance to work. It may take several minutes of nursing for the let-down reflex of a new mother to take effect. Taking a baby from the breast before the milk lets down is frustrating for the baby who doesn't get the milk and for the mother who is left with full breasts, a situation that can lead to painful engorgement, clogged ducts, or infection.

Other advice sometimes given is to "let the baby empty the breast." But your breasts are never empty. Even though they may feel soft after a feeding, they are constantly producing milk. In fact, some women who want to build up their milk supply switch breasts more than once during the same feeding session, and their babies obtain more milk that way.

One study of two thousand babies aged two to three weeks found that feeding sessions lasted from ten to sixty minutes, averaging half an hour. Every baby is different, and yours may want to nurse for either shorter or longer periods of time. However, you want to watch out for extremes in either direction. Although some babies can get most of the milk from the breast in the first five minutes of nursing, at least ten to fifteen minutes per breast provides more of a safety margin, and will go a long way to assure that your baby ingests the calorie-rich hind milk necessary for adequate weight gain. If, in the very early weeks, your infant nurses less than ten minutes or more than fifty minutes in one nursing session, he may not be getting enough milk.

As your baby gets older, he'll become more efficient and may get all the nutrients he needs in only five to seven minutes per breast. In Chapter 10 we'll talk more about nursing sessions *after* the newborn period and about how to tell whether your baby is getting enough to eat.

BURPING YOUR BABY

The loud burps that erupt from the mouth of a tiny baby can be startling. They are also satisfying to both mother and baby, since it signals you that your baby has emitted gas or air swallowed during a feeding. If she can bring this up in the form of a hearty burp, she'll be more comfortable and ready to nurse some more.

When to Burp Your Baby

After your baby has finished suckling from one breast it's time to burp him. Breastfed babies usually swallow less air than do bottle-fed infants, and some nurslings hardly ever burp after a feeding. Others invariably do, especially if you produce a great deal of milk so that your baby has to gulp to keep up with the supply.

Babies often spit up milk when they burp. This is normal. However, if your baby vomits forcefully, so that the milk spurts vigorously out of his mouth for some distance, call your doctor, since this may indicate a problem.

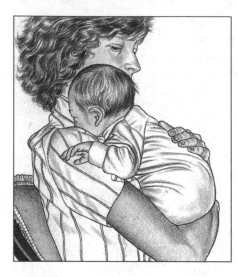

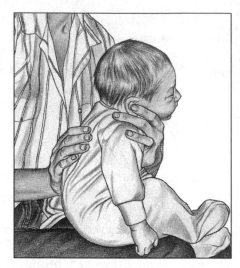

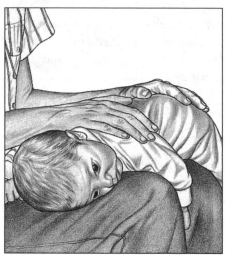

These illustrations show the three best ways to effectively burp your baby. Babies feel much better when they bring up bubbles of air after feedings. Amazingly loud burps sometimes erupt from the mouths of tiny infants.

How to Burp Your Baby

There are three equally effective burping positions:

- holding him vertically with his head over your shoulder;

- sitting him on your lap, supporting his head with one hand; or

- laying him on his stomach across your knees.

Put a diaper in front of your baby's face to catch any spit-up milk and then gently rub or pat her back. Don't pound her hard! She won't like it and she won't bring up her burps any faster for being thumped. If she hasn't burped in a few minutes, don't be concerned. You can diaper her, put her to the other breast, and then let her drift off to sleep as she finishes nursing.

When your baby has finished nursing and been burped (whether he obliges or not), you can put him in his bed. The American Academy of Pediatrics no longer advises parents to lay their babies down to sleep on their stomachs. Instead, the Academy recommends that the safest sleep position for most babies is on the back. If you have questions about this, discuss it with your baby's doctor, since there are some circumstances in which some babies should be placed on their stomachs.

BOWEL MOVEMENTS

While your baby was still cradled in your womb, her bodily organs began to function. At about the sixth month of fetal life, a mass of cast-off cells from her liver, pancreas, and gallbladder began to form in her intestines, remaining there until birth. This dark-green tarlike substance called *meconium* is excreted in her bowel movements during the first couple of days after birth. Its elimination seems to be speeded up by the colostrum she gets.

Once the meconium is out of your baby's system, her stools will range in color from a golden daffodil yellow to a yellow-green to a brownish tint. The bowel movements of a breastfed baby are usually looser and more frequent than those of a formula-fed baby. They're milder-smelling, too.

When you're changing your baby daughter's diapers a few days after birth, you may notice some pink staining from the vagina. This "false menstruation" is due to hormones secreted by the placenta just before birth. It will stop in a day or two and is nothing to worry about.

YOUR BABY'S WEIGHT AFTER BIRTH

Most newborn babies lose weight in the few days after birth, mainly because of their elimination of birth fluids and meconium. Breastfed babies tend to lose weight for the first two to three days, until the mother's milk becomes more plentiful. Women who have borne previous babies usually produce a large supply of milk more quickly.

A loss of 5 to 7 percent of birth weight is not uncommon, although the occasional breastfed baby may lose a bit more than that. We used to believe that breastfed babies regained birth weight more slowly than bottle-fed babies, but now this seems to be more a result of restricting nursing sessions, making them too short and too far apart. Your baby will gain weight faster if you nurse frequently and as long as your baby wants to stay on the breast.

Phone your doctor within a day or two after you leave the hospital, to report on the number of stools and feedings your baby is having in a twenty-four-hour period. Depending on this information, the doctor may want to see you and your baby right away, or may refer you to a lactation specialist, or may ask you to come in a week to ten days after delivery to weigh and examine your baby and to observe your nursing technique. If your doctor is not providing the information you need, ask for a referral to a private lactation consultant in your community.

If your baby is not back at birth weight by two weeks of age, seek help in seeing whether she is nursing properly.

Do not weigh your baby yourself. This activity is anxiety-provoking and usually not necessary. Babies' weights fluctuate greatly, and many home scales are not accurate. Mothers are sometimes tempted to weigh a baby before and after a feeding to find out how much milk he drank, but controlled experiments with formula-fed babies have found that baby scales tend to underestimate milk intake.

And don't compare your baby's weight gain with that of other babies. Different babies gain weight at different rates of speed. In the past, formula-fed babies seemed to gain weight faster than breastfed babies, but recent research has shown little or no difference between the two groups. Still, there is a considerable range among normal, healthy infants.

You can check to see whether your young baby is getting enough nourishment, using the criteria that follow. This information focuses primarily on the very young baby, but also is applicable to babies several months of age.

Is My Baby Getting Enough Milk?

This is the big question to which every nursing mother wants a resounding YES! answer. Fortunately, there are some solid criteria so you may be able to answer the question yourself. The following checklist is the one that I (Dr. Eiger) have suggested that my patients follow.

Your baby is probably getting enough to eat if you can answer yes to all of the following questions. If you cannot, call your baby's doctor right away.

Your Baby's Urine and Stools   The evidence in your baby's diapers is the most important sign of his or her adequate milk intake.

Judging Intake by Output

DAY OF BABY'S LIFE	STOOLS PER DAY	COLOR OF STOOL
1 to 2	1 to 2	blackish, tarry
3 to 4	3 to 4	brownish-blackish
4 to 6	4 to 6	brownish-yellowish
6 to 30	8 to 10 (normally 1 after each feeding)	yellowish
30 and later	may be infrequent (up to 7 to 10 days without a stool)	yellow

• Does your baby have the number, color, and size of stools described in the box above at the appropriate ages?

Your baby should be having regular bowel movements in a quantity of at least one tablespoon (one-half ounce) or more. After the first few days, they should be yellow and loose, with small curds. They may smell and look like yogurt, or like a mix of cottage cheese and mustard.

If a baby over five days old is passing dark stools or fewer than those listed in the table, this is a sharp warning that she is probably *not* getting enough nourishment. If your baby is two weeks old or younger and goes two days without having a bowel movement, call your doctor since this may signal a problem.

However, if your baby is one month or older, is nursing well, and shows no change in appearance or behavior, there is no cause for alarm if he goes several days without a bowel movement, even if he has been having them every day. In this situation, you can wait for three or four days before calling your doctor, and the likelihood is that the doctor will reassure you that healthy babies of this age often change their bowel habits abruptly and that there is nothing to worry about.

• By the third or fourth day, does your baby have six or more wet diapers per day, with colorless or very pale urine?

Today's disposable diapers are so absorbent that they rarely feel wet. To check for urination, pinch the bottom of the diaper; if the padding does not spring back to its original shape, the diaper is wet. Also, if it's wet it will feel heavy. Or you could use cloth diapers for the first few weeks. (You could let it be known that diaper service would be a wonderful baby present.)

Your Baby's Appearance and Behavior

• Does your baby seem satisfied and content for an *average* of two to three hours between feedings in the first month or two?

• In the first month or two, does your baby nurse eight to twelve times in every twenty-four-hour period, for ten to twenty minutes on each breast?

• After three days of age, when you open your baby's mouth during a nursing session, can you see milk inside and is the inside of your baby's mouth pink and moist?

• Is your baby's skin soft and supple?

• Does your baby have bright eyes and an alert manner?

• By the third month, is your baby nursing six to eight times in a twenty-four-hour period, and does the baby seem contented for up to five or six hours at least once during the twenty-four hours?

Your Baby's Weight

• At your baby's first doctor's visit, was her initial weight loss less than 7 percent of birth weight? (Breastfed babies should normally have an office visit within twenty-four to forty-eight hours after early hospital discharge, then at seven to ten days of age, again at three weeks, and again at six weeks.)

• Did your baby regain birth weight by two to three weeks of age?

• Is your baby gaining an average of from 4 to 6 ounces a week (about one-half ounce a day) in the first month?

Your Nursing Experience

• Can you hear swallowing sounds when your baby is at the breast, in a ratio of one or two sucks per swallow for the first five or ten minutes of nursing?

• Do your breasts feel fuller before a feeding and softer afterward?

• When you nurse from one breast, does milk drip from the nipple of your other breast? Can you feel the tingling of a let-down reflex as you begin to nurse? The presence of either of these signs affirms that your milk is flowing, but their absence does not mean that it is not.

NOTE: Do not test for hunger by offering your baby a bottle after a nursing. Many infants have such a strong urge to suck that they'll often take milk from a bottle even when they are not hungry. (Doing this may sabotage the course of breastfeeding, since some babies enjoy the ease of getting milk from a bottle and are less motivated to work a little harder at the breast. Furthermore, offering a bottle too soon can cause temporary nipple confusion, which you may need professional help to reverse.)

JAUNDICE IN INFANTS

Jaundice is extremely common in newborn babies and is almost always harmless. Very nearly all jaundiced babies can continue to be breastfed. In people with jaundice the skin, the mucous membranes, and the whites of the eyes take on a yellowish tint because of deposits of *bilirubin.*

Bilirubin is a substance that results from the breakdown of red blood cells. It is normal for red blood cells to be breaking down in our bodies slowly and steadily all the time. The breakdown products of the red blood cells are converted in the liver to bilirubin, which is then excreted into the small intestine, and from there into the large intestine, from which it leaves the body.

Babies are born with a surplus of red blood cells; this surplus was necessary to supply oxygen to the growing fetus in the uterus. After birth, the infant's body must quickly break down this surplus of red blood cells, which, as explained above, is then excreted from the body through the intestinal tract as bilirubin.

Jaundice occurs when bilirubin accumulates in the body for one of three reasons: because the red blood cells break down too quickly, because the liver does not process the bilirubin as fast as it should, or because a large amount of the bilirubin that is excreted by the liver into the intestine is then reabsorbed by the intestine and returned to the bloodstream.

The two reasons to be concerned about jaundice are first, that it may signal another problem, and second, that very rarely the bilirubin levels rise so high that they can damage the brain. Therefore, it is important to treat jaundice when the bilirubin count approaches high levels.

Types of Infant Jaundice

Four basic kinds of jaundice appear in young babies.

Physiologic Jaundice: Normal jaundice is common in both bottle-fed and breastfed infants. In fact, nearly every newborn has an increased bilirubin level in the blood, and about 60 percent become clinically jaundiced (visibly yellow). The rate, intensity, and duration are higher among babies born before thirty-seven weeks of gestation. The yellowness of eyes and skin usually appears about the third day after birth. This kind of jaundice is harmless and does not need to be treated; it will go away by itself, usually by one week of age in the full-term baby, three or four weeks in the premature.

There is no reason to suspend or stop breastfeeding, and there is no benefit to giving supplemental formula or sugar water to jaundiced breastfed babies.

Breast Milk Jaundice: This is apparently caused by the presence of an unidentified substance in most mothers' milk that increases the rate of re-absorption of bilirubin from the intestine. This type of jaundice is a normal extension of physiologic jaundice of the newborn. It shows up in about two-thirds of normal, exclusively breastfed infants. It appears five to seven days after birth, peaks around days nine to twelve, and remains for several weeks or even as long as two to four months. In fact, current medical opinion is that instead of being considered a disease, this is normal and expected—and that formula-fed babies' lower bilirubin concentrations are the abnormal situation.

In almost all cases, there is no need to stop breastfeeding. If bilirubin levels are very high, some doctors advise supplementation of breastfeeding with formula (using a nursing supplementer*), phototherapy (see "Treatment," below) while continuing to breastfeed, and occasionally, in severe cases, temporary interruption of breastfeeding for twelve to thirty-six hours. If the bilirubin concentration in the blood drops, the baby probably has breast milk jaundice. However, current medical opinion maintains that breastfeeding should never be interrupted only for the purpose of establishing a diagnosis. The diagnosis can be made by ruling out known causes of pathologic jaundice with a few simple laboratory tests on the baby's blood.

Breastfeeding Jaundice: Some breastfed babies develop an abnormal type of jaundice in the first week of life. This seems to be due not to the breastfeeding itself but to the fact that the baby is not receiving enough nourishment. The mother may not be nursing frequently enough, the baby may not be suckling properly, or the hospital's practice of giving water or glucose water to the infant may be reducing his stimulation of the mother's breasts, and as a result, decreasing her milk production. This, then, is the equivalent of adult "starvation jaundice," which appears in most animals that fast for twenty-four hours or more.

To see whether your baby is getting enough to eat, review the section earlier in this chapter, beginning on page 118. Improved management of breastfeeding and increased frequency of feeding are usually all that is necessary to

---

*These devices are described in Chapter 15.

bring down the bilirubin level. Occasionally, supplementation of breastfeeding with formula may be needed while the mother's milk supply increases. A nursing supplementer device may be helpful in this situation as well.

Pathologic Jaundice: This kind of jaundice differs from physiologic and breast milk jaundice, both of which are harmless and not symptomatic of any illness. This type of jaundice results from the too rapid breakdown of red cells, which occurs in some conditions, such as ABO or Rh incompatibility in mother-child blood types,* an enzyme deficiency, and certain other disorders.

This kind of jaundice may appear on the first day of life and persist for several weeks. Both the condition itself and the jaundice need to be treated. These babies may need breast milk even more than healthy babies do, and they should continue to be breastfed while they are being treated.

Another type of rare pathologic jaundice results from inherited or infectious diseases of the liver and other organs. The blood bilirubin test will often suggest this as the cause if a certain type of bilirubin (direct) is found when the test is performed.

Diagnosis

You can learn how to recognize signs of jaundice. Look at your baby under natural daylight or fluorescent lighting. Press your fingertip on the tip of your baby's nose, forehead, or thigh for a few seconds. His skin should look white after you take your finger away—even if your baby is Asian or African American.

If the skin looks yellowish, take the baby to the doctor. Chances are that it will be just physiologic jaundice, but it's always better to err on the side of caution.

The doctor will have the baby's blood tested to measure the bilirubin levels. These tests may be repeated, sometimes as often as several times a day to monitor the bilirubin levels. If the doctor determines that these levels are very high or if the levels are rising quickly, the doctor will institute quick treatment.

Treatment

We now have two excellent ways of treating severely jaundiced babies. In *phototherapy*, babies are put under high-intensity fluorescent lights called *bili-lights*. The babies are clad only in a diaper and their eyes are covered to protect them from the lights.

---

*Rh factor incompatibility, which can be very severe, is, fortunately, quite rare these days; ABO blood-type incompatibility is milder and commoner.

The other therapy is *exchange transfusion;* this is most often done in extreme cases of mother-baby blood-type incompatibility.

At one time jaundiced babies were given water to flush out their bilirubin, but we now know that is unnecessary.

You can—and should—continue to breastfeed during the testing and treatment periods. If your doctor recommends phototherapy for your baby, find out how your hospital manages this. The baby does not need to be under the lights all the time, so your breastfeeding schedule need not be disrupted. You can continue to nurse on cue, except for the periods when your baby is under the lights. If you have rooming-in, you may be able to have the lights brought into your room. If this is not possible, see whether you can stay with your baby in the nursery. The lights tend to make babies lethargic, so you may have to wake your baby every two hours to nurse. In fact, increased frequency of nursing may help to lower the bilirubin level.

If your jaundiced baby is healthy in every other respect, you should be able to take her home with you at the normal time of discharge, even though you may have to bring her into the hospital for blood tests to monitor her bilirubin levels. Although home phototherapy has been widely used in recent years, it is rarely necessary to undergo the expense and the effort. If your baby's bilirubin levels are high enough to need phototherapy, she will need to be in the hospital.

In almost all cases you can continue to nurse your jaundiced baby. Even if your baby needs to remain in the hospital, you will probably be able to go there to nurse him for some feedings and to leave your expressed milk for other feedings. The only time your doctor might want you to interrupt giving your milk to your baby would be in the presence of very high bilirubin levels, especially when the previous bilirubin levels were not known and the rate of rise of the bilirubin in the blood is uncertain. If such an interruption is called for, pump or express your milk to maintain your milk supply during this brief, temporary break. You can freeze this milk for later use. (See Chapter 17 for suggestions on expressing and storing breast milk.)

As we said earlier, today, when mothers and babies generally leave the hospital twenty-four to forty-eight hours after birth, it's important to take your baby to your health care provider on the third to fifth day of life. This allows a trained observer to check for jaundice—as well as for breastfeeding progress, to determine whether your baby is eating enough. The most important sign of adequate nutrition is the number of bowel movements and wet diapers your baby is having.

When to Seek Immediate Help

If you experience any of the following, do not wait to seek help. The sooner you deal with problems like these, the better your chances for solving them quickly. Call your doctor, midwife, or lactation consultant if you experience:

• *Painful nipples.* Breastfeeding should not hurt. There is a difference between tenderness and pain; some temporary tenderness is not uncommon, but painful, bleeding, and cracked nipples are signals that something is wrong. In almost all cases, with help, you can heal very quickly.

• *Fever and/or chills.* This is an almost certain sign of an infection, possibly mastitis. If caught and treated early, you do not need to stop nursing.

• *Signs of dehydration in your infant.* Although dehydration is relatively rare in babies, if it does occur, it can be extremely dangerous. But again, if this situation is caught early, it can almost always be resolved so that you can continue to breastfeed. *You must seek immediate medical help if your baby shows any of the following:*

> Has gone more than twenty-four hours in the first few weeks without the number of urinations and stools described in the section on page 119. Breastfed babies are *never* constipated, so too few movements in the early weeks represent a very important early warning signal.

> Repeatedly falls asleep soon after going onto the breast.

> Regularly sleeps longer than four hours between feedings.

> Is not gaining weight as indicated on page 118, or even continues to lose weight after the first few days.

> Seems listless, sick, or drawn, and has a weak cry.

> Is less active than previously.

> Does not have resilient skin: when you pinch it, it does not spring back.

> Is running a fever.

> Has a sunken fontanel (the soft spot) on the top of the head.

> Has dry mouth and/or eyes and fewer tears than usual.

• *Your intuition tells you that something is not right with your baby or with you.* If you think something is wrong, trust yourself and keep checking it out. If your baby is acting strangely, but doesn't do it at the doctor's office, videotape the behavior and show the doctor the tape. If you don't feel right but you can't put your finger on the problem, consult someone who should be able to help you.

Don't ignore a problem hoping it will go away. It's always better to nip something serious in the bud than to look back and say, "I should have done . . ."

IF PROBLEMS OCCUR

During the first few weeks, both you and your baby are learning what to do. You may have many more questions than answers, and your baby can't even ask the questions. You should not be suffering; neither should your baby. Most of the difficulties you may have in the very beginning will resolve themselves, but if you encounter any of those listed in the box on page 125, **do not wait to seek help.**

Now you'll continue to do all you can to ensure your baby's well-being—by taking good care of yourself (which we talk about in Chapters 7 and 8), by taking only those medications or drugs that will not interfere with nursing (see Chapter 9), and by enjoying breastfeeding and your relationship with your baby over the next months (discussed in Chapter 10). You're ready to continue on the great adventure of parenthood.

Eating, Exercising, and Your Weight

*I can't believe the junk I used to put into my body. Nursing gave me the moti-
vation to reform my eating habits. After all, I'm still eating for two, and I don't
want to put junk into my baby's body.*

—GLORIA, PHILADELPHIA, PENNSYLVANIA

As a nursing mother you take it for granted that you need to take
care of your baby. You may not realize, however, how much taking
care of your baby depends on taking care of yourself, as well. Your
health, your energy level, your comfort, and your state of mind all affect
your ability to give milk.

In this chapter, we talk about how your diet, your activity level, and
the activity of breastfeeding affect your postchildbirth weight. In Chapter 8
we'll talk about how you look, how you can get some rest (really!), and how
you feel emotionally. And in Chapter 9, we'll talk about how the various
substances that you might take recreationally or for medical reasons could
affect both you and your baby.

DIET: WHAT YOU EAT, WHAT YOU DRINK

Just as you "eat for two" during pregnancy, you continue to "eat for two"
during the time when most or all of your baby's food intake comes from
your body. This does not, of course, mean that you eat twice as much as you

normally eat. It does mean that for your baby's optimal development, both before and after birth, your diet should contain essential nutrients.

The first three months of pregnancy constitute the crucial period for the formation of your baby's organs. During the next three months, the baby's body continues to grow and develop. The final trimester (three-month period) is a period of remarkably rapid growth. A lot is happening in your baby's development, and all of this growth requires nutrients from you. The way your baby is nourished during these last months determines whether or not she or he will have enough stores of energy after birth.

Most of your vitamins and minerals should come from the grocery store (in the form of food), not the drugstore (in the form of pills). So take the vitamin supplements your doctor may prescribe, but do not make the mistaken assumption that they can replace a well-balanced diet. Supplements do not supply the necessary carbohydrates, proteins, fats, fiber, and other nutrients that are found in food.

If you were eating well before you became pregnant, you won't have to make any significant changes during the first three months of your pregnancy. You will only need to eat a little bit more for the rest of your pregnancy and for as long as you are breastfeeding exclusively, that is, feeding your child nothing besides your breast milk. If your eating habits have been catch-as-catch-can, this is a good time to improve them. You'll benefit yourself, and your baby will be off to the best possible start.

Over the past few years American eating habits have undergone a number of changes. Many of us have become more nutrition-conscious, and in line with our new awareness we have been eating more fresh vegetables and fruits; more fish, pasta, dried beans and peas, and grains; more lowfat milk and yogurt; and less red meat, whole milk, and eggs. All these changes are in line with current guidelines for sound nutrition during pregnancy and lactation.

Probably the easiest way to judge whether you're following a basically sound diet is to go by the Food Guide Pyramid developed by the United States Department of Agriculture (see the illustration). The pyramid graphically demonstrates the key aspects of a healthy diet. At the wide base of the pyramid are the foods you should eat the most of, and at the narrow point on top are those you should eat the least of.*

The pyramid emphasizes an overall healthy eating pattern, with vari-

---

*To order a copy of *The Food Guide Pyramid* booklet, which gives more details about dietary guidelines, send a $1.00 check or money order made out to the Superintendent of Documents to Consumer Information Center, Dept. 159-Y, Pueblo, CO 81009.

Food Guide Pyramid

A Guide to Daily Food Choices

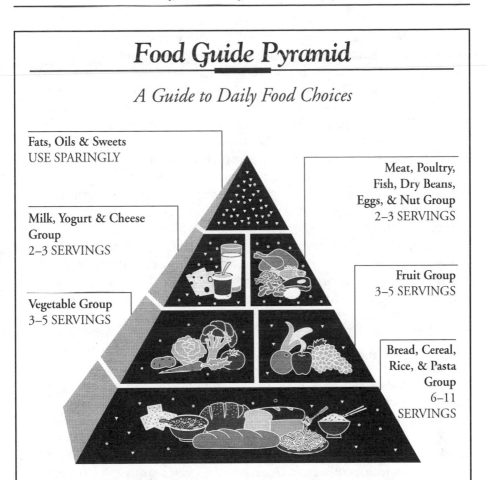

Fats, Oils & Sweets
USE SPARINGLY

Milk, Yogurt & Cheese
Group
2–3 SERVINGS

Vegetable Group
3–5 SERVINGS

Meat, Poultry,
Fish, Dry Beans,
Eggs, & Nut Group
2–3 SERVINGS

Fruit Group
3–5 SERVINGS

Bread, Cereal,
Rice, & Pasta
Group
6–11
SERVINGS

Use the Food Guide Pyramid to help you eat better every day . . . the dietary Guidlines way. Start with plenty of Breads, Cereals, Rice, and Pasta; Vegetables; and Fruits. Add two to three servings from the Milk group and two to three servings from the Meat group.

Each of these food groups provides some, but not all, of the nutrients you need. No one food group is more important than another—for good health you need them all. Go easy on the fats, oils and sweets, the foods in the small tip of the pyramid.

KEY

☐ FAT NATURALLY OCCURRING AND ADDED   ▽ SUGARS ADDED

These symbols show that fats and added sugars come mostly from fats and oils, and sweets, but can be part of or added to foods from the other food groups as well.

Source: U.S. Department of Agriculture/U.S. Department of Health and Human Services

ety and balance. Its message: Eat anything you want, as long as the amount you eat of any particular food or type of food is in proportion to its place in a healthy diet. And the key word in *proportion* is *portion*. When following the pyramid's recommendations, focus on portion sizes, not platefuls. For example, a portion size of pasta is one-half cup; but your local spaghetti palace will probably load three or four portions onto a plate for one.

Your pyramid diet will consist of a large percentage of complex carbohydrates (bread, cereal, rice, and pasta); and smaller amounts of fat (in many foods); and protein (meat, poultry, fish, dried beans, eggs, and nuts). The pyramid recommends lots of fruits and vegetables, and small amounts of animal foods and processed foods high in fat, salt, and sugar. This way, you get a healthy mix of nutrients, along with fiber.

To figure out how much food you need, you have to calculate your own calorie requirements. Figure out the amount that keeps you at a stable, normal weight, and then add 500 calories while you're nursing. For example, a woman 5 feet 4 inches tall, who normally weighs 120 pounds, probably needs about 2,200 to 2,700 calories a day while she's breastfeeding. The box on page 136 presents a healthful Pyramid-based food plan describing serving sizes of typical healthy foods and recommended daily servings.

Eat foods that have a high proportion of nutrients for the calories contained. "Empty calories"—foods that fill you up without fulfilling your nutritional needs—deprive both you and your baby. You can eat the right kinds of foods and enjoy them, too, with flexible dietary guidelines. You need, of course, to make wise selections. Thus your cereal choice should not have sugar as its first or second ingredient and you won't top your vegetables with gobs of butter. To be sure you're eating well for *you*, consult your doctor (or a registered dietitian or a nutritionist with a graduate degree in nutrition—to find one, see the Resource Appendix) and become knowledgeable about nutrition in general.

Components You Need to Pay Special Attention To

Calcium: Calcium is vital in the diets of all women, to prevent *osteoporosis*, a thinning of the bones that causes widow's humps and fractures later in life. The National Academy of Sciences' new recommendations for adequate intake of calcium, issued in 1997, recommend 1,000 milligrams (mg) daily for eighteen- to fifty-year-olds of both sexes. Currently, the average

Foods Containing Calcium

CALCIUM SOURCES	SERVING SIZE
Milk (may be whole, skim, evaporated, dry or buttermilk. Skim is the best source. May be used in soups, vegetables, or puddings)*	1 cup
Yogurt (low-fat is best)	1 cup
Calcium-fortified orange juice	1 cup
Cheddar cheese	1½ ounces
Canned salmon or sardines (with bones)	3½ ounces
Tofu	1 cup
Kale, mustard, collard, or turnip greens†	1 cup cooked
Broccoli	1 cup cooked
Cottage cheese‡	2 cups
Ice cream‡	1¾ cups
Dried beans‡	3 cups cooked

*Milk is an excellent source of both calcium and protein. If you don't like or can't tolerate milk, you can obtain both these nutrients from other sources. However, if you don't drink the amount of milk recommended here, you need to increase your intake of protein above the amounts recommended in the chart on page 133.

†The calcium from plant foods is better absorbed than that in dairy foods.

‡These foods are not good sources of calcium; you would have to eat the large amounts shown here to get the same calcium as in 1 cup of milk.

American adult gets only 500 to 700 mg per day. These new recommendations are also appropriate for pregnant and nursing women of the same ages. In the past, women in these categories were advised to consume extra calcium; now, higher intakes are recommended for everyone.

As a nursing mother, you especially need your 1,000 milligrams of calcium a day, since so much leaves your body in your milk. However, since recent research shows that *extra* calcium has no protective effect, you can probably get enough in your well-balanced diet, especially if you eat the foods in the Food Guide Pyramid that are rich in calcium. The Pyramid recommends at least three servings of dairy foods per day for nursing women. For other calcium-rich foods, see the box above.

As the estrogen levels in your body build up (shown by the resumption of your menstrual periods), your bone mass will rebuild itself, a process that continues for several months. So a really good calcium intake should also continue for some time, probably for about six months after your menses resume.

If your intake of calcium from foods is good, you should not need to take extra supplements, which would only result in your excreting the extra calcium in your urine. Furthermore, some calcium supplements contain lead in excess of 0.5 micrograms, which is an inadvisable level for pregnant and lactating women. At this writing, the United States Food and Drug Administration is considering setting a mandatory lead level in calcium supplements. Meanwhile, if you do need to take a calcium supplement, look for one that is lead-free.

While nursing mothers lose some bone mass during lactation, by one year after weaning, their bone mass is completely restored. In fact, as we pointed out earlier, women who have ever breastfed have half the risk for bone fractures as women who did not nurse babies. The longer a woman's lifetime lactation lasts, the lower her risk of fracture. This seems to be one more piece of evidence that nature really wants women to breastfeed.

Iron: To be sure you get enough iron, eat some of your protein in the form of lean red meats and organ meats (liver and heart). Meats are very rich sources of zinc and iron in readily absorbable forms. You can improve your iron intake by eating iron-fortified cereals, cooking acidic foods like tomato sauce in cast-iron pots, choosing darker cuts of fish and poultry, eating an acidic or vitamin C–rich food or beverage with iron-rich foods to improve iron absorption (in combinations like orange juice and iron-fortified cereal or meatballs with tomato sauce). If you drink a lot of tea, take it between meals, since large quantities taken at mealtimes may interfere with the absorption of iron.

Protein: The recommended servings in the Food Guide Pyramid provide generous amounts of protein, needed during pregnancy and lactation. Note that the serving portions for meat, poultry, and fish are much smaller than those served in most restaurants. The recommended two-and-a-half- to three-ounce servings go far toward providing you with protein, while letting you save money, calories, and fat intake.

Next to human milk, eggs contain the most usable protein in the human diet. More than half the protein is in the white, which has no fat or cholesterol; both fat and cholesterol are abundant in the yolk. While you can eat as many egg whites as you want, it's probably best not to eat more

Sources of Protein*

PROTEIN SOURCE	SERVING SIZE
Lean cooked fish, meat, or poultry (after cooking)	2½ to 3 ounces
Eggs	2 to 3
Dried beans or peas	1 cup cooked
Cheddar cheese	2 ounces
Cottage cheese	½ cup
Macaroni and cheese	1 cup
Chili with meat and beans	¾ cup
Cheese pizza	¼ of 14-inch pie
Peanut butter	¼ cup
Nuts	½ cup
Seeds	½ cup
Tofu (soybean curd)	1 cup

*There is some overlap between the charts in this chapter, and also between the sources of various nutrients. For example, some foods provide calcium as well as protein. The charts for specific nutritional sources, such as this one, should be used in conjunction with the chart on page 136 for the pyramid-based food plan. Thus, each day you would choose two or three servings from one of the protein-rich foods listed in the left-hand column, with each serving of the size indicated here.

than four yolks a week, including those you use in cooking. In some recipes, for half the eggs called for, you can substitute two whites for one whole egg. For other sources of protein, see the box above.

Vitamin D: Be sure to get enough vitamin D, either through 15 minutes of direct sunlight (without a sunscreen) a day on your face, hands, and legs; from vitamin D–enriched milk; or from a supplement. You will need a supplement if you do not drink at least twenty-four ounces of vitamin D–enriched milk a day. This is especially important if you're African American, since recent research has found that some black women excrete less vitamin D in their milk than do white women. Aside from the other important benefits of this vitamin, it helps you to absorb the calcium in your diet.

DHA: The long-chain fatty acid DHA (docosahexaenoic acid) is essential for your baby's brain and eye development and is also thought to raise IQ scores in childhood. DHA occurs naturally in breast milk—*if* the mother's diet contains fish, red meats, organ meats, and eggs.

DHA is also important for adults—especially for mental health, cognitive functioning, and vision. You give your DHA stores to your baby during pregnancy and lactation, and it takes more than nine months after giving birth to return to your normal DHA levels. For this reason, some physicians and nutritionists have begun to encourage pregnant and nursing women to take a DHA supplement, which is available over the counter from pharmacies and health food stores. However, such supplementation is still controversial, because so far there is no scientific evidence of actual benefits for mothers or their babies.

Folate (Folic Acid):   This B vitamin is crucial in the diets of women of child-bearing age, especially for women who are considering pregnancy, and also for those who are already pregnant or lactating. The vitamin is important for ensuring the health and normal development of both mother and infant; it is especially important for preventing certain birth defects. Recent research also suggests that it may reduce the risk of heart attack.

Food Sources of Folic Acid (Folate)

FOOD SOURCE	SERVING SIZE
Citrus fruits and juices	¾ cup
Cooked spinach	½ cup
Raw spinach	1 cup
Cooked cauliflower, broccoli, asparagus	1 cup
Lentils, black-eyed peas, pinto beans, red kidney beans	½ cup
Beef or calf liver	3 ounces
Chicken or turkey liver	½ cup diced
Fortified dry cereals	1 ounce
Other fortified grains and breads	See bread group serving sizes on page 136

Current folic acid recommendations from the National Research Council, the U.S. Public Health Service, and the Food and Drug Administration range between 180 and 400 micrograms (mcg) for nonpregnant, nonlactating sexually active women; 800 mcg during pregnancy; and 400 during lactation. To obtain the essential amounts of folate in food, a breast-feeding woman needs to consume at least 2,000 calories daily or take a multivitamin pill with 400 mcg of folic acid.

A good folate intake can be obtained by following the U.S. Food Guide Pyramid guidelines, and eating just a few more servings than the bottom of the range for each food group. All products made with "enriched" flour or grain products like bread, rice, and pasta now contain added folic acid, making it easier to take in enough folate. However, the U.S. Public Health Service still recommends a supplement for women of childbearing age. For good sources of folate, see the box on page 134.

The Vegetarian Diet

A meatless diet can provide a healthful eating pattern if you choose your foods carefully. However, two aspects of a vegetarian diet provide challenges: first, you need to be sure you get enough calories from your diet, and second, you need to take in enough protein. You would do well to consult a dietitian or nutritionist to be sure that you're meeting your baby's nutritional needs, as well as your own. To find a professional, contact the American Dietetic Association (see the Resource Appendix).

• *Getting enough calories.* Since plant products are lower in calories than animal foods, it's sometimes harder to take in enough calories. This is especially true if you are a *vegan,* a very strict vegetarian who eats no animal-based foods of any kind. If you eat no meat, fish, or poultry, but do eat eggs and dairy products *(ovolactovegetarian)* or dairy products alone *(lactovegetarian),* you'll have an easier time getting all your nutrients. Be aware, though, that if you're eating large quantities of cheese as meat substitutes, you may be taking in too much fat.

• *Obtaining enough protein.* Your needs for protein, vitamins, and minerals are higher when you're pregnant and nursing. Therefore, you have to be especially aware of your food choices and the way to combine plant-food proteins to make them "complete," that is, containing all the essential amino acids.

Most cultures in which people do not regularly eat meat have developed favorite combinations of plant foods that provide complete proteins.

Serving Sizes of Foods in Pyramid Groups

FOOD GROUP	SERVING SIZE	SERVINGS PER DAY
Breads and Grains (whole-grain preferable)		**6–11**
Bread	1 slice	
Cooked rice, pasta, or grits	½ cup	
Cooked cereal	½ cup	
Ready-to-eat cereal	1 ounce	
Corn bread	1 square	
Dinner roll	1	
Hot dog or hamburger roll	½	
Corn tortilla	1	
Pizza crust	2½-inch wedge	
Muffin	1 small	
Wheat germ	1 tablespoon	
Crackers	4	
Vegetables		**3–5**
Chopped raw or cooked vegetables	½ cup	
Leafy raw vegetables	1 cup	

Latin Americans, for example, eat beans with either rice or corn, and in Nepal, villagers typically eat rice with lentil sauce at every meal.* However, you don't have to eat these foods at the same time; eating them over the course of a day is fine.

A Healthy Vegetarian Diet

For You.   While you're eating for two your daily needs will include six or more servings of grains, two to three servings of dried beans, nuts, seeds, eggs, or meat substitutes; three or more servings of vegetables (one or more

*A comprehensive guide to combining plant foods to provide complete protein is *Diet for a Small Planet* by Frances Moore Lappe (New York: Ballantine twentieth anniversary edition, 1991). Good information is also given in *What to Eat When You're Expecting* by A. Eisenberg, H. Murkoff, and S. Hathaway (New York: Workman, 1986).

FOOD GROUP	SERVING SIZE	SERVINGS PER DAY
Fruits		3–5
Melon wedge (¼ cantaloupe)	1	
Piece of fresh fruit	1	
Fruit juice	¾ cup	
Canned fruit	½ cup	
Dried fruit	¼ cup	
Dairy Foods		2–3
Milk or yogurt	1 cup	
Cheese	1½ to 2 ounces	
Meat and Protein		2–3
Cooked lean meat, fish, or poultry	(after cooking) 2½ to 3 ounces	
Cooked beans	½ cup*	
Egg	1*	
Peanut butter	2 tablespoons*	
Fats, Oils, Sweets		
Limit these items, especially if you need to lose weight.		

*These amounts are equivalent to 1 ounce of lean meat, or ⅓ serving.

of dark leafy greens); two to four servings of fruit (at least one citrus); and two to three glasses of milk or its calcium equivalent. You may need supplements that include modest amounts of vitamin B_{12}, vitamin D, calcium, iron, zinc, and folic acid.

The above servings are minimums; you will need more food than described here to reach an adequate calorie count. If you are of average height and build, you should be eating at least 2,200 to 2,700 calories during lactation. If you are smaller or larger than average, adjust your intake accordingly.

If you have been a vegan for several years, you and your breastfed baby should be taking vitamin B_{12} supplements. Your baby will also need vitamin D if you live in a climate in which you or your baby do not get enough exposure to sunshine.

For Your Child. You need to be especially careful that your infants and young children obtain enough protein to stay healthy and grow properly—especially after weaning. They also need reliable sources of vitamin B_{12}, vitamin D, calcium, iron, and zinc.

You may want to modify your diet temporarily to eat eggs and dairy products throughout your pregnancy and lactation. You should also add extra protein sources to your children's diet after six months of age (even if you continue to breastfeed) until they're about five or six years old. In infancy they can obtain protein through pureed tofu, cottage cheese, and pureed and strained legumes.

What You Drink

Liquids are important in your diet, especially while you're nursing, since you give up fluid to your milk. A good rule of thumb is to drink to satisfy your thirst. This usually turns out to be about six to eight glasses of fluid a day. Include milk, juice, and other beverages.

Pay attention to what your body tells you. No matter how busy you are, you don't want to disregard your body's signals. You'll probably find that you become thirstier while you're nursing. Besides thirst, another measure is the color of your urine. If your urine is dark in color, showing that it is very concentrated, you probably need to increase your fluid intake. On the other hand, if you are feeling overfull or bloated, you may be drinking too much. Actually, too much fluid (more than twelve glasses a day) may decrease your milk production.

One way to get enough fluids is to keep a full pitcher of water and a glass close by your favorite nursing place throughout the day. A cup of water, milk, soup, caffeine-free drink (carbonated is okay), or fruit juice should become part of your routine before each nursing. While you may drink coffee, tea, caffiene-containing sodas, and alcoholic beverages in moderation, they are not able to meet your body's needs for fluids, since they have a diuretic effect. That is, they stimulate your kidneys to excrete more fluid, and so less liquid stays in your system. Experts recommend offsetting the loss of hydration by drinking extra water for every diuretic drink consumed. Also, caffeine-containing beverages that you drink may come through your milk and make your baby more wakeful.

Nursing women are sometimes urged to drink large quantities of liquids, but recent research on the effects of supplemental fluids doesn't show that they have any effect on increasing milk production. Experts currently recommend six to eight glasses of hydrating liquids per day for all adults—nursing or not.

Should You Avoid Any Foods While You're Nursing?

If you have no food allergies yourself, most of the foods you eat won't cause problems for your baby. Some foods eaten by a nursing mother do, however, seem to affect her baby adversely.

Cow's milk is an offender for some women. Some nursing babies who have shown symptoms of colic (more about colic in Chapter 10) experienced fewer symptoms when their mothers stopped drinking cow's milk or eating cow's milk products for a while. The same kind of result has been exhibited by babies who have symptoms other than the typical signs of colic: inconsolable crying and apparent sharp intestinal pains, usually accompanied by gas. Such symptoms as vomiting, diarrhea, runny nose, wheezy bronchitis, and eczema have all, in some cases, disappeared when their breastfeeding mothers gave up dairy products.

If your baby is colicky, and if, when you stop drinking cow's milk for a while, your baby's symptoms go away, you might try drinking milk again a couple of weeks later. It's possible that your baby's digestive system will have matured, and you will no longer need to deprive both of you of the good nutrients in milk. If you do give up dairy products for a while, you may want to check with a nutritionist to be sure that you are still receiving adequate nutrients from other foods or, if necessary, from supplements.

Other foods that are implicated to a lesser extent include eggs, citrus fruits, wheat, and chocolate. Some allergists have commented that the foods babies react to are often those that the mother had eaten in large amounts while she was pregnant, giving rise to the possibility that the baby may have been sensitized to them in the uterus.

Nursing babies sometimes suffer from gas after mothers eat foods from the cabbage family, such as broccoli or brussels sprouts. Others become crampy after their mothers drink herbal teas or wakeful after their mothers drink coffee or other caffeine-containing beverages such as tea or cola drinks, or eat chocolate. One nursing mother found that her baby got sick whenever she had eaten something with garlic in it, and then she remembered that her husband suffered cramps after eating garlic, making her think that they both might have the same kind of reaction.

One case reported in the medical literature was that of a three-month-old baby whose urine was periodically a bright pink. After the mother noticed that she had trouble removing an orange-pink stain from a plastic glass from which she had drunk orange soda, she tried abstaining from this drink—and then trying it and watching the baby's urine. There seemed to be a definite connection, and so the mother eliminated the soda from her diet.

All foods eaten by a mother flavor her milk, and an occasional baby with a discriminating palate may or may not like a distinctive taste. He may either nurse happily—or reject the breast milk. However, as you'll find throughout your parenting career, children are unpredictable. In one study, a group of infants nursed longer, sucked more, and drank more when their mothers' milk smelled like garlic, compared to when that flavor was absent. These pint-size gourmets may have become accustomed to their mothers' garlicky diets while still in the uterus.

It takes an estimated four to six hours between the time you eat a food and the time it affects your milk. If you can establish any relationship between certain foods that you eat and reactions from your baby, it's easy enough to avoid these foods.

You'll also want to avoid certain foods to minimize the risk of passing on any environmental pollutants in your milk (as detailed in the section "Protecting Your Baby and Yourself from Pollutants"). For the most part, however, you can eat any nourishing food you want without fear that your baby will be affected.

Do Some Foods Make Milk?

Virtually every culture in the world has recommended certain foods to nursing mothers, in the belief that they help to make milk. In China, nursing mothers have been urged to eat "a mixture of pork fat and red gram (a type of bean), cuttlefish soup, shrimps' heads in wine, and a special sweet wine made from glutinous rice, given together with the larvae of the blow-fly." In India, garlic, tamarind, and cottonseed are customarily offered to breastfeeding women. In France, doctors prescribe a powdered form of fennel to increase women's milk supply. All over the world, herbal preparations are freely given to nursing women.

Dr. Derrick B. Jelliffe, the late director of Population and Family Health at the University of California at Los Angeles, concluded that the effects of such potions are largely psychological. The mother thinks that a certain food will increase her milk supply, so she relaxes and has a good let-down reflex, thus "proving" the value of the food.

The best way to build up your milk supply isn't what *you* eat, though. It's what—and how much—and how often—your baby eats. The more often you nurse your baby and the more vigorously she nurses, the more milk you're likely to have. For other suggestions on building up your milk supply, see Chapter 10.

Avoiding Chemical Pollutants

- Do not eat freshwater fish from waters known to be contaminated. (For information about suspect waters and fish species, call your state's Department of Environmental Conservation.)

- Peel or thoroughly wash fruits and vegetables to get rid of pesticide residues.

- Cut away the fatty portions of meats, poultry, and fish (dark sections and skin), since pollutants tend to be concentrated in the fat.

- Avoid dairy products rich in butterfat.

- Avoid using pesticides and stay away from places where they are used, but if you *must* use them, use the nonspray kind.

- Put continual pressure on governmental agencies to monitor the use of new chemicals that may be just as pervasive, and to continue to study their effects on human beings.

- Remember that research consistently shows that even in a world contaminated with many pollutants, human milk is still the best food for human babies.

Protecting Your Baby and Yourself from Pollutants

Many women have been alarmed by "scare" reports that imply that the presence of chemical residues in mother's milk makes it dangerous for babies. The truth, as we stated in Chapter 2, is that *there is absolutely no medical evidence that breastfed babies suffer any ill effects from such chemicals* except for a few rare cases of heavy occupational or accidental contamination.

Since DDT and the PCBs have been banned or restricted since the 1970s, the levels of these chemicals are declining, although they are still in the atmosphere to some degree. One study of Canadian women who live on the Akwesasne Mohawk Reservation near an industrial plant where large amounts of PCBs had been dumped concluded that any effect of PCBs on babies was the result of polluting substances that had crossed the placenta during pregnancy and birth, rather than having been transmitted in their mothers' milk.

What, then, should a nursing mother do? Under ordinary conditions it's not necessary to have your milk tested, even if you live in an area where these chemicals are at high levels. The Committee on Environmental Health of the American Academy of Pediatrics recommends breastfeeding for infants up to one year old and does not recommend testing breast milk for PCBs because, as one doctor wrote, "neither the experts nor local physicians can decipher the results."

The only time it might make sense to have your milk analyzed would be if you were exposed to a highly concentrated dose of chemicals, either through an industrial accident, exposure at work, or massive ingestion of contaminated foods, *and* if you or your baby showed any symptoms of chemical poisoning. Fortunately, this kind of experience is extremely rare.

For special precautions that pregnant and nursing women should take, see the box on page 141.

Important Points to Remember

• The normal diets of many Americans are low in fruits and vegetables. As a nursing mother at the 2,200-calorie level, you should eat a minimum of seven servings a day, including one citrus fruit (a rich source of vitamin C) and one serving of a vitamin A–rich fruit or vegetable. (The darker the green vegetable or the deeper the orange of the squash, the more potential vitamin A.) Increase your intake of leafy greens.

• Most American diets are too heavy in fat and added sugar, and too light on complex carbohydrates (breads, grains, fruits, and vegetables). You should be getting about 50 percent of your calories from carbohydrates, about 25 to 30 percent from fat, and 25 to 30 percent from protein.

• No one food is indispensable. If you're allergic to eggs, substitute an ounce of meat or Cheddar cheese, or one-fourth cup of cottage cheese, or two tablespoons of peanut butter.

If you dislike or are allergic to milk, are lactose-intolerant, or find that milk seems to make your baby colicky, you can get equivalent nutrients by eating yogurt or cheese, along with calcium-rich foods like broccoli and bone-in canned sardines or salmon.

• You may want to give milk a try, even if you don't ordinarily drink it. Many women find it thirst-quenching during pregnancy and lactation. You should be able to handle the lactose in milk by gradually increasing your intake (to reasonable amounts), or by drinking lactase-treated milk, or both. You may end up really enjoying this nutrient-packed food.

• To save money, substitute nonfat dry milk for liquid milk, take more of your protein in low-priced beans and grains than in meats, get the cheaper cuts of meat, which are just as nutritious, and buy fruits and vegetables in whichever form is cheapest at the time—fresh, frozen, or canned.

• An extra 500 calories a day in your diet, in addition to calories drawn from your body fat stores, should last you through your course of breast-feeding. If you're nursing twins or a very big baby, you may need to eat more.

• By and large, you can be guided by your own body. If you're under-weight to begin with or if you're very active, you will need more calories. If you're very overweight, you probably have enough fat stores so that you can make do with fewer calories. After you start to nurse, you should not be putting on weight—if you are, you're probably eating too much. If you're losing a great deal (more than half a pound a week or two pounds a month), you're probably not eating enough. You should not be losing weight rapidly.

LOSING WEIGHT: HOW MUCH, HOW SOON?

There's a paradox about nursing and women's weight. Breastfeeding does not make women gain weight. In fact, it uses up calories and therefore helps to get rid of extra weight. Nature's way of providing the extra calo-ries needed for milk production is to store up fat during pregnancy. Then lactation helps to use up these fat stores. Therefore, as a nursing mother, you are more likely to lose the fat you gained (especially the lower-body fat) during your pregnancy than is the woman who does not nurse her baby.

According to one recent study, four out of five nursing women who do not restrict their diets lose up to one and a half pounds a month for the first four to six months after delivery, with a smaller loss afterward. An-other study found that six months after delivery, breastfeeding women are, on average, closer to their prepregnancy weight than are formula-feeding mothers.

After six months, the more frequently you nurse and the more time you spend breastfeeding, the more weight you are likely to lose. However, some women who decrease their physical activity and think they must eat more to make milk do gain weight. This can be minimized by this rule: "Eat when you're hungry and stop when you're full." Meanwhile, watch for grad-ual weight loss.

In sum, every woman is different, and some nursing mothers retain at least some of the weight they gained during pregnancy longer than others do. The question then is what to do about it.

Strenuous Dieting Is Not the Answer

While you're breastfeeding, you should not be dieting strenuously. You should not be following a liquid diet, taking any weight-loss drugs, or cutting your calories below the recommended amount for your height and build. Here's why:

• First, your body needs to have enough nutrients to produce milk. If you cut down too drastically on what you eat, you'll be robbing yourself. Your body will maintain the quality of your milk at your expense by cutting into your lean tissues (your muscles) and your bones. This means that you could lose muscle tone and bone density, and become anemic.

• Then, if you become very undernourished, you'll produce less milk, so you'll be robbing your baby of her essential nutrients.

You Can Lose Weight Without Strenuous Dieting

A modest weight loss will not affect your production of milk, and you will serve yourself and your baby best by *gradually* dropping any excess weight left over from your pregnancy. If you are not losing weight gradually while nursing, the two effective ways to do this are by exercising regularly (more about this later in this chapter) and by cutting down without cutting out. For example, you can:

• Substitute skim milk and nonfat yogurt for whole milk products.

• Broil, boil, roast, or bake meats and potatoes instead of frying them.

• Eat more fish and poultry and less red meat.

• Eat smaller amounts of fatty meats and fish.

• Snack on raw vegetables and fruits instead of potato chips and cookies.

• Eat fresh fruits rather than sweetened canned ones.

• Eat more bread, pasta, and rice, seasoned with spices or fruits rather than with butter, margarine, or oil.

• Go lightly on high-calorie fruits like avocados and cherries.

• Eliminate or eat very little of high-fat cheeses, rich sauces, fatty salad dressings, sugared soft drinks, sugary cereals, cookies, cakes, pastries, and candy.

• Read the food labels (see the box on page 145).

What the Labels Usually Mean*

The following descriptions give information for a single serving:

   Calorie free = no more than 5 calories

   Sugar free = less than ½ gram of sugar

   Salt free = fewer than 5 milligrams (mg) of sodium

   Low sodium = no more than 140 mg of sodium

   Fat free = less than ½ gram of fat

   Low fat = no more than 3 grams of fat

   Light = ⅓ fewer calories than, or half the fat in, the regular version or a similar food

*This information was provided by the Center for Science in the Public Interest, Washington, D.C.

Monitor Your Weight

A safe rule of thumb is to plan to lose no more than two pounds per month while you're nursing. Thus, in six months you'll have lost twelve pounds, and by eight months you'll have lost sixteen. This, in addition to the weight you lost with your baby's birth, will probably bring you back down to or close to your prepregnancy weight. After all, it took nine months to put on all those pounds, so it's not unrealistic to expect it to take about the same amount of time to take them off.

This may happen without any special effort on your part—many nursing mothers who eat normally lose about one to one and a half pounds a month for the first four to six months after delivery without making any special effort to shed pounds. However, about one in five nursing mothers does *not* lose weight while breastfeeding. So the best approach seems to be to wait for two or three months after childbirth to see how *your* body responds.

If you're losing steadily, even if it's only one pound a month, you don't have to do anything special about your eating habits. If not, you can start to cut back gradually. Then by the time your baby is nine months old and is taking less milk in proportion to other foods in her diet, you can begin your plan to lose one to two pounds per week.

Losing weight slowly by changing your eating and exercise habits is better than dropping weight quickly, since you're more likely to keep the pounds off. A well-planned exercise schedule is extremely important in your weight-loss program for a number of reasons, which we'll talk about in more detail later in this chapter.

If You're Considerably Overweight: The advice against losing a great deal of weight during lactation does not necessarily hold for women who are very overweight. One new mother we know had put on thirty excess pounds before she got pregnant and then gained another fifty pounds during her pregnancy. With the help of her doctor, she worked out a calorie-restricted but balanced diet and over a period of eight months lost sixty-five pounds, or two pounds a week, while continuing to breastfeed successfully. In this case both mother and baby did well. However, most women are not carrying this much excess weight, and such a large weight loss should not be undertaken *unless* it is medically indicated for your health.

A New Look at Your Body

As we said, some women do lose the weight they gained during pregnancy very soon after their babies are born and remain quite slender throughout lactation and afterward. You don't have to be plump to be a good milk producer. However, as we also said, other women keep their more rounded contours for a longer time.

You may need to think about your weight in a new way. When did you ever see a thin fertility symbol? Just as breastfed babies grow differently from formula-fed babies, the bodies of breastfeeding mothers tend to follow a different schedule from those of non-nursing mothers. A substantial weight gain during pregnancy helps to assure a healthy baby, and part of that weight seems to be nature's way of providing energy for milk after your baby is born.

If you're a typical contemporary American woman, you'll probably have no more than two or three children. Recognizing that during pregnancy and lactation your nutritional status has to support two lives—yours and your baby's—and recognizing the very small proportion of time in relation to your total life span that you will spend breastfeeding, you need to ask yourself: "Can I stand being a few pounds heavier after the birth of each baby, with the assurance that after I've stopped nursing I'll lose this extra weight?" Since you recognize the value of breastfeeding, you can probably answer this question with a ringing "yes!" You may want to talk this issue over with your husband or partner to help him understand and support you.

If you want to feel beautiful now, go to your closest art museum and find paintings featuring breastfeeding mothers. Chances are that most of them will be ample in size—and you'll have a lovely standard of maternal beauty to identify with. Meanwhile, you can enjoy your baby, enjoy your food, and enjoy your life.

EXERCISE: HOW MUCH, HOW SOON?

You may love to exercise or you may hate it. You may have barely fitted in time between your workouts to give birth to your baby. Or you may be the kind of person who has always reacted to the thought of exercise by immediately lying down. Most probably, you're somewhere in between. Whichever place on the fitness spectrum you fall into, you can tailor a routine to your inclinations and your abilities.

The right kind and the right amount of exercise can bring you many benefits, not only now but throughout your life. As Dr. Robert Butler, director of the International Longevity Center at Mount Sinai Hospital in New York, has said, "If doctors could prescribe exercise in pill form, it would be the single most widely prescribed drug in the world." This is particularly good news for nursing mothers, for both short-term and long-range reasons.

Assuming you're in good health, following an active, well-planned exercise schedule during lactation can do wonders for you—especially now. In the weeks and months after giving birth, exercise can help by:

• Toning up sagging postpregnancy muscles, so that you'll feel and look better.

• Assisting you to lose the weight and fat you gained in pregnancy, usually being even more effective in losing fat than dieting. Exercise actually tends to diminish appetite while using up calories, so it's a vital element in maintaining desirable body weight.

• Helping to heal the backache that plagues so many new mothers, as you find yourself bending and lifting more than you've probably done in your entire life. It may even allow you to avoid it in the first place.

• Boosting your energy level—although it's not, unfortunately, magical enough to completely overcome the fatigue that comes from not getting enough sleep.

• Speeding your sexual recovery by tightening muscles that were stretched during childbirth.

Furthermore, exercise isn't only for the postpartum period. Throughout life it helps you build your muscles, strengthen your heart and lungs, lower your blood pressure, protect against heart attacks and cancer, improve your emotional state, and possibly lengthen your life.

Weight-bearing activities like walking, running, skating, and jogging are effective in controlling fat. They also help to increase bone density, thus serving as an important aid to preventing osteoporosis. Exercise reduces stress and anxiety better and more safely than tranquilizers and therefore contributes to your mental health. One reason exercise boosts your morale is that it releases endorphins, brain hormones that give a feeling of well-being.

The best news is that when you find an activity you like, it should actually be fun. You can share the pleasure, too, as bicycling, skating, folk dancing, and other vigorous activities form a good basis for lively family and other social outings. And you can serve as a wonderful role model for your children, thus offering them one more tool for forging a healthy life.

A well-planned exercise program should not have any adverse effects regarding breastfeeding. Research has shown that moderate to strenuous aerobic exercise has no negative effects on either your supply of milk or the quality of breast milk. It *is* thought to change the taste temporarily among women who exercise to *exhaustion*.

Postpartum Exercise

You can begin to do some exercises within twenty-four hours after your baby is born if you start easy, build up gradually, and use common sense. If you had an episiotomy, you may want to wait until you are no longer sore before you undertake vigorous exercise. To find a program, check your bookstore for a book about exercise before and after childbirth—and check with your doctor before starting.

You can begin by doing pelvic tilts, deep breathing, and Kegel (pelvic floor) exercises (see the box on page 253 in Chapter 13). Kegels will also help if you find you have minor incontinence after childbirth. All of these are safe to do right after delivery. In a few days, you can move on to head and leg lifts, leg slides, and a variety of stretching and bending exercises.

Do not overdo! Pregnancy-related changes in your body persist for about four to six weeks. Pay attention to what your body tells you. Warm up slowly, rest between exercises, and stop before you feel tired. Fatigue is an enemy of successful breastfeeding. At the beginning it's more important to establish your milk supply than to preserve your reputation as an athlete. If you develop any unusual symptoms, such as pain, increased vaginal bleeding, dizziness, faintness, or shortness of breath, stop what you're doing. Call your doctor if the symptoms persist after you stop.

The amount of exercise you do will vary, depending on how active you were before you gave birth. If you were very sedentary or if you're now anemic or very overweight, do only limited exercise, and be sure to get your doctor's approval.

One way to monitor your progress is to keep a chart of the number and kinds of exercises you do each day. You'll be able to see how much more you can do as the days go by, and you'll feel proud of your efforts. If you feel good about an hour after exercise, you know that you have not overdone it. However, if you do feel tired, drink some extra fluid. The next day, cut back your exercise level, and build up more slowly.

Developing a Regular Exercise Schedule

One thirty-nine-year-old woman we know, who had been running regularly for fourteen years, ran eight miles a day before she became pregnant and continued to run during her pregnancy, cutting down her distance to two miles a day in late pregnancy. She even did one last short run as her labor was beginning. Within one to two weeks after the birth of each of her five children she began running again. She has breastfed them all and has always produced plenty of milk. Why does she do it? Here's what she says:

"I feel better overall if I exercise regularly. I run to stay fit and have a chance to be outdoors every day. Running helps control my appetite and weight but lets me eat more! It also sets a good example for my kids; they run and participate regularly in various activities."

This woman, of course, may not remind you of anyone you know, least of all yourself! While just reading about this vigorous a schedule will exhaust most of us, it's heartening to see that it can be done. It clearly shows that less ambitious exercise programs are eminently feasible.

You need to figure out what you like to do and what's comfortable for you to do—and then keep doing it on a regular basis. It's better to exercise three or four days a week than to work out every day. It's also good to vary your activity rather than do the same exercise every day. And it's better to work out a routine than exercise on a sporadic, catch-as-catch-can basis. Some research suggests that breaking up your routine into three ten-minute sessions is just as valuable as exercising for a straight half hour. It might be easier for you to find these ten-minute segments of time than to find an uninterrupted half hour.

The most important thing for you to realize is that you're doing the best thing you can for your baby by breastfeeding, and that, as one mother said, "I know that everything else I do is gravy." Eventually you'll lose your extra weight, you'll go back to your former measurements, and you'll be able to resume your previous exercise program. For the duration of nursing, do what you feel good about doing—and feel good about yourself. For suggestions for exercising while breastfeeding, see the section that follows.

AN EXERCISE GUIDE FOR THE NURSING MOTHER

• Schedule your exercise around your breastfeeding. Working out immediately *after* nursing your baby is best for several reasons.

1. Your breasts are not full and uncomfortable and your baby won't be hungry for a while. Some women nurse first thing in the morning (sometimes even before the baby is fully awake), put the baby back to bed, and then exercise.

2. Extremely strenuous exercise can change the taste of breast milk, making an occasional baby reject it. Any flavor change may be caused by a normal, short-term rise in lactic acid concentration after extremely vigorous exercise. Lactic acid levels are less likely to rise after moderate exercise, and in any case are not harmful to infants. Most babies are not bothered at all. However, some who don't like the taste may want to nurse again a short time later.

3. If you choose an activity for which you don't have to meet anyone's schedule but your own, you'll be much more flexible in fitting exercise into your day. One working mother told us about her late-night schedule: Three nights a week, after nursing her daughter at about 10:00, she runs for half an hour with a friend (along a well-lighted course).

• You may not always be able to exercise immediately after a feeding. If you do find that you'll need to nurse your baby soon after a strenuous workout, take the time to cool down, drink a glass of water, shower or rinse off your breasts (if your baby does not like the salty taste of perspiration), and perhaps change your clothes. You may be able to postpone the feeding long enough to avoid any temporary change in the flavor of your milk.

• Choose an activity that you enjoy doing, so that you'll keep on doing it. Among the wide range of activities to choose from are walking, running, jogging, cycling, folk-dancing, inline- or ice-skating, cross-country skiing, yoga, and jumping rope. Swimming is excellent for building muscles and body tone, but it may not be as effective as weight-bearing exercise for controlling fat and building bone density. Its effectiveness depends partly on the individual person and partly on the amount of swimming you do.

• Strenuous arm exercises can sometimes have a negative effect on breastfeeding. So if you regularly lift weights or do other demanding exercises involving repetitive arm movements, resume slowly and see how it

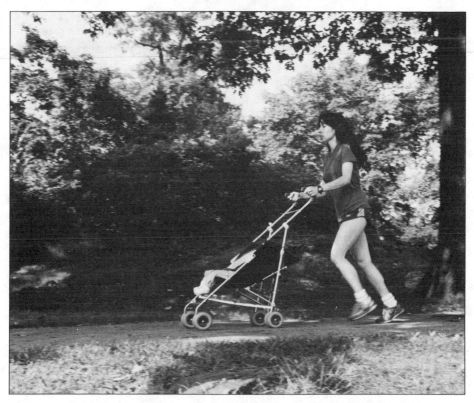

Jogging while pushing a stroller gives this mother her exercise and the baby her fresh air.

goes. If all goes fine, keep going. However, if you notice the beginning of a clogged milk duct or any other problem, cut back and try again later.

• Start your exercise program with very short sessions of a few minutes at a time, three times a week, and gradually increase the frequency and duration of your exercises. If you're exhausted one hour after stopping, cut back—you're doing too much.

• Warm up and stretch before doing aerobic exercise, and cool down and stretch afterward. The after-exercise stretch is the more important one, so if you have to skimp on time, shorten the before-exercise stretching.

• Drink a glass of water before beginning to exercise, and another glass afterward. A good rule of thumb is to drink four to six ounces of water for every fifteen to twenty minutes of exercise. It's important for everyone, but especially for a nursing mother, to replace the fluid lost while exercising. You need to drink more in hot weather.

- Find an "exercise buddy," a friend you can work out with two or three times a week. Although this does compromise the flexibility of your schedule, the benefits of exercising with a friend may be worth the extra planning. For one thing, you'll stimulate each other to keep up with the program, and for another, your workout will do double duty as a social get-together. But don't fall into the trap of judging yourself by what your friend can do. This is *your* personal program, and you need to exercise according to *your* own rhythms.

- Concentrate on activities that you can do without leaving your baby or at times when someone else can be with the baby. You might work out on a stationary bicycle or other at-home equipment, jump rope, or follow a videocassette. One mother's at-home routine includes low-impact aerobics three mornings a week with a videotape and nightly ten-minute spot-toning exercises. She even persuaded her husband to join her in the spot-toning.

- Walking is excellent exercise, and if you carry your baby in a backpack while you walk, the extra weight will use up more calories. This is another activity that can do double or even triple duty: As you walk with your baby, you're both getting fresh air. And if you meet a friend, you'll also have adult company. Or you might run or fitness-walk early in the morning or at night when your partner or older children are home to watch your baby.

- If your favorite exercise program involves going out to a gym or class, treat yourself to a sitter or barter baby-sitting time with a friend or neighbor. Some gyms and health clubs provide child care, a service that can accustom your baby to being with other people and that can help you make friends with other mothers. Again, this will do double duty as a social outing as well as a physical one.

- Dress comfortably. Wear a supportive bra. If you're full-figured, a nursing bra may not provide enough support, so invest in a sport bra in the larger size you need now, and change into it for your exercise sessions. Wear underpants that don't ride up, rub, or constrict. Cotton or polypropylene absorb sweat best. If you get overheated when wearing leotards and tights, switch to shorts and a T-shirt.

- Invest in the equipment that will encourage you to keep exercising— whether it's a baby jogger, a treadmill, a set of steps, or whatever.

- Incorporate exercise into your daily life by taking the stairs rather than an elevator whenever you can, walking to do errands instead of driving, and doing active chores at home.

- Most of all, enjoy your exercise as a time to care for yourself!

How You Look, How You Feel

I believe in rewarding myself—we women don't reward ourselves often enough. So I treat myself by buying clothes that feel good and look good, keeping up my exercise schedule, getting my nails done on my lunch hour, and enjoying those precious times with my baby.

—EMMA, NEW YORK, NEW YORK

You are not living *solely* for your baby even during these months when so much of your time is spent with this newest member of your family. You still have other people in your life, like your husband or partner, your other children, other family members, and friends. Furthermore, you're still a person with your own life and your own needs. Ignoring those needs can have negative ramifications for you and for those you love, both now and in the years to come. For all these reasons, you want to pay attention to your own care even as you're caring for your baby. You need to care for yourself, physically, mentally, and emotionally. And yes, this means looking out for your wants, as well as your needs.

CARE OF YOUR BREASTS

Fortunately, your breasts are a sturdy part of your body, so you don't need to treat them like fragile china. In fact, as we noted earlier, while you're pregnant or nursing, you don't need to do much of anything special to take care of your breasts. You don't need to bother with any special nipple-care rituals, and you don't need any special salves or ointments.

But your breasts do need to feel comfortable, which for many women involves wearing a good nursing bra. Later in this chapter we talk about finding bras that will do just that, while making it more convenient for you to breastfeed. And you do need to let your body's natural moisturizers work on your breasts by not putting any drying agents on them, including soap.

If you splash water over your breasts during your daily shower and change your bra at least once a day (or more often, if you're leaking a great deal of milk), your breasts and your nipples will be clean. Furthermore, disposable or washable breast pads worn inside your bra will help protect your nipples while they help to prevent leakage of milk onto your clothing.

Although breastfeeding women were for years advised to apply a soothing cream or ointment to the nipples after feedings to prevent or treat nipple soreness, research does not show any evidence that any of these creams or salves help. In fact, some can even do harm.

If a substance needs to be wiped off before a baby nurses, the friction on the mother's breasts may contribute to soreness. Also, some salves contain ingredients that some women are allergic to; the more ingredients a product contains, the greater the possibility of a reaction.

If you do use anything on your nipples and they become sore, stop using it immediately. If it was a prescription item (for treating thrush, for example), ask your doctor to prescribe a substitute.

One over-the-counter balm that some women find soothing is purified lanolin. It does not have to be wiped off before you nurse, and it will not hurt you or your baby. However, since lanolin is a fatty substance made from wool, don't use it if you are allergic to wool. Lansinoh for Breastfeeding Mothers® is a safe, pure brand of USP-modified lanolin.*

A more effective practice is keeping your nipples free of surface wetness. You can do this by changing your bra or breast pad if they get wet from leaking milk.

Your breasts should feel good during lactation. Because they are doing something they never did before, however, they may feel somewhat tender on the second or third day of nursing, and possibly even later. *However, you should not be hurting. Painful, cracked, or bleeding nipples are not normal.* If you develop soreness that's more than mildly uncomfortable and if it doesn't go away in a day or two, take care of it immediately. You may need to change your breastfeeding technique (see Chapter 6) and also treat your nipples (see Chapter 15). One way to take care of your breasts is to wear a comfortable bra.

---

*If you cannot find this product in your local pharmacy, you can obtain it from La Leche League or from distributors for Ameda/Egnell breast pumps.

Wearing the Right Bra

Your bra is the single most important item in your wardrobe these days. Even if you're small-breasted and don't ordinarily wear a bra for support, you may want to wear one now—if for no other reason than to hold breast pads or to prevent milk from leaking through your clothes. While you don't need a bra specially designed for breastfeeding, it usually makes life easier.

You'll need at least three bras—one on you, a clean one in the drawer, and one hanging up to dry. If you're leaking a great deal of milk, you'll want to change bras or liners often to keep your nipples from getting sore and your clothes from getting stained.

Nursing bras come in a wide variety of styles and fabrics, from no-nonsense sturdy to lacy and sexy. Some are soft; some have underwires for added support. Some have a row of hooks down the front; others have a hook at the top of each cup. You may find the front-closing style easier to put on and take off.

The nursing bra you bought at the end of your pregnancy may still fit during lactation if you allowed a little extra room. If it's too tight, though, *do not wear it.* A tight bra can cause clogged milk ducts and a great deal of discomfort. If you find, after wearing a style for a couple of weeks, that you like

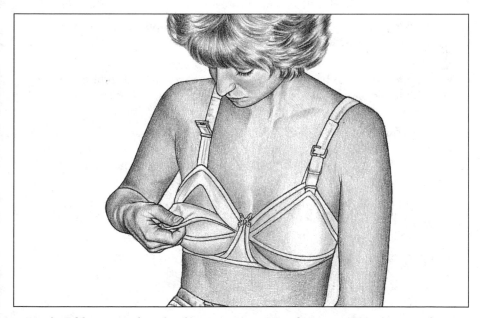

A comfortable nursing bra that lets you uncover one breast at a time, using only one hand, makes life—and nursing—easier. Some bras come with a front clasp rather than one in back, which can make it easier to put on and take off.

Finding the Right Nursing Bra for You

A bra that fits right may help to maintain your breast contours; one that is designed for function will simplify the process of breastfeeding. Keep the following points in mind when you go shopping:

• Be sure you can uncover your breast generously enough so that the fabric of the bra puts no concentrated pressure on any one spot on your breast, and so that your baby can latch on well.

• Look for a style that lets you uncover one breast at a time, using only one hand.

• All-cotton or another breathable, absorbent fabric is best.

• The straps should be broad and adjustable, preferably padded or cushioned, and preferably not elastic.

• Do not buy a garment with plastic-lined cups; they will trap moisture, which may lead to nipple problems.

• The cup should support the entire lower half of your breast in a natural position, and should completely and comfortably cover your entire breast. Put the bra on and hold your arms straight down at your sides. If it fits properly, your nipple line will be level with a point midway between elbow and shoulder.

• The band should fit snugly, neither binding nor slipping up and down. To test this, put your hands on your hips and look at yourself, front and back, in the mirror.

• The bra should not be so tight that it leaves marks in your skin under your arms, under or across your breasts, or over your shoulders. If it has underwires, be sure the ends of the wires do not dig into your breast tissue.

• Stay away from low-cut push-up bras. These tend to cut across the fullest part of your breast and put pressure on the tissue. Also, with these bras, the temptation is to lift your breast out of the cup instead of lowering the cup completely for nursing.

• When buying a bra before your baby is born, allow for some growth afterward. You'll want a little bit of extra room in the cups and in the band. Do not buy a size that you already have to wear on the loosest hook.

• If you are small-breasted and don't need the support of a structured bra, you may prefer to wear a simple stretch bra that can be easily pulled up for nursing rather than a garment designed specifically for breastfeeding.

it, order more by phone or e-mail, or ask someone else to pick them up for you. If not, look for a style you like better. For tips on bra shopping, see the box on page 156.

Protect Yourself from Leaking Milk

You may feel a wonderful sense of abundance when your breasts produce so much milk that it issues forth even when you're not feeding your baby. You may also not want to walk around with nice round spots where your breasts meet your blouse. Although you need not feel embarrassed by public evidence of this wonderful way of nurturing your baby, you may not feel like announcing your lactational status to the world. (See the suggestions beginning on page 159 on clothing that is least likely to show marks from leaking.) Most important is the fact that excess wetness that stays next to the skin of your breasts can cause problems.

You can protect your breasts and your clothing from leaking milk by putting some type of lining inside your bra. You can buy disposable nursing pads in the pharmacy. If you do, get the kind with no gauze lining, since this can stick to your breasts and cause hairline cracks and painful tenderness. If you want to save money or if you find that any disposables you try stick to your skin, you can buy washable, reusable pads. Look for all-cotton ones, since synthetic fibers are not absorbent.

Or you can make your own. Insert a folded man's all-cotton handkerchief in each cup of your bra, or cut out four-inch circles from all-cotton diapers or old T-shirts and stitch three or four thicknesses together. They're very absorbent, fold to the size you need, wash and dry quickly, and don't show through. Do not use synthetic fabrics and no-iron finishes; they are not as absorbent and may be irritating.

Change breast pads often enough to keep your breasts dry. Milk-soaked pads that remain next to your skin form an ideal place for bacteria to grow, possibly causing sore nipples or a breast infection.

Some women like to use plastic breast shells, the kind used to bring out inverted nipples as described in Chapter 4, for catching leaking milk. However, the shells have been known to *promote* continued leaking because of the constant pressure they exert upon the breasts. Occasional use should cause no problem. If you do use them, keep them dry and empty them often.

Leaking is usually common in the early weeks, but even though you continue to produce ample supplies of milk, leaking generally stops being a problem within a couple of months. If you're still leaking through your clothes, try stopping the leak by pressing your breast with the heel of your hand or your forearm when you feel the tingling that signals let-down.

Lumps in the Breast

Your breasts will feel different, and possibly lumpier, during lactation. If you discover a lump in your breast while nursing or in your monthly breast self-examination, chances are that it is related in some way to the fact that you're breastfeeding. If the lump is red, swollen, or painful, it may signal a plugged duct or an infection, which you'll treat by the methods suggested in Chapter 15.

However, if you develop any lump that remains unchanged for more than three days, you should call your doctor. It may be a tumor. Nursing mothers are no more likely to develop breast tumors than are women who do not breastfeed. The only risk that nursing mothers run is the possibility of overlooking a tumor by attributing a lump in the breast to a nursing-related cause. Fortunately, almost all tumors in young women are benign.

If you need to have a breast examination, you do not need to wean your baby. In the unlikely prospect that you have to have the lump removed surgically, you may still be able to continue nursing on the other side and eventually to resume nursing on the affected side.

HOW YOU LOOK

Since how you look affects the way you feel, it's worthwhile to invest a little time, effort, and money into looking good.

A Few Beauty Tips for the Nursing Mother

There is a grace in motherhood that can make this among the loveliest times of your life—much more beautiful than any Hollywood notion of glamour.

This is the time to make life as easy for yourself as possible. Find a few simple self-care routines you can stick to, and make them yours. On a busy day, just running a comb through your hair and washing your face can make you feel good, as well as look good.

Custom-tailor your routine to your own priorities. Since you can't do everything you did before, pick the parts of you whose looks you care the most about—and take care of them. One woman may feel messy if she doesn't wash her hair every day; another can't stand seeing unpolished toenails; a third feels unkempt with unshaven legs.

Your Hair

• This is not the time to make a radical change in the way you wear your hair, unless you're going from a very elaborate coif to a "wash-and-wear" one.

• Don't have a style that you need to set.

• You may want to wait a while to get a permanent, since it may not take during or soon after pregnancy, probably because of the changes in your hormonal balance. However, permanents and hair coloring agents appear to be safe for your nursing baby. There's no evidence of any harmful effects.

• If you hate the way your hair looks, put on a sweatband or a cap with a visor that matches your clothing.

Your Skin

• Your skin may become coarser and blotchy during and soon after pregnancy. Be patient. This, too, will change.

• Whenever you think of it, put some hand or body lotion or baby oil on your body. A loving way to ease back into intimacy with your husband is to give each other body massages. You can do this even if you don't feel ready to become sexually active.

Your Nails

• You'll be more comfortable if your nails are short and pale rather than long and dark. Aside from the danger of scratching your baby, long nails are more likely to break. When bright red nail polish chips, it's more obvious than when a light-colored one does. You may want to buff your nails now instead of polishing them.

• The fun place to apply polish these days is on your toenails. For one thing, it's wonderful to know that you can reach them again. For another, they won't chip so fast, and you might enjoy the undercover glamour.

Your Clothes

You probably don't need to buy anything special to wear while you're nursing. Most likely you already have enough suitable clothing to wear as is, or with minor alterations. However, now that you can put away your maternity clothes (at least most of them), picking up a few extra wardrobe items may give your spirits a lift.

• Do pick garments that are washable and wrinkle-resistant and that don't need ironing.

• A number of companies specialize in making clothes for nursing women. These are generally equipped with disguised slits in strategic places that make them convenient for breastfeeding.

You can find ads for these clothes in the pages of parenting magazines, and you can order from catalogs by phone, mail, or e-mail. This is an easy way to shop, and almost all mail-order houses make it easy to return items if they don't fit right or don't look as good in person as they did on the page.

• Warm-up suits or sweatsuits are ideal for your first postpartum wardrobe. They come in a range of wonderful colors and fabrics from terry to velour; the waistlines are adjustable; the pullover tops hide your middle and can be easily pulled up to nurse; you can keep them on while you sneak in a nap; and they're easy to throw into the washer and dryer.

With coordinated socks, sneakers, barrettes, and/or headband, you can have a put-together look—and you'll look like an athlete even if you don't feel like one. Buying three or four in different colors will give you a basic everyday wardrobe, which you'll probably still be wearing after you've weaned your baby.

• Another easy and comfortable choice is an outfit of leggings and a long shirt or pullover. However, if you had a cesarean birth with a midline incision, neither of these would be a good choice, since you won't want anything elastic around your waist until the incision heals. So you probably don't want to go overboard on shopping until after your baby is born, since there's always the possibility of an unplanned cesarean.

• Some women like wearing a loose jumper made of some no-iron material. If it doesn't already come with nursing slits, you can make them yourself.

• For more formal occasions, separates—blouses, T-shirts, and other tops worn with skirts or pants—are easier to manipulate than dresses. Wraparound skirts or skirts and pants with elasticized waists are especially good, since your former waistline will be only a fond memory for a few months.

• Button-front blouses are convenient, but so are knit pullovers, which can be easily pulled up to allow for modest nursing. When you're wearing a button-front blouse, you can nurse more discreetly if you unbutton from the bottom up rather than from the top down. When you wear a pullover, your baby's body will cover your midriff and the pullover will cover your breast.

• Choose prints rather than solid colors; prints are less likely to show milk that may leak through. Avoid white, pale colors, and clingy materials. Remember that breast pads that fit into your bra will absorb leaking milk and help to prevent your clothes from getting stained.

• Ponchos and loose-fitting cardigan sweaters and jackets are good cover-ups for unobtrusive nursing.

• You may want to have one pretty scarf or shawl that you can keep handy to drape around your shoulders when an unexpected caller comes to the door while you're in the midst of feeding your baby.

• Nursing nightgowns, which also come in a range of styles and fabrics, are also good for both comfort and morale, although two-piece pajamas work well, too.

• Don't make the mistake of trying too soon to squeeze into too-tight prepregnancy clothes. It's bad for your morale, as well as your comfort. Besides, tight blouses rub against your nipples and can trigger a let-down at the most inconvenient times. More important, they have occasionally been implicated as the cause of a clogged duct or breast infection.

• If you sew, you can make your own clothes or adapt those you already own. You can, for example, make horizontal seams across the bustline of a blouse or dress, or open darts under it where you can insert invisible zippers or Velcro. Or you can put zippers under the armholes of sleeveless dresses. You can attach fake pockets over each breast with Velcro. A flip of your wrist will lift a corner of the pocket to make the breast accessible to your baby but protected from public view. However, remember that Velcro makes noise when you open it and factor this into your decision.

• If you work outside the home, see the suggestions in Chapter 12 for clothes for the working nursing mother.

GETTING ENOUGH REST

Weariness seems to be the lot of every new mother. Right after your body has undergone the aptly named experience of labor, you have more responsibility but get less sleep. If stress and fatigue kept women from breastfeeding, none of us would be here today, because our mothers, grandmothers, great-grandmothers, and more distant forebears certainly had their share of both. However, the better you feel, the easier the breastfeeding will go, so it makes sense to get as much rest as possible.

Finding Help

If you can hire someone to help you in the house right after you come home from the hospital, the money you spend will be an investment that will yield dividends for the entire family.

• Maybe you can find a high school or college student or an older person who can come in for a few hours each afternoon, straighten up the house, take your older children out, and cook and clean up after dinner.

• One new mother told us, "The best thing I did for myself was hire a neighbor to come in for just one hour every afternoon. She runs the washing machine or puts away the clean laundry, hangs up clothes, takes out the garbage, and washes whatever dishes are piled up in the sink."

• Another helpful—and inexpensive—option is to hire a youngster (age nine to fourteen) to be a "limited-responsibility" sitter. You wouldn't leave a baby or even an older child alone in the house with this young a sitter, but children this age often love babies and small children, and would almost pay *you* to let them stay with your youngsters.

Such a sitter can play an important role. The sitter can, for example, play with an older child while you're busy with your baby. During the "witching hour," that hour or two before dinner or bedtime when babies are often fussy, the sitter can hold your baby while you're fixing dinner or reading to your older children.

Ways to Guard Your Rest

THE TELEPHONE

Telephones are wonderful lines of communication, but they can also be invaders of privacy and disturbers of rest. They don't have to be, though, if you take precautions like the following:

• When you and your baby want to rest, turn off the bell on your telephone.

• Hook up an answering machine with a message along the lines of the following: "I'm sleeping or busy with the baby right now. Please leave your name and number and I'll call you back when I can." Or indicate when someone else will be home to answer the phone.

• Return your phone calls while lying in bed at a time when it's convenient for you to handle them.

THE DOORBELL

To prevent being disturbed by unexpected callers or solicitors, hang a notepad and pen on your door, next to a sign that says something like this: "Please do not ring the doorbell. We cannot be disturbed now. Please leave a note."

As one mother who took this route said, "The young neighbor I hired to be a 'big sister' to my three-year-old was more mature and useful as a sitter when she was nine than she turned out to be when she hit her teen years!"

• If your budget doesn't allow this, perhaps the person or persons acting as your doula, or special helper, can help out, for which you can reciprocate at some time in the future. Grocery shopping, bringing a cooked meal, and taking out your older children are all tasks that friends and family members will often do cheerfully.

HOW DO YOU FEEL—AND WHY DO YOU FEEL THIS WAY?

As the mother of a new baby, you are in one of the most intense periods of your entire life. You're likely to be swept up by a dizzying array of emotions, including excitement, joy, and a deep sense of inner satisfaction—as well as worry, disappointment, and possibly even depression.

You may look at your baby sometimes, perhaps when you have just been roused from a deep sleep or when your nipples are tender or when you turn down yet another invitation because you can't or don't want to get a baby-sitter, and think, "Motherhood isn't all it's been cracked up to be." If you do, you are not alone. Practically every mother alive has at one time or another had this thought. For no matter how much you longed to have a child and how much you love him, he has wrought vast changes in your life.

The birth of a baby marks a major transition point in both parents' lives, but it's usually much more marked for the mother, since your life is apt to change more than the new father's. Even in these "liberated" times, in most homes most of the responsibility for raising children falls to the mother. Even if you will be working full-time, you'll probably still be the parent who finds the child care and takes your child to the caregiver, who stays home when your child is sick, who keeps track of what needs to be done. Studies show that married working mothers generally handle 70 to 80 percent of child-care and household duties in addition to their paying jobs.

As a breastfeeding mother, you are apt to be particularly conscious of your involvement in your baby's care, and your primary responsibility for that care. No matter how much you love your baby, you may chafe at her complete dependence on you. And as you become aware of these feelings, you're likely to be overwhelmed by shame because you *know* that mothers are supposed to love their babies *all* the time, twenty-four hours a day, seven days a week. This is one of the things that we *know* that is not necessarily so.

Many new mothers are guilt-ridden when they realize that they feel no great surge of love when they first see their babies. But maternal love sometimes takes time to develop. In one classic study, only half of a group of fifty-four new mothers said they had had positive feelings when they first saw their babies (and only 13 percent identified these feelings as love); about a third reported having had no feelings at all. It took most of the mothers about three weeks to begin to love their babies; by three months the loving tie was usually firmly set.

Are You Feeling Blue?

You may find yourself losing your temper over little things, or crying at the slightest provocation. You may have problems eating, sleeping, or getting up in the morning. In a severe case, you might even lose interest in everything and everybody. To make matters worse, you may worry and feel guilty about the depression itself.

The first thing you need to know is that your reaction is not abnormal. The low feeling that about half of all new mothers feel soon after their babies' birth is generally called the "baby blues." It used to be called "milk blues" or "milk fever," because it often comes a few days after birth, along with the first appearance of milk. Then there is a more troubling—and fortunately, less common—reaction known as "postpartum depression."

About half of all new mothers have these "baby blues," and second-time mothers are more vulnerable than mothers of first babies. What causes these low feelings?

Some experts feel that the changed hormonal balance in the body is to blame, especially in light of the sudden change in hormone levels brought by the delivery of the baby and placenta. This explanation, however, doesn't explain why only half of new mothers experience these blues even though they all experience similar hormonal changes. And second-time mothers don't experience more hormonal changes than first-timers. Furthermore, nursing women have higher levels of prolactin, which often is a calming influence, and yet they're just as likely to have the blues.

The answer probably lies in the combination of changes in your body and changes in your life. If this is your first baby, you have to transform the entire rhythm of your days to fit your baby's needs. Both you and your husband are suddenly catapulted into new feelings of responsibility, and your relationship with him is affected.

In addition, your new baby's own personality may be a factor. If your baby cries a lot, sleeps little, and is slow learning how to nurse, she will pose special challenges. Even if you already have other children, the arrival of a new

Differences Between Postpartum Blues and Postpartum Depression*

	"BABY BLUES"	DEPRESSION
Time of Onset	3 to 10 days after delivery (sometimes after a helper goes home)	Any time in first year after delivery
Duration	A few days, up to 2 weeks	At least 2 weeks, but often longer
Incidence	From 30 to 84% of new moms; average, 56% of them	10 to 40% of new mothers
Symptoms	Mood swings, crying easily, headaches, forgetfulness, restlessness, irritability, negative feelings toward baby and other family members	All those experienced with the blues, plus anxiety, despair, problems with sleep and eating, feelings of helplessness and hopelessness, irrational fears about baby and self
Treatment	Balanced diet, vitamin and mineral supplements, exercise, help in caring for the baby, emotional support from family and friends, brief psychotherapy or counseling (especially cognitive therapy, which helps you to think positively)	All those recommended for the blues, plus antidepressant medication if prescribed by doctor and not harmful to baby (see Chapter 9)
Prognosis	Good!	Good!

* This chart is adapted, with permission, from one prepared by Kathleen A. Kendall-Tackett, Ph.D., of the Family Research Lab of the University of New Hampshire, Durham, New Hampshire.

baby means new financial responsibilities, new room arrangements, and new routines for the entire family. On top of that, you're probably wondering how you can handle your older children's reactions to the new baby. All this when chronic fatigue is likely to make all your other problems seem worse.

Ways to Boost Your Postpartum Morale

Many new mothers find the following measures help them to feel better:

• Take care of yourself. You can't meet your baby's needs if you don't meet your own.

• Eat a healthy diet comprising foods you enjoy. Whenever possible, try not to rush your eating. Take vitamin and mineral supplements as suggested by your doctor.

• Get as much rest as you can. Nap during the day when your baby sleeps to make up for losing sleep at night. Set a schedule whereby your partner brings the baby to you during the night, if the baby is not sleeping in or near your bed.

• Develop an exercise routine. If you haven't followed one before, this is a good time to start. You need those endorphins!

• Forget about housework for now. The Board of Health won't come for you if there are dustballs under the bed or full wastebaskets in every room. Do what you absolutely have to do, and let the rest wait.

• Ask for help—all kinds of help—from your husband or partner, your relatives, your friends—and don't forget how much help your older children can be.

• Work out an arrangement so that your partner can spend more time at home and do more in the home, at least for a while.

• Pay for as much help as you can afford. It's a sound investment in your comfort and peace of mind.

• Cut back on outside responsibilities. Let someone else collect the union dues, bake the cookies, staff the hot line, chair the meeting.

Before you have a baby, it's impossible to know what life with one will be like. Most women—including adoptive mothers—find that taking care of a newborn is more exhausting and time-consuming than they had ever imagined. Your sleep is constantly being interrupted to feed your baby and your body is working to recover from your labor.

In our society the typical new mother tends to lack self-confidence in her maternal ability. You *know* motherhood must be difficult because there are so many books telling you how to handle your children's psyches, how to raise their IQs—even how to feed them at your breast! And if the professionals disagree about the best theories of child rearing, how are you to have confidence that you know what's best?

- Take some time for yourself every day, even if some days it's only fifteen minutes to read a magazine or listen to music. Or you could set aside a few minutes every day for meditation, or playing the piano, or writing in your journal, or just taking what one mother calls her "ten-minute sanity walk."

- Pay attention to your appearance; you'll feel better if you look better.

- After the first week, get dressed every day. At first, staying in your nightclothes may help you get your rest, since people won't expect too much of you. After this time, though, it can be dispiriting to find yourself still in your bathrobe at 6:00 P.M.

- Join a mothers' group (such as those sponsored by La Leche League, a childbirth education group, or a local family service agency). Other mothers have similar problems and feelings and can help you with yours.

- See a mental health professional who will give you short-term counseling or cognitive therapy to help you deal with stress and think more positively.

- If your symptoms are especially troubling, see a psychiatrist (an M.D.) who can discuss options such as personal psychotherapy or the use of antidepressant medication. Be sure the doctor knows you are breastfeeding. If the medication is not listed among those in Chapter 9 that are safe for your nursing baby, check it out with La Leche League International (see the Resource Appendix).

- Also, check with La Leche League before taking any herbal, homeopathic, or other alternative remedies. Not all substances that grow naturally are safe for breastfeeding mothers to take.

You may look at this list and groan, thinking that any or all of these suggestions are too much trouble. But exerting yourself to take care of yourself may well make you feel better.

Although the "baby blues" are not a new phenomenon, new stresses around motherhood may provide a fertile soil for them to develop. Having idealized both childbirth and breastfeeding, some women find that neither experience has lived up to their expectations. They're disappointed with the experience and disappointed in themselves, feeling that they have not quite measured up. Women who had planned to have a completely unmedicated delivery and then needed anesthesia, women who had practiced their breathing exercises and then needed a cesarean delivery, and women who have a rocky start with breastfeeding are apt to forget that the ultimate goal of childbirth and child rearing is a healthy baby and a healthy mother.

Then, in an age when women are urged to have it all, many women learn that having it all at the same time can be overwhelming. Combining career with motherhood is much harder than most women expected it to be. As a result, you may feel that there's something wrong with you—rather than with the unrealistic expectations that only Supermom could fill.

Ideally, as a breastfeeding mother, you should feel empowered that your milk is helping your baby bloom. However, because of cultural pressures your confidence may be actually undermined by the fact that you're the exclusive supplier of your baby's food. When a bottle-fed baby cries, or has frequent or sparse bowel movements, or sleeps too little or too much, a mother (and the people around her) will blame the formula or the baby's personal inclinations. When the same thing happens with a breastfed]baby, the first reaction is often to blame the breastfeeding. You worry that your baby's not getting enough milk or that your milk isn't good enough or that you're doing something wrong. The unhelpful remarks of other people often feed this anxiety. No wonder your confidence is shaky and your feelings can run away with you!

If you're having major problems with breastfeeding—if your baby isn't gaining enough weight or if you have developed a medical condition that makes it very difficult to continue nursing—it's not surprising that you should be upset. Almost always, with the right help you will be able to overcome such difficulties and to move beyond them.

Similarly, almost always, the blues will leave as suddenly as they came. To help them go away, you may want to try some of the suggestions in the box on page 166.

If, however, you are still feeling depressed more than two weeks after your baby is born, you may benefit from speaking with a mental health professional. Some of the differences between the milder "blues" and the full-blown clinical depression are listed in the box on page 165. The most important difference is that the "blues" are temporary and will pass within a couple of weeks after they appear, without doing anything in particular about them. A clinical depression, on the other hand, does need more attention and treatment.

What You Need to Tell Yourself

You may be feeling blue if you have to or decide to wean your baby earlier than you had originally planned to. If so, it's only natural to feel sad and disappointed, to mourn the loss of an experience that was highly meaningful. There is no reason, however, to feel guilty or like a failure as a mother. By nursing for whatever time you did, you gave your baby more benefits than he would have received if you had never breastfed him at all.

Be reassured that you are doing the best you can for your baby. Then accept your negative feelings along with your positive ones and realize that you're neither bad nor inadequate for having them.

We can't help how we *feel* about things, even though we can control what we *do* about our feelings. You'll learn to live with these mixed feelings as you learn to live with mixed feelings about every other aspect of life—your marriage, your work, your schooling. So it is with parenthood. We learn to take the bad with the good—the dirty diapers with the joyous gurgles, the waking up at three in the morning with the bright smile that rewards us as we go to our baby, the burdens of responsibility with the all-embracing love of a child.

When you come right down to it, most parents feel that the joys of having and raising children far outweigh the demands they make.

The thought and care that you put into both the inner and the outer you will pay off in many ways. The better you feel, the happier your breastfeeding—and parenting—experience is likely to be. And the better cared for *you* are, the more both you and your baby will benefit.

Drugs and the Nursing Mother

Is there any new information on the Pill and breastfeeding? What about other medicines? I ask health care providers a lot of questions and they say it's okay to take this or that, but I wonder!

—FRANNIE, CENTRAL, SOUTH CAROLINA

F rom time immemorial people have taken a variety of drugs for a variety of reasons—to cure their diseases, to ease their pain, to drown their sorrows, to achieve new levels of consciousness. During the past half-century, however, our pharmacopoeia has mushroomed incredibly: 90 percent of all the medicines available today were unknown fifty years ago. In addition, with advances in medical research we now know that any drugs that you take can affect the fetus you carry in your womb and the baby you breastfeed.

While you're nursing your baby, you're justifiably concerned about anything that you take into your body. Your major questions are whether a particular agent will pass through your milk, and if it does, whether it will affect your baby.

It's comforting to know that, in general, you can safely take most commonly used drugs and continue nursing your baby. Most drugs do cross into breast milk, but in most cases they do so in such small amounts that they will not hurt your nursing baby. All too often, physicians unnecessarily tell mothers not to breastfeed if they are taking any medicine, for fear that the substance will hurt the baby.

In this chapter we will focus on the effects of drugs on nursing babies. We will not be discussing the effect of any drugs that you take during your pregnancy. If you are pregnant while you are reading this, we want to emphasize how essential it is for you to consult your doctor before you take *any chemical agent*. Some drugs—over-the-counter, prescription, and recreational—can have harmful effects on the fetus when taken by a pregnant woman. So can some herbal preparations.

Basically, whether you're pregnant or nursing, you should not take *any* drug unless you have a sound medical reason for it. This is the best course for both you and your baby. However, if there is some medical indication that a particular agent is important for your physical and emotional well-being, in *most* cases you can take it.

There are three basic scenarios in situations like this:

1. In most cases you can take the prescribed medication and continue breastfeeding.

2. In some cases you can temporarily interrupt breastfeeding—which we'll explain how to do later in this chapter.

3. In a very few cases, you will have to make a hard decision because you cannot take some drugs and continue nursing.

The boxes in this chapter list drugs that would fit into each scenario, according to criteria that are accurate at the time of this writing. The drugs are divided into the following categories:

• those you can take without fear while you are nursing (in the box on page 174);

• those that, if you need to take them temporarily, require a brief interruption of breastfeeding (in the box on page 176);

• and those that, if you need to take them, will require that you wean your baby (in the box on page 178).

However, these lists are only guides at best, since new drugs are coming on the market every day and new findings are emerging about many established ones. Before we discuss chemical agents taken while you are already breastfeeding, we want to look at the effects on nursing of drugs taken during labor and delivery.

DRUGS DURING CHILDBIRTH

Biblical scholars still debate whether God's injunction to Eve, "In travail shalt thou bring forth children," implied labor or sorrow. In any case, most societies have evolved ways to speed delivery, make the mother's work easier, and lessen her discomfort. General anesthesia, which renders the woman completely unconscious, is rarely used today. More common is regional (local) anesthesia, which blocks the nerve pathways that would carry the sensation of pain to the brain.

If you receive medication during labor and delivery, some of it will pass through the placenta and enter your baby's blood supply and tissues. The effect of the anesthesia in your body will wear off in a few hours, but it may take several weeks for all the drugs to be eliminated from your baby's immature system.

Babies whose mothers received *a great deal* of pain-killing agents during childbirth are likely to be quite sleepy the first few days of life. While this does not seem to have a permanent effect on full-size, full-term babies, it does affect their early activities, including their interest in nursing. Since the vigorous suckling of a hungry baby is vital for establishing an ample supply of milk in the mother, if your baby is sleepy and not interested in nursing, both you and she are at a definite disadvantage in building up your production of milk.

What About Epidurals?

The most commonly administered regional anesthesia today is the epidural block, in which an anesthetic agent or a narcotic, or a combination of both, is injected into the space between the spinal cord and its outer covering to deaden sensation in the lower half of the body during delivery. This method of childbirth medication has increased dramatically over the past twenty years—especially for urban first-time mothers who are attended by obstetricians and covered by private health insurance.

The use of epidural blocks, especially for mothers who plan to breast-feed, is controversial. Some research reports ineffective early suckling by infants whose mothers received epidural anesthesia, and other research shows no effects on these babies. The controversy is still not settled as of this writing.

Epidural blocks are relatively safe in that less anesthesia is needed to lessen discomfort, and it can be stopped temporarily to let the mother have full control over pushing, and then restarted after delivery. However, problems with epidurals may include prolonged labor and a temporary lessening of the ability to nurse.

What Should You Do?

There is no simple answer to this question. If you can avoid anesthesia during childbirth, you should. However, you are the only person who can gauge your pain, and you are also the person who is most concerned about your child's well-being. Therefore you, in consultation with your physician, should be the one who decides which, if any, obstetric medication should be used. And if you do need anesthesia, there is no reason for you to feel guilty. Most mothers who have received obstetric anesthesia have gone on to breastfeed long and happily.

You have to weigh the relative risks and benefits of pain relief. If you're in so much pain during childbirth that you're worn out and overstressed, your ability to nurse will be affected. The best thing, then, is to educate yourself ahead of time about your options, including nonchemical means of alleviating discomfort, such as breathing and relaxation techniques, either alone or in combination with lower doses of anesthesia. Many of the negative effects of drugs are dramatically dose-related, so keeping down the amount you take minimizes the risk.

It's extremely important for you to discuss with the doctor who'll be attending you during the birth what kind of medication will be ordered for you while you're in labor. You have to be very clear about what you want. You might say, perhaps, something like: "I want to have the least amount of medication possible. I want to avoid general anesthesia. But what if my prepared childbirth techniques are not enough and I'm in a lot of pain? How can I feel more comfortable while posing the least amount of harm to my baby?"

You and your doctor can discuss your situation, in light of your medical history and physical condition, and the two of you can arrive at a possible course of action. You should feel confident that both your needs and those of your baby are carefully considered and that you are getting the best care possible for your own individual situation.

After you and your physician have agreed upon the probable procedures to be used in your situation, ask the doctor to make a note of the plan on your chart, so that if she or he is not available when you go into labor, whoever is there will be guided by your wishes.

MEDICINES

There is a world of difference between pregnancy and lactation, regarding the ability of drugs to affect the infant. The drugs you take can have very different effects, depending on whether your child is still in the womb or is being breastfed. A number of medicines taken by the pregnant woman that can cause serious birth defects in the developing fetus may cause no harm to the infant when ingested in the mother's milk. However, it's possible that some drugs that may be safe for a fetus, because they are detoxified by the mother's kidney and liver, are not safe for a newborn baby whose own sys-

Medicines That Can Safely Be Taken by Nursing Mothers*

Medicines that breastfeeding mothers can generally take with safety in the usual doses while they continue to nurse their babies are:

Acetaminophen (Tylenol)

Acyclovir (for herpes)

Most antibiotics

Antiepileptic drugs

Antihistamines

Antihypertensives, except for some drugs in the "beta blocker" category

Aspirin (one or two tablets a day for occasional short-term use, i.e., just a few days, after the newborn period—although ibuprofen is preferred)

Caffeine (moderate coffee drinking is not harmful to a nursing baby)

Cimetidine (Tagamet)

Codeine

Cold remedies (over-the-counter)

Decongestants

Fluconazole (Diflucan; for thrush in milk duct and on breast or vaginal yeast infection)

Ibuprofen (Advil; one or two tablets a day for occasional short-term use, i.e., just a few days)

Loperamide (Immodium)

Phenobarbital (in small amounts; doses large enough to put the mother to sleep can make the baby sleepy, too)

Drugs that enhance thyroid function

Tolbutamide (for diabetes)

Vaccines

*Sources for this box and the boxes on pages 176 and 178: American Academy of Pediatrics Committee on Drugs, 1994; Cheston Berlin, M.D., personal communications, 1998; Sia, 1985; Govoni and Hayes, 1985. Names in parentheses after generic names of drugs are common trade names.

tem is too immature to do this important task. We cannot, therefore, apply what we know about one situation to the other.

The problem is that there's so much we don't know. We don't, for example, know about the long-term effects of a baby's receiving drugs through her mother's milk. We don't know whether receiving drugs now in infancy might cause a hypersensitivity to certain components later on. Nor do we know whether a buildup of the drug in the baby's system could cause problems now or later.

What Should You Do?

As the most important rule of thumb (even for people who are not nursing an infant), it's best to take the least amount of medicine possible. If you don't need it, don't take it. If you do need it, take it in a way that will minimize its effects on your baby.

You should not be taking large amounts of *any* medicine, even the most innocuous-seeming over-the-counter or herbal preparation, without your doctor's knowledge. Nor should you take anything for more than three or four days without checking with your doctor. This is important for your own health, as well as your baby's; you might be masking symptoms of a serious nature. You can take an occasional ibuprofen (which would be better to use than aspirin), acetaminophen, antihistamine, or other over-the-counter preparation, such as the ones listed in the box on page 174, without checking with your doctor first.

In some rare cases your medical situation might require a course of treatment that could have an adverse effect on your baby. Should this occur, you will have to make the best of a less-than-ideal situation and wean your baby. If this becomes necessary, you need to remember that for whatever length of time you have breastfed, you have given your child a good start in life. Now, you can still provide warmth and comfort and nurturance in many other ways, and the most important gift you can give your child is a healthy mother.

Whenever possible, it's better to continue breastfeeding than to wean your baby prematurely because you are taking a drug that might harm your baby. This is especially true if weaning would be abrupt. Sudden weaning is painful for the mother and upsetting for both mother and baby. Early weaning also deprives the baby of the benefits of breastfeeding. Therefore, it makes sense for mother and doctor to work together to solve medical problems within the context of breastfeeding, whenever this is possible. The only drugs that would require early weaning are those listed in the box on page 178.

Ask Your Doctor

Before taking any new drug, check with *your baby's* doctor, as well as with the one prescribing the medicine for you. Tell your doctor or dentist—whoever is treating you—that you are nursing your baby. Ask the following questions:

1. *Will this drug pass through my breast milk?*
    Most drugs do, but the baby is generally exposed to less than 1 to 2 percent of the mother's dosage. The baby's absorption may be even lower. In any case, this small amount is usually not harmful.

Medicines That Require a Temporary Cessation of Breastfeeding

One of the more common situations in which a mother should stop breastfeeding for a little while because she needs to take a drug that might harm her baby is when she undergoes a diagnostic procedure requiring her to take a radioactive compound (like Gallium-67, Iodine-123, -125, or -131, or Technetium-99m). While the drug is in her system, radioactivity is present in her milk and will reach her baby. Should you need this type of procedure, you could protect your baby by doing the following:

• Ask your doctor to consult a nuclear medicine physician who can prescribe the agent with the shortest half-life in breast milk.

• Discontinue breastfeeding for twelve hours to two weeks, depending on the compound. The long-lasting types of these medicines are hardly ever given anymore. Most often, two or three days is the longest one needs to suspend breastfeeding.

• Before the procedure, pump your breasts and freeze enough milk to feed your baby for the period of time you are not breastfeeding. Or you can use formula for this short-term interruption of breastfeeding if your baby is not at risk for allergy.

• Continue to pump your breasts (to maintain milk production) during the time the radioactive agent is present in your body. In fact, you can pump and freeze your milk, and use it later, since the radioactivity disappears from it within hours or days, depending upon the medication and the dosage. You might want to label the milk with the date, so you will know when it is safe to use.

• Modern radiology departments can measure milk for the presence of radioactivity. You can resume nursing when the radioactivity has disappeared. This is the safest step of all.

---

2. *Is this drug potentially dangerous to my baby?*

A mother on continuous or long-term medication for some medical condition needs to pose this question to her doctor and her baby's doctor, since the possible cumulative exposure to the drug must be considered in evaluating its effect on the baby.

3. *What complications or discomfort would I experience if I do* not *take this medicine? Would they be acceptable, from both medical and comfort standpoints? Would it be safe for me to forgo treatment?*

You could probably put up with a few aches and pains, but if your health is at stake, being a martyr will benefit neither you nor your child.

4. *Can I safely postpone treatment until my child is older and his more mature body systems are better able to detoxify chemicals in the milk?*

Sometimes a compound that would be dangerous for a one-week-old or one-month-old poses no problem for an older baby. And sometimes it's possible to wait.

5. *Can I monitor my baby for possible symptoms and stop taking the medicine in time? If not, can another agent be substituted?*

6. *Is this a new medicine about which little is known, and if so, can another, more established one be substituted?*

7. *Why am I being advised to stop nursing? Is it because the maker of the medicine does not know what the effects would be? Or because there are known ill effects?*

Among the considerations your doctor will have to weigh are whether this medicine is one that can safely be given to a baby of your baby's age, whether the dosage you need will send too much of the drug into your baby's system, and for how long a period you'll need to be taking the compound.

If You Must Take a Prescribed Medicine

If your doctor determines that it is medically necessary for you to take a drug, you and your baby's doctor will have to decide whether you can continue to breastfeed during your course of treatment, whether you should interrupt breastfeeding temporarily and then resume nursing, or whether you need to wean your baby.

Even if the medicine you're taking is considered safe for your baby, you still want to minimize its effects as much as possible. One way to do this is to take it immediately after a feeding and to delay the next feeding as long as you can so that the medicine will have as much time as possible to work its way through your system before the baby's next nursing.

If you have a question about a medication you've been prescribed, call La Leche League International (see the Resource Appendix). Between the reference texts and research studies in the League's Center for Breastfeeding Information and the physicians on the League's Health Advisory Council, help is available to guide you and your doctor.

Meanwhile, watch your baby closely for any unusual symptoms— fever, sleepiness, vomiting, unusual crying, loss of appetite, diarrhea, rash, irritability, and so forth. Call your baby's doctor if you notice these or other possible signs of drug effects.

Medicines That Should Not Be Taken by Nursing Mothers

MEDICINE	REASON FOR NOT USING IT WHILE NURSING
Bromocriptine (Parlodel)	Inhibits prolactin secretion, decreases milk supply.
Chemotherapeutic agents used to treat cancer: Cyclophosphamide (Cytoxan, Neosar, Procytox) Doxorubicin Methotrexate (Amethopterin)	These drugs are given precisely because they kill cells in the body. There is a danger, therefore, that even a tiny dose may have harmful effects on the cells in the baby's system. They may suppress a baby's immune system, and their effect on growth is unknown.
Ergotamine (Ergomar, Ergostat, Gynergen)	Doses used in medicines for migraine headaches can cause vomiting, diarrhea, and convulsions in baby. May decrease milk supply.
Lithium	Can cause irritability and poor feeding.
Antidepressants (Prozac, Zoloft, and tricyclic agents)	Can cause drowsiness and irritability in infant. Unknown long-term effects on child's central nervous system.
Atenolol	This drug, which is given to prevent migraine headaches and also to lower blood pressure, may cause slowing of a baby's heart rate, especially in preterm infants or those with impaired kidney function.

If you have to take a medicine that is thought to be harmful to your nursing baby, and if you need to take it for only a short period of time (say, a week or two), you can pump or express your milk during that time and discard it, while feeding your baby formula or previously expressed milk. This way, you'll be keeping up your milk supply and you'll be able to resume nursing as soon as the medicine is no longer in your system. If breastfeeding has been well established, the baby will probably be eager to go back to the breast.

Regarding antianxiety, antidepressant, and antipsychotic agents, the only negative effects that have shown up in nursing infants whose mothers have taken them are that the babies seem to be somewhat sedated and to show some symptoms of colic during the first two weeks of life. However, since these compounds do appear in human milk, there is a concern that if a breastfeeding mother takes them for significant periods of time, her baby's central nervous system function, which is developing rapidly, might suffer. So far we do not know what the long-term effects on the central nervous system might be.

So what should you do if your doctor advises you to take one of these medications? The safest course is not to take these drugs while you are nursing. However, if you do take the drug and do continue to breast-feed, be sure to monitor your baby closely for the first signs of drowsiness or irritability.

BIRTH CONTROL PILLS

If you take oral contraceptive pills, they may inhibit your production of milk, especially if you take them early in lactation. Birth control pills contain hormones, either estrogen or progesterone or a combination of both.

Studies done in the 1960s and 1970s suggested that estrogen was the hormone most responsible for this decrease in milk production. However, those studies were done with pills containing larger amounts of estrogen than are in the contraceptive pills on the market today. Contraceptives containing only progesterone (the progestin-only minipill), including the long-acting injections (like DepoProvera) and under-the-skin implants (Norplant), do not appear to be associated with a decrease in milk production if taken after six weeks after delivery, when the milk supply is established.

Neither estrogens nor progesterones have been associated with any change in the quality of breast milk. Furthermore, long-term studies have failed to find any effect on growth in children up to eight years old whose mothers took estrogen-based birth control pills while nursing. Also, no effect on growth or the onset of puberty has been found up to seventeen years of age in children whose mothers took progesterone compounds.

It is probably safe, then, to take the low-dose-estrogen birth control pills, but if you are comfortable with another form of birth control, you might want to use it temporarily. The various kinds of contraceptives are discussed in Chapter 13.

HERBS AND OTHER NATURAL REMEDIES

Many people today turn to herbal, homeopathic, or other alternative remedies to avoid taking artificial chemicals into their systems. However, not all substances that grow naturally are safe for pregnant or breastfeeding mothers to take. Quite a few are not safe for anyone to take. Strong infusions of licorice, for example, can increase blood pressure; large quantities of sage can reduce the supply of breast milk; and the sale of other commonly used herbal preparations has been outlawed because illness has been traced to them.

Aside from the fact that very little hard scientific research has been conducted on these substances, they are not uniform and as a result their effects are not predictable. That is, the herbal tea or preparation you buy in one health food store may have a very different strength from one that you make yourself, or that you obtain from a different source.

Many herbs are very powerful and can produce serious side effects. Therefore, you should not use them any more casually than you would take an unknown drug. You should treat herbs as potent substances and should use them only under the direction of someone who is extremely knowledgeable about the herb in question and its effect on a breastfeeding mother and baby.

The only herbal preparations that are generally considered quite safe are major brands of herbal tea. However, even with these, you need to use good sense. Moderation is the key. If you drink two or three cups of herbal tea a day, and if you steep them for a fairly brief time to keep the infusion mild, you probably won't run into trouble. Just avoid drinking too much or drinking a very strong mixture.

Avoid private brands of herbal tea or home-brewed potions. Poisonous alkaloids may make them toxic.

RECREATIONAL AGENTS AND HARD DRUGS

A number of substances that are commonly ingested for nonmedical reasons can also have effects on breast milk and breastfed babies. With these, you have more choices about your level of use, or any usage at all.

Tobacco

If you smoke, is breastfeeding still best for your baby? Yes. Would it be better for your baby if you did not smoke, or at least cut down while you're nursing? The answer here is a more emphatic yes. It would also be better for you and everyone else in your household.

Nicotine, the main substance released when you smoke a cigarette, passes through your milk to your baby, but most of it is altered in your baby's liver and kidney. Since gastrointestinal absorption is slow, you would expect few if any severe toxic reactions in the nursing baby of a smoking mother.

However, nicotine does interfere with milk production, and therefore babies of smoking mothers gain weight more slowly. It's also possible that nicotine absorbed through breast milk can make babies fretful. The main reason given by mothers who discontinue breastfeeding is that they "don't have enough milk," or that their babies "don't seem satisfied." It may be possible to avoid both these problems by not smoking.

Also, a great deal of evidence is accumulating about the adverse effects of "passive smoking," that is, inhaling the smoke of other people. Babies are especially vulnerable, especially to upper respiratory infections, when the person closest to them is the one breathing smoke on them. This is true whether a baby is being fed by breast or bottle.

If you're pregnant now, you probably already know that smoking causes a wide variety of prenatal complications. The most well-documented finding related to smoking is the tendency of pregnant smokers to bear smaller babies, and it's harder to establish breastfeeding with a premature or low-birthweight baby. The good news is that women who stop smoking by four months of pregnancy do not experience these complications.

If you feel that you can't stop smoking even for the duration of your pregnancy and lactation, you can still take some steps that will lessen the risk to your baby to some extent:

• You can avoid smoking while you're nursing. Aside from the danger of the tobacco smoke, there's the very real risk of dropping hot ashes on the baby.

• You can cut down, smoking as little as possible, especially around your baby.

• You can make special efforts to smoke in another room or outdoors.

• And you can do your smoking immediately after a feeding rather than shortly before one.

Minimizing the Effect of Alcohol on Your Nursing Baby*

A 120-pound woman will need about two and a half hours to metabolize the amount of alcohol in one drink. One drink consists of 1.5 ounces of 86-proof alcohol, 5 ounces of wine, or 12 ounces of beer.

If you do drink, safeguard your baby's health by doing the following:

• Before drinking, express or pump and store your alcohol-free breast milk to feed to your baby if insufficient time has elapsed between your last drink and the baby's feeding. Express or pump your postdrinking milk and discard it until enough time has elapsed.

• Do not drink more than your self-imposed limit.

• Choose drinks low in alcohol (like a champagne punch or small glass of wine or beer) or drinks diluted with water or juice.

• Drink slowly. Sip from one drink all evening.

• Eat before and during drinking.

• Be sure your drinks are measured when poured.

• Order juice or a soft drink instead of taking an alcoholic drink you don't want. You can always tell friends that your baby is under the legal age for drinking.

---

*We are indebted for these suggestions to Pat Schulte, R.N. See the bibliography.

Alcohol

Alcohol in moderation is a relaxant; in excess it acts as a depressant. In recent years most health care professionals have advised women not to drink any alcohol during the entire duration of pregnancy. What about during lactation?

Moderate amounts of alcohol—a couple of glasses of beer or wine in a week, or a cocktail—will probably not have any ill effects on your nursing baby. For years, nursing women were advised to drink alcohol, especially beer, to produce more milk. However, research has contradicted this bit of folklore.

One study found that when nursing women drank a small amount of alcohol, their babies sucked more frequently during the first minute of a postalcohol feeding but they consumed less milk during subsequent feedings over the next three to four hours. Since adult panelists could smell a difference in the milk produced by the alcohol-drinking mothers, it's possible that the babies didn't like the taste of the alcohol-containing milk, and therefore took in less. Also, the babies slept more fitfully when their mothers drank alcohol; they took more frequent naps during the day, but slept for shorter periods of time. They may, then, have drunk less milk because they were sleepy. Still, no permanent harm seemed to have been done to these babies.

Heavy drinking, however, is another story altogether. It can affect your ability to care for your baby, and it can make your nursing baby drowsy by depressing the nervous system. Even daily social drinking is questionable. If, at any time while you are lactating, you expect to attend an event where you may engage in social drinking, you can minimize the effect on your baby by following the suggestions given in the box on page 182.

Marijuana

We know less about marijuana than about any other intoxicant. We do know that its most active ingredient is fat-soluble and does appear in breast milk. It's also capable of being stored in the body for one month or longer, even after a single exposure. Since studies of nursing animals have shown structural changes in brain cells and drowsiness in nursing babies after their mothers used this drug, it certainly seems prudent for pregnant and nursing women to abstain from using marijuana.

Cocaine

Pregnant and nursing women should not use cocaine at all in any form, and women who cannot abstain should not breastfeed for their baby's sake—and enroll in a treatment program for their own sake.

Many reports have described serious behavioral and health problems in babies born to women who used cocaine during pregnancy, which underscores the dangers inherent in this drug. Many people underestimate the risk of cocaine, feeling that an occasional use at a party will do little harm. Aside from the fact that we don't know that such a pattern is indeed safe, we also don't know which people who begin as social users will become addicted. Anyone using cocaine is playing with fire, and a pregnant or nursing woman risks injuring her baby in the flames.

Amphetamines

These powerful stimulants can cause irritability and poor sleeping patterns in a breastfed baby. Therefore, pregnant and nursing women should not use them.

Barbiturates

While these drugs can apparently be taken safely by nursing mothers in the usual small medical doses, overuse of them can be dangerous to both mother and baby. For the user they can be addictive or even fatal. They're particularly dangerous when taken with alcohol, and nearly one-third of accidental drug-related deaths are caused by barbiturate overdose. If a mother takes enough barbiturates to put her to sleep or to make her drunk, her baby will almost always be adversely affected. Again, this is a class of drugs to stay away from, especially when you're nursing.

Heroin

Women addicted to heroin are more likely to bear premature babies who have become addicted to the drug within the womb. If a mother is in a detoxification program after the birth, continuing to breastfeed will help her baby rid its system of the drug, as well. If she is going to continue to use heroin, however, breastfeeding can be dangerous to her baby. The heroin does go through the milk and may affect the baby even more than it does the mother, causing tremors, restlessness, vomiting, and poor feeding.

Other Drugs

Phencyclidine (PCP) is a potent hallucinogen that is dangerous to both mother and baby. Methamphetamine seems to be transmitted through breast milk, and at least two cases in which babies died allegedly from overdoses of methamphetamine in their mothers' milk have led to criminal indictments of the mothers.

As a nursing mother, you have many choices to make. Your decision about the substances to which you will expose both yourself and your baby is one of the most important ones you will make for the well-being of both of you.

You Are a Nursing Family

One of the nicest things about the first few weeks after my baby was born was that nobody expected me to do anything. And even if they did, I would just say, "Oh, I couldn't do that—I'm nursing the baby, you know."

—GINA, VANCOUVER, BRITISH COLUMBIA

No matter how much you've read, how many classes you've taken, or how many friends you've spoken to, you get a whole new understanding of what parenthood is all about when you and your baby are together at home.

Many new mothers impose unrealistically high expectations on themselves. In their eagerness to look upon childbirth as natural (which it is), they forget that recovery from it is natural, too, and that most societies around the world decree a period of rest for the new mother while she is cared for by others in the community. In their belief in their own strength and competence (which is justified), they deny themselves the means to restore that strength and enhance that competence.

You're probably more tired now than you ever thought you could be, and you wonder whether you'll ever be back to your old energetic, self-confident self. You *will*. And you'll get there sooner if you give yourself what we routinely grant our newly elected public officials—a settling-in time for establishing new routines and responsibilities. You need *your* "first 100 days," too. No one is ever prepared for the time and the energy needed to care for a new baby, but over the next few weeks you'll develop your routines, enjoy your baby, and forget how hard life seemed to be such a short time before.

If you can, take the first two or three months after birth as an orientation period. You'll have the time you need to let your body recover from

A Visit to a New Mother

One mother of a one-month-old baby embarrassedly told me (Sally Olds) when I visited her, "The baby was up a lot last night and I didn't even get dressed to-day until three o'clock." She apologized for not being up to date on her thank-you notes and for having a messy apartment. She fretted because she hadn't resumed her professional contacts. She's a prime example of the modern mother who pushes herself too hard and too fast.

I reassured her and told her to treat herself the way a loving grandmother would—to keep telling herself how well she was doing, what a beautiful baby she had, and how she had the right to enjoy him without worrying yet about the outside world.

pregnancy and birth and initiate lactation, and to let your psyche get used to the idea of being a mother. Meanwhile, your baby will use this time to get used to the world, to make the big adjustment from having everything done for her in your womb to learning how to do things for herself. The more you can smooth the transition for both of you, the sooner the fun part of mothering and breastfeeding will take over.

Your husband or partner can be enormously helpful at this time. His involvement can go far toward cementing the two of you as a parenting team, and the three of you as a family. Because of work commitments he may have, however, and because at this time a woman (especially one who has breastfed herself) may be able to give a special kind of help, this is the time to call upon one or more people who can serve as your *doula*, as de-scribed in Chapter 4.

These first few weeks are crucial for the nursing family. You don't want to—and you don't have to—shut out the rest of your family and the rest of your life. It's especially important for your baby to bond with your partner, for the two of you to nurture your own adult relationship, and for you both to be attentive to the needs of any older children. However, your primary commitment right now is to your nursing baby and to yourself. You have to feed your baby when he is hungry; you have to get enough rest to help your flow of milk; you have to work at becoming a twosome.

Happily, allowing yourself to focus on your baby this way can free you to enjoy him more. By not feeling pressured by other demands, you can give your all to this courtship period. You can consider the worries and the anxieties of these early weeks as akin to the same kinds of tension that often accompany the period of falling in love. Because that is, after all, what parents and babies do.

BREASTFEEDING AT HOME

Probably the first thing you'll want to do after coming home from the hospital or birthing center is to climb into bed and feed your baby. This is natural and normal—and the best thing you can do for both of you. Your transitional milk may not have come in yet if you leave the hospital within forty-eight hours of birth. If your baby seems fussier and hungrier than she was for the past day or two, this is natural since she has used up some of the body stores she was born with and is now feeling pangs of hunger. Don't worry: Just rest and nurse frequently, and your milk supply will increase.

The concept of "supply and demand" is expressed nowhere more elegantly than in the relationship of the nursing mother and baby. Remember: The more your baby nurses, the more milk you will produce. *The single best thing you can do to ensure successful breastfeeding is to be available to nurse when your baby wants you.*

Still, this is easier said than done. How do you know when your baby wants to nurse, instead of wanting something else? How do you know when your breasts are supplying enough of the milk that your baby needs? How can you continue to meet your own needs as an individual and as part of an adult couple? We'll talk about these questions in this chapter and also in the next two.

When to Nurse Your Baby

Does feeding "on cue" mean nursing a baby every time he whimpers? It can, but it doesn't have to. As the other half of the nursing duo, you'll learn how to read your baby's signals.

You'll learn to distinguish different kinds of cries—the rhythmic pattern that often means your baby is hungry, the sudden onset of loud crying followed by breath-holding that may indicate pain, or the long, drawn-out wails that communicate frustration.

You'll learn when your baby's restless stirring in the crib means that she's about to awaken and when it's just an interlude in sleep. You'll also learn when a smile means that your baby is happily enjoying solitary play, and when one that appears as you walk into the room means that your company is wanted.

This learning is not instinctual; it comes through getting to know your baby and through trial and error. You'll take your cues from your baby and you'll interpret those cues. You'll recognize that your baby's healthy growth depends not only on satisfying his hunger for food and his longing to be held and cuddled, but also on his coming to realize that he has the power to influence his world. Responding to signals that your baby sends lets him appreciate this power and build on it in the future. By answering his needs as well as you can when he is small, you'll be setting your child on the road toward becoming secure and independent.

On the other hand, sometimes you'll know what your child needs better than she does. You'll recognize those times when your baby might accept your breast if you offer it, but when she might need some other kind of care, like cuddling or rocking, even more. And sometimes you'll have to take other considerations, like your own needs and those of other family members, into account. You know that caring for a baby goes far beyond offering your breast.

In general, you'll have confidence in your baby's ability to set the pace for nursing and in your ability to keep up with him. You'll nurse your baby whenever he seems to want the breast. He'll want it for the milk, of course. But he'll also appreciate the warmth of your body, the rhythms of your breathing and heartbeat, the comfort of your arms, the feel of your skin on his face.

In the early weeks your baby will probably want to nurse on an average of every two or three hours. She may sometimes sleep for four or five hours between feedings—and at other times want to be fed almost hourly for several feedings. To stimulate your breasts as much as possible and help your baby go a little longer between feedings, offer both breasts at each nursing (see page 110.) You need to remember that this period of frequent nursing won't go on forever.

Babies vary greatly in the feeding schedules they seem to want. Some average ten to fourteen feedings during a twenty-four-hour period for the first month; others are content with eight or even fewer. By one month, six to ten feedings in twenty-four hours constitute a typical range, and by three months, some babies cut back to between five and seven feedings in a day, sleeping through the night, while many others still want to nurse around the clock. Then, just as you seem to see a pattern in your baby's schedule, it's likely to change, possibly because of a spurt in appetite.

How to Tell When Your Baby Is Getting Enough Milk

One of the biggest problems of nursing, in the minds of many women, is that they cannot tell how much milk their babies are drinking. This is actually one of its biggest advantages, since the nursing mother is not tempted to urge her baby to drain the last drop, thus taking more than he needs. If you feed your baby on cue, your supply of milk should keep up with his appetite. If you're well and if you take reasonably good care of yourself (see Chapter 7), you're virtually assured of having plenty of milk—especially if you don't worry too much about it.

After you've been nursing for a while, you'll notice that your breasts are no longer hard and full the way they were at first. This does not mean that you're producing less milk. The glandular changes in your breasts and the increased blood circulation caused their initial fullness. Once your milk production is fully established, your breasts may become softer and smaller, even while producing copious amounts of milk.

The section beginning on page 118 lists ways to tell whether your baby is getting enough to eat. If you're worried about this for any reason, or if you're having trouble with nursing, call a health professional (doctor, nurse, midwife, or lactation consultant), a friend or relative who has breastfeeding experience, or another breastfeeding support person. The person you consult may be able to reassure you over the phone or may want to see you and your baby in person.

Appetite Spurts

Very often babies who have been on fairly regular schedules that everyone seems happy with suddenly begin to clamor for more food. This seems to occur most often at about three weeks, six weeks, three months, and six months of age. Your baby may be undergoing a "growth spurt," a period of rapid growth that makes her especially hungry. Or you may be in an "activity spurt," doing so many other things that you get overtired and produce less milk. Whatever the reason, the best way to satisfy your baby's expanded appetite is to nurse more frequently for a few days to increase your milk supply. More suggestions on building up your milk follow.

Ways to Build Up Your Milk Production

New mothers sometimes fear that they won't have enough milk to feed their babies. They hear stories about other women who "didn't have enough milk," and they worry that they might be in this category. But when you look closely at the situations of these other women, the problem can almost always be ascribed to lack of information, lack of encouragement, or faulty nursing technique by either mother or baby. You need to tell yourself that millions of other women nurse their babies, and you can, too. Following one or more of the suggestions below should increase your milk supply within a few days.

• Nurse your baby more frequently for several days, using both breasts at each feeding. This is the *single best way* to enhance your flow of milk.

• Wake your baby, if necessary, to feed him more often, or pump or express milk between feedings.

• See a lactation specialist if your baby is not suckling well or nurses only a few minutes at a time.

• Cut back on your schedule. Do less. Rest more. Nap at least once a day, more often if you can manage it. Ask someone else to help with marketing, cooking simple meals (or getting take-out food), and doing basic laundry. Most people like to help a new mother, so take advantage of this willingness now. You can always reciprocate later on. Ask visitors not to come for a few days unless they're people who will wait on you, not expect you to entertain them.

• If you can, take an occasional day or two off from work or from other obligations (by, for example, having someone come in to care for your other children) so that you can focus only on nursing your baby.

• Check your diet. Are you eating enough? Are you eating the right foods? Are you drinking enough fluids? Some women find that eating or drinking more seems to produce more milk.

• Take extra vitamin B complex. Some nursing mothers have found that one to three teaspoons a day of brewer's yeast helps.

• Make a special effort to relax, as suggested in the box on page 192. Of course, this is hard when you're concerned that your baby isn't getting enough milk—but the more you can relax, the more milk your baby is likely to receive.

• Believe in yourself and trust your body. The most effective milk producer of all is the stimulation of your breasts by a nursing baby.

Note: Do *not* offer your baby formula. A few ounces soon turn into a full bottle, which soon turns into several bottles, until you find that you're producing even less milk. If your baby is drinking from a bottle, he is not stimulating your breasts and thus not doing the most effective thing that will increase your supply of milk. In most cases, a breastfed baby should not be offered a bottle until nursing is well established—by at least six weeks of age.

The only exception to this is if your baby is sick or so small that his health is endangered, and if your baby's doctor (not your friends or relatives) feels that he absolutely needs a supplement. If so, offer it through a nursing supplementer (see Chapter 15 and the Resource Appendix), a dropper, or a spoon.

Waking Your Baby

Babies are so angelic looking while they're asleep that this is a favorite time for parents to slip into the room, gaze on them with adoration—and express thanks for these precious, peaceful hours. There are some occasions, however, when you may want to gently awaken a sleeping baby (for ways to do this, refer back to the box on page 111):

• *If your baby confuses night with day.* Some babies regularly sleep for five or six hours during the day and cry to be fed almost every hour after you have gone to sleep. You may be able to change the inner "body clock" of a baby like this by waking him at two- or three-hour intervals during the day; he'll eventually realize that daytime is for nursing and nighttime is for sleep.

• *If your baby is not gaining enough weight.* Some premature babies and others who are unusually docile nurse obligingly when they're awake but don't wake up often enough to take in the nourishment they need. In these cases it's sometimes advisable to wake them to increase the number of feedings. For more on the slow-gaining baby, see Chapter 15.

• *If you have scheduling conflicts.* If you expect other children home from nursery school, if you have to go to work, or if something else is going on that would make feeding time hectic and rushed, you may be doing both you and your baby a favor by waking her half an hour or an hour early so that the two of you can enjoy a relaxed quiet nursing.

How Long Should Feedings Be?

We are a clock-watching, number-counting, measuring, and quantifying society. We were this way even before watches with sweep-second hands and digital clocks came into common use, and now many of us have to fight the urge to run our lives like train timetables. You can learn from your baby—who does not tell time—and you can use your breastfeeding experience to overthrow minute-hand monarchy and digital despotism.

There is no hard-and-fast rule for establishing the lower or upper limits of a nursing session. Some babies are goal-oriented efficiency experts who milk one breast in five minutes, go on to do the same with the other, and promptly fall asleep. Others nurse and rest, nurse and rest, and want to linger at the breast for an hour or more at a single feeding.

Tips on Relaxing Before and/or During Feedings

BEFORE A FEEDING

- Lie down for a few minutes.

- Take an herbal bath or hot shower.

- Do deep breathing (like the kind you learned in your childbirth class), yoga exercises, visual imagery, meditation, or other relaxation techniques.

- Develop a few affirmations that you can repeat to yourself, such as: "I am a bounteous supplier of milk for my baby"; "I am doing the best thing I can as a mother"; "My baby is growing fit and healthy from my milk."

- If your nipples are tender, take an occasional ibuprofen or acetaminophen about thirty minutes before you plan to nurse. If you are in real pain, see a lactation specialist. (See Chapter 15 for suggestions on healing sore nipples.)

- Telephone a reassuring friend, preferably another mother who is currently nursing or has recently breastfed her baby.

BEFORE OR DURING A FEEDING

- Eat a healthful snack, such as a small sandwich, piece of fruit, or raw vegetables.
- Drink a glass of water, milk, or juice.
- Listen to calming music before and during the feeding.
- Read something light and enjoyable.
- Watch a favorite television show.

DURING A FEEDING

- Nurse in a quiet room.
- Nurse lying down.
- Sit in a comfortable rocker with arms.

Most babies seem to need at least half an hour. Some research indicates that an actively suckling baby (past the newborn stage) will milk each breast in five or six minutes, getting only a trickle the rest of the time. Other research points to multiple let-downs at a single feeding session, with the breasts making milk as long as the baby nurses.

The best way for you to decide when it's time to put your baby down is to watch the baby, not the clock. As we pointed out in Chapter 6, you can tell when your baby is actively nursing. Listen for swallowing sounds, and look for the working of jaws and temples. If you're holding your baby properly and if your nipples are used to the suckling, you can nurse for as long as you and your baby want to stay with each other.

These feeding sessions can be wonderful opportunities to relax, put up your feet, and enjoy being with your baby. Once your nursling is latched on, you might want to watch television or read, or read to a toddler who nestles on one side of you while your baby nurses at the other. If your schedule dictates time limits for some nursings, you can provide a balance by letting other feeding sessions be leisurely.

If your baby never wants to stop nursing, you will want to have her evaluated by a doctor or a lactation consultant, or both, to be sure that she is taking in enough nourishment. If you are reassured that she is developing normally, and if she just needs a lot of sucking, you may want to offer her a pacifier after nursings—as long as she is at least six to eight weeks old. (As we said earlier, giving babies pacifiers sooner, before breastfeeding is well established, carries the risk of nipple confusion. Too frequent pacifier use can also result in a baby's doing too much nonnutritive sucking and not enough at the breast.)

Pacifiers have a long history in baby care: They're good tools for providing extra sucking time for babies who need it, for soothing a baby at times when you can't nurse her, for cheering up one twin while you're nursing the other one, and for comforting a colicky baby. But if you use them to "plug" your baby's mouth closed every time she opens it or to put her to sleep, you may be covering up other needs and creating a hard-to-break habit.

You know your baby best, and you need to trust yourself to know when a pacifier makes sense and when it doesn't. Different babies prefer different shapes of pacifiers, so see what's available in your community, try one, and if your baby rejects it, try other kinds.

IF YOU HAVE "TOO MUCH" MILK

Abundance is wonderful, but occasionally a woman has such a forceful letdown that her milk flows too quickly into her baby's mouth. The baby will gulp noisily, gasp, choke, gag, and sputter during the feeding. He may stop nursing after only a few minutes, only to burst into loud wails of hunger and frustration. A baby forced to drink too quickly in this kind of situation will swallow air, have uncomfortable air bubbles, hiccup, spit up, and be unable to satisfy sucking needs. Ironically, with all this abundance, he may not get enough suckling comfort.

This is easy to correct in one or more of the following ways:

• Express the first torrents of milk until it starts to come in a steady drip.

• Try lying on your back or leaning back in a recliner, with your baby lying on top of you. This allows the force of gravity to reduce the flow of milk from your breast and lets your baby control her intake more easily.

• If your baby starts to choke or spit up during a feeding, remove him from the breast, express a little milk into a cup, and once he has calmed down, bring him back to the breast.

• Be sure your baby is latched on and properly positioned. Some babies slide down a firm full breast and clamp down on the nipple, resulting in sore nipples for the mother.

• To cut down a too copious supply of milk, offer just one breast at a feeding. If your other breast becomes uncomfortably full, express or pump your milk, and save it for relief bottles. Over the next few days, your milk supply should decrease to a level your baby can handle more easily.

WHEN YOUR BABY CRIES

Crying is the most powerful way—often the only way—that babies can let the outside world know they need something. It's a vital means of communication and the first way that infants establish any kind of control over their lives.

Research shows that babies whose cries bring relief seem to become more self-confident, seeing that they can affect their own lives. By the end of the first year, babies whose cries have brought tender, soothing care cry less and communicate more in other ways, while babies of punitive or ignoring caregivers cry more. So don't be afraid of spoiling your baby by going to him when he cries. An infant cannot be spoiled by being picked up and held; the holding itself may be what he's crying for.

When your baby cries two or three hours after the last feeding, you immediately know what to do—bring her to the breast. But suppose she cries an hour after a feeding? Or the minute the feeding ends? What should you do? First, you might check to be sure she has not shown earlier signs of hunger (as listed in the box on page 75, number 8). Then you might think of other reasons why she might be crying, and try one of the suggestions in the box on page 200.

If your baby only occasionally cries soon after being nursed, offer her

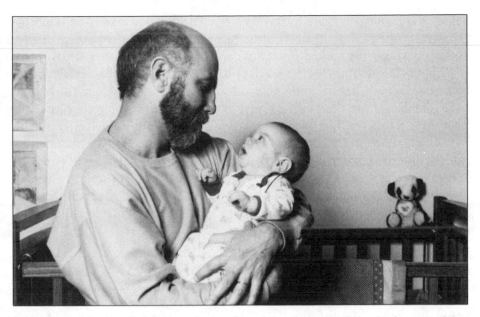

Carrying babies is a time-honored way of soothing them—and the mother isn't the only person who can comfort a crying infant.

your breast and don't worry about the timing. But if he is regularly waking and crying oftener than every two hours, or if he often cries right after feedings, you'll want to try other ways of comforting him.

You cannot, of course, expect to keep your baby from ever crying at all. Frustration and discomfort are a part of life, and part of growing up involves learning how to deal with problems. Babies often fuss in their sleep, find a more comfortable position, and in a few minutes go back to sleeping peacefully. Furthermore, every baby is different. Some babies seem to need to cry lustily for a few minutes before they can let go of the waking state and fall asleep. Unnecessary handling at times like these sometimes overstimulates babies, interferes with their falling asleep, and makes them cry even more from fatigue. Constant parental management can get in the way of babies' solving their own problems.

Babies do cry less when they're carried around, however. Both child-care professionals and casual observers have noticed that babies in cultures where their mothers carry them around most of the day cry less than babies in Western countries. In industrialized societies (in which babies are generally carried the least), they tend to increase their crying until six weeks of age, then gradually cry less up to four months of age, crying mostly in the evenings.

A team of Canadian researchers conducted an experiment that has helped to change baby care in the Western world. They asked some mothers to carry their babies in their arms or in a baby carrier for at least three hours a day, and they asked others to carry their babies as they usually did (which was less than three hours a day) but to change their babies' environment by placing a mobile and an abstract picture of a face where the babies could see them from their cribs. The results: The babies who were carried at least three hours cried less than the ones who were not carried this much.

If your baby seems to be crying "all the time," or for long, unhappy periods at all different times of the day, and nothing that you do will comfort her, call your doctor. The crying may stem from a problem serious enough to merit medical attention. Most likely, you'll be reassured that your baby is healthy, and you may receive some suggestions for making her—and the rest of the family—more content.

THE COLICKY BABY

Some infants become fussy practically every day, often for hours, and usually in the late afternoon or early evening, and nothing you do can quiet them. The catchall term for this kind of behavior is *colic,* and often it's hard to know why this happens.

What Is Colic?

Colic is defined in one medical dictionary as "paroxysms of pain, crying, and irritability, due to such causes as swallowing air, overfeeding, intestinal allergy, and emotional factors." The truth is that no one seems to know what makes certain babies subject to extreme fits of crying, during some of which they do seem to be in pain but during others there's no obvious reason for their unhappiness. Some people ascribe it to the baby's getting tired late in the day, or to his responding to the fatigue of other family members, or to late-day tension in the household, or to some kind of stomach upset.

Most babies magically outgrow this daily crankiness sometime between six weeks and three months of age. "Tincture of time" seems to be the best prescription for most of these babies—that, and knowing that there's nothing that you're doing or not doing that's causing all that crying. Meanwhile, even when your baby doesn't seem to respond to your efforts to cheer her up, it's worth continuing to try, since she's at least getting a sense that the people around her care about how she feels and are there for her—and that the world is a friendly place.

What Causes Colic?

Often this kind of regular crying stems from physical discomfort, possibly due to an immature gastrointestinal tract. You can see this in the baby who draws up her legs and screams, apparently in severe pain. It's paradoxical that the typical colicky baby is an eager nurser who's gaining well, who feeds quickly, and who spits up a little bit of milk after every feeding.

It's noteworthy that colic does not seem to be related to personality, since many babies who cry a lot in early infancy turn out to have cheerful, sunny dispositions later on.

If your baby seems to suffer the stomach upset typical of colic, you might try exploring *how* the baby eats and *what* you eat.

How does he eat? Does he gulp furiously so that he swallows air? If so, this may be causing gas and fretfulness.

Does your milk come too quickly? If so, your baby may be taking in too much and becoming too full. Or, despite the fact that he is taking in large amounts of milk, he may not be getting enough calories and may actually be hungry *even though* his stomach is full. Babies who spend too little time at one breast before being switched to the second breast tend to ingest a great

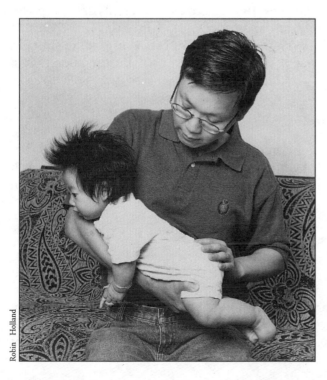

Robin Holland

This father soothes his uncomfortable baby daughter by holding her in the "colic hold." This hold lets mom or dad walk around and help a baby with tummy pains in two ways: the warm pressure of the adult's arm against the baby's belly and the upright or semi-upright position of the baby's body.

deal of the high-lactose fore milk rather than the higher-fat-containing, more satisfying hind milk. Lactose, because it is rapidly digested, may produce intestinal gassiness, green watery stools, and a very fussy baby.

To remedy this situation, try offering only one breast at a feeding and let your baby suckle at that breast until she seems satisfied. At every feeding, then, your baby will drain your breast enough to take in the hind milk.

What are you eating? Research points to substances that a nursing mother eats, especially cow's milk, as a cause of some colic. When mothers eliminate cow's milk products from their own diets, their babies' symptoms sometimes go away. Other foods in the mother's diet that may cause trouble are eggs, citrus fruits, wheat products, nuts, peanuts, and chocolate. None of these foods is indispensable. As the charts in Chapter 7 show, many different foods are good sources of essential nutrients.

If you do remove dairy or other foods from your diet, try them again a couple of weeks later. It's possible that your baby's digestive system will have matured, and you will no longer need to deprive both of you of the good nutrients in those foods. If not and if you decide to stay away from these foods, check with a nutritionist to be sure that you are still receiving adequate nutrients from other foods or, if necessary, from supplements.

Most cases of colic, though, do not seem to be linked to anything the mother eats or anything she does. In many cases the parents are relaxed (at least until the crying jags begin) and experienced (since this isn't their first baby). Yet still their babies cry. So do what you can, don't blame yourself, and look forward to that happy day when the colic will be just a notation in your child's baby book.

What Can You Do?

Besides all the ways to soothe a crying baby listed in the box on pages 200 and 201, two particularly helpful techniques for helping one who acts as if the problem is a stomachache (the baby draws up his legs and cries as if in pain) are:

• Laying him on his back and gently bicycling his legs to help him release gas; and

• Holding her in the "colic hold": Stretch her out horizontally on her tummy along your arm, with her head at your elbow and your hand cupped between her slightly dangling legs, holding her by her buttocks or thigh. Holding a baby this way allows you to walk around, and two things help the baby: the warm pressure of your arm against the baby's belly and the upright or semi-upright position of the baby's body.

And don't forget that other help is often available. Historically, mothers have turned their crying babies over to another loving caregiver for a little while so that the mother can get some relief from her baby's crying. In some cultures, early evening, when many babies have their longest crying period, is known as the "grandmother's hour." This is one great benefit of having other hands to rock the cradle. As the noted anthropologist Margaret Mead told me (Sally Olds), in calling for a system by which several people take turns caring for a baby: "The worst thing is just having the mother boxed up with the baby twenty-four hours a day, which nobody ever meant to have happen in the whole history of the human race."

NIGHT FEEDINGS

It's the middle of the night, and everyone, including the family dog, is sleeping peacefully. Everyone, that is, except your new baby, whose lusty bawling pierces your sleep. You wonder when that happy day will come when you can once again know a night of uninterrupted sleep. This is hard to say.

The age at which babies give up night feedings seems to be an individual characteristic unrelated to size at birth, weight gain afterward, the amount of food eaten in a day, or whether this food comes from breast, bottle, or jar. Babies seem to be born with differing needs for sleeping and eating. While the average newborn sleeps about sixteen hours a day, one healthy baby may sleep only eleven hours, while another sleeps twenty-one. After three months babies become more wakeful in late afternoon and early evening, and by six months more than half their sleep takes place at night.

An occasional baby gives up middle-of-the-night feedings as early as six weeks; many give it up at about three months; and many others need it for several months longer. In the early weeks you need those night feedings as much as your baby does, so that your breasts will continue to be well stimulated and will not become engorged and uncomfortable by morning.

Gradually your baby will go longer between night feedings until one morning you'll wake up, breasts full, wondering what's the matter and dashing to your baby's side. Nothing is wrong; your baby has just slept through the night for the first time.

Night feedings are a little easier if you don't bother changing the baby's diapers unless he's absolutely drenched or seems uncomfortable. If a diaper change is necessary, your partner can do this. Meanwhile, you'll be getting your rest.

Ways to Comfort a Crying Baby

Babies cry for a limited number of easy-to-figure-out reasons: If he's hungry, you can feed him. If her diapers are soiled, you can change her. If he has gas, you can burp him. If none of these actions solves the problem, you can dig into your bag of maternal tricks, try one at a time, and see which ones your baby is most likely to respond to.

• Pick him up and hold him. Your baby may miss the rhythms of life in the womb, when he felt your heartbeat and breathing all day long. He may be filled with vast unnameable yearnings to be held close and cuddled.

• Sit with her in a comfortable rocking chair. A little rocking and cuddling can help you to relax, too.

• If you're nervous and upset, your baby may be responding to your mood. At times like this, it's sometimes helpful if someone else can hold your baby for a while. Meanwhile, making extra efforts to put your own cares out of your mind and to relax will help you—and may also help your baby.

• Hold him to your chest vertically with his head over your shoulder, and walk him around.

• Change her diaper. Some babies are uncomfortable with wet or soiled diapers, although most don't seem to mind.

• Try switching positions, perhaps moving your baby up so he's lying over your shoulder, his stomach resting on the top of your shoulder.

• Pat or rub her back.

• Burp him. A bubble of air may be causing discomfort.

• Change her position in the crib—maybe putting her head where her feet had been.

• Wrap him snugly in a small blanket; some infants feel more secure when firmly swaddled from neck to toes, with their arms held close to their sides.

• Make your baby warmer or cooler, either putting on or taking off clothing or changing the temperature in the room by thermostat, space heater, or air conditioner.

• Lay her on her stomach on your chest so she can feel your heartbeat and breathing.

• Give him a massage. You can learn infant massage from a certified instructor who will teach you gentle exercises, songs, games, and specific strokes to help relieve a baby's discomfort from congestion, gas, or colic. See the Resource Appendix for help in finding a massage teacher.

- Give her a warm bath. You may even want to get into the tub with her. If you do, you will, of course, be very careful holding her, especially while getting in and out of the tub.

- Put him in a sling or other baby carrier next to your chest and walk around or sit with him. While you're holding him this way, you can get some of your work done at the same time (like desk work, vacuuming, marketing, etc.). Some of these carriers are designed so that you can nurse without taking your baby out of the carrier.

- Sing or talk to your baby.

- Provide a continuous or rhythmic sound, like music from the radio or stereo, a simulated heartbeat, or "white noise" from a whirring fan, vacuum cleaner, or other appliance. You can make a tape recording of one of these sounds.

- Lay him tummy down across your knees and jiggle your legs up and down. This helps many a parent get through dinner. (Of course, you won't be drinking hot coffee while doing this.)

- Put her in a windup swing seat or cradle. (Some go for as long as forty minutes.)

- Turn your baby's crib into a rocker by putting springs on the crib legs. At first you can gently rock your baby in it; when he gets bigger he'll be able to do it himself. Or get a device that will make the crib vibrate. One commercial system simulates the motion and sound that a baby feels during a car ride.

- Take your baby out of the house—for a ride in her stroller or the car—at any hour of the day or night. In bad weather you can walk around in an enclosed mall. The distraction will help you, as well as your baby.

- Lay your baby on top of a folded towel or put him in an infant seat on top of a washing machine or dryer that's been running for a few minutes. Some babies like the warmth and the motion. If you do this, be sure not to leave his side for even a moment.

- If someone other than yourself is taking care of your baby, it sometimes helps if the caregiver puts on a recently worn item of your clothing (robe, sweater, etc.) so your baby can sense your familiar and beloved smell.

- "Dance" with your baby to music from the radio or stereo.

- If all else fails, and if your baby is at least twelve weeks of age, try a pacifier as a last resort. Some babies can't work up any interest in pacifiers, but others find them soothing.

- Remember this mantra, and repeat it over and over to yourself: "I am not a bad mother because my baby cries a lot."

Sleeping Arrangements

Different families handle sleeping arrangements and nighttime feedings in different ways. The following are the most common:

• For the first month or so, when the baby is waking up several times a night, he sleeps in a crib or cradle next to the mother's bed. As soon as she hears him begin to stir, she reaches over, brings him into bed with her, nurses him, and puts him back in his crib. After about a month the baby sleeps in a separate room.

• The baby sleeps in her own room right from the start. If the parents are afraid they won't hear her cry, they use a baby monitor or rig an intercom system between their room and the baby's. As soon as she starts to cry, the father gets out of bed and brings the baby to the mother. After the baby has been nursed, the father takes her back to her own bed.

• The baby sleeps in the same bed with the parents. Whenever he wakes up, the mother reaches over, nurses him, and both go back to sleep without getting out of bed. There are significant health benefits in the shared sleeping pattern, which in many parts of the world is the norm, partly because it

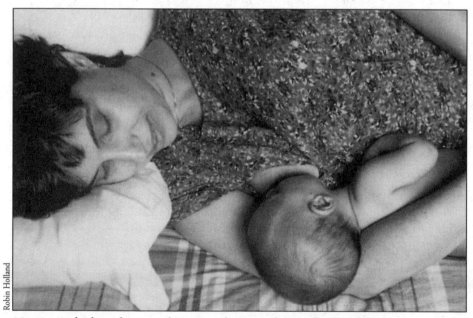

Robin Holland

Nursing in bed can be a good way to take a rest during the day and to enjoy a cozy "midnight snack." During middle-of-the-night feedings babies get both contact and comfort as well as food while resting. Mom rests too.

enables mothers to respond to their babies most comfortably and easily during the night. One research team found that mothers and their three-month-old infants who sleep together tend to wake each other up during the night, and that this may prevent the baby from sleeping too long and too deeply. Other research has found that co-sleeping promotes breastfeeding. Infants who sleep in their mothers' bed nurse about three times longer during the night than infants who sleep separately, both because they nurse more frequently and because each feeding lasts longer. While some critics warn against parent-infant co-sleeping for fear that mothers or fathers will roll over on their babies, this is a rare occurrence. Parents can do much to make co-sleeping safe for their baby. If you do bring your baby into your bed to sleep, you need to observe the following cautions.

First, closely examine the structure of the bed to ensure that the baby cannot get trapped between the mattress and the wall, bed frame, headboard, footboard, bed railings, other furniture, or anything else. Parents often move the bed against a wall in the belief that this will prevent a baby from falling onto the floor, but the danger of the baby's getting wedged between the mattress and the wall still exists because parents may fail to notice when the mattress has come away from the wall. Babies who learn how to rock from side to side, roll over, or move up onto hands and knees and propel themselves by pushing against a flat surface can often move to a corner of the bed, but if they become wedged between two objects they may not have the strength and coordination to free themselves.

Do not let your baby sleep with you if you have had alcoholic drinks or any drugs (medicinal or recreational) that could make you sleep heavily, if either you or your spouse is usually a deep sleeper, or if you are very heavy. Do not let older children—including toddlers—sleep next to the baby. Do not put the baby to sleep on a waterbed or a sofa. Do not smoke in bed or near the sleeping baby. Be sure that the bed is low enough and the floor is covered with a firm but soft covering so that if the baby does fall out of bed, she or he will not be injured. Do not use heavy quilts, comforters, or blankets in the bed. Do not let the baby sleep on or near a pillow. Remove all other soft items, including stuffed toys, from the bed. Be sure that no objects can topple or collapse onto the bed. Be sure that the baby cannot get tangled up in his or her clothing, and that there is nothing in the bed that can catch the clothing and ensnare the baby. Do not put the baby to bed with a pacifier on a cord, or with anything around his or her neck. Do not put the baby in a bed close enough to a drapery or Venetian blind cord that she or he could reach or get caught in. Do not put the baby on a plastic mattress or sheet covering. Do not let any plastic bags remain on the floor, on the bed, or nearby where the baby could roll over and fall into them.

Encouraging a Baby to Give Up Nighttime Nursing

If you don't really mind getting up at night, there's no age by which your baby *has* to sleep through, so you can just wait until he gives up night feedings him-self—and try to catch up on your own sleep by scheduling a nap during the day.

But if your doctor says your baby is growing well, if he is nursing often and well during the day, if he's at least twelve weeks old, so your milk supply is well established, and if getting up with him leaves you exhausted and irritable, you may be able to encourage him to sleep for longer stretches at night. Sometimes one of the following will work:

• Try nursing later at night, maybe at midnight, to see whether this will hold your baby till morning.

• Let your baby fuss (not scream) for five or ten minutes when he wakes during the night; if he's not too hungry, he may go back to sleep.

• If your baby sleeps separately, let your partner go to comfort the baby, maybe by rubbing her back or rocking her in her crib. From a very early age, your baby associates your looks and your smell with feeding; if you go to her side, she'll ex-pect to nurse. This is why the father or someone else is often more successful in getting her back to sleep.

• If your baby is on a "night shift," sleeping during the day and up a lot at night, reorient him by waking him up and nursing him every two to three hours during the day, and keeping him awake by taking him out, bathing him, play-ing with him, or sitting him in an infant seat where he can see interesting things and people.

• Although some parents feed their babies solid foods in the belief that this will help them go longer between nursings at night, there's no evidence that this does any good. You should follow the AAP recommendations and continue giving your baby breast milk alone for six or more months. (Suggestions for starting solids are given in Chapter 18.)

• Offer a pacifier, if your milk supply is well established and your baby is at least twelve weeks old.

When both parents sleep in the same bed with the baby, each one needs to mentally acknowledge before falling asleep the presence of the infant in the bed. This consists of a mental notation like the car stickers that say "Baby on Board"; but in this case the message is "Baby in Mind." This can virtually guarantee that the parents will not overlie the baby during sleep, since almost all healthy, clear-headed parents sleep lightly when they know that the baby is in the bed with them.

Whichever way you decide to arrange your family life is up to you. Babies grow up happy and healthy under all of the above and a variety of other sleeping arrangements, as well. Basically, your choice will depend on your own views of parenting and marriage, and on your own personal preference.

The Joys of Nighttime Feedings

It's hard for an exhausted new mother to think of night feedings as being anything but a burdensome sleep-robber to be ended as soon as possible. Yet many women have found that they welcome and enjoy them more than they ever thought they would—especially if they're able to nap during the day.

Women who like night feedings talk about the warm feeling of nursing in bed, surrounded by the people they love. They talk about the special feeling of being the only two people awake in the house. They talk about the serenity of being alone with their babies. They talk about the slightly illicit feeling of slipping out of bed in the middle of the night and sitting with the baby and a snack in front of a late TV show. Other mothers who long for these nighttime feedings to end often find with some surprise that years later they look back upon them with nostalgia. Still, if you're in the latter group, you may find the suggestions in the box on page 204 helpful.

DIAPERS, REVISITED

Remember that your breastfed baby's bowel movements and habits are quite different from those of a bottle-fed baby. A grandmother or friend used to bottle-fed babies may look at your baby's stools, become worried about his health, and alarm you. So put their minds and your own at ease.

Your baby may move his bowels quite frequently, possibly after every feeding during the first month. After the first month, his pattern may change abruptly to infrequent movments. He may even go more than ten days without a movement, as discussed in the table on page 119. Breastfed babies tend to excrete less waste than formula-fed infants, because human milk is digested so completely.

The bowel movements of a breastfed baby are usually soft, seedy, and yellowish. They've been described as being like soft-scrambled eggs with a little water around them or like a mixture of cottage cheese and mustard. Sometimes there's only a stain on the diaper; this is not diarrhea. Sometimes your baby strains a bit; this is not constipation. All these patterns are normal and healthy.

Your baby's stools may become looser in response to something you have eaten—large quantities of fruit juice, for example, or certain foods in the cabbage family. Try to discover the offending food and avoid it. Do not take any strong laxative, because this can give your baby diarrhea.

While constipation is rare among breastfed babies, some babies do go a long time without moving their bowels—*after* the first month or two, never before this time. If your baby goes a week or even two weeks without moving her bowels, this is nothing to worry about. But be forewarned: When the baby begins again to move her bowels, a great deal of soft, unformed stool may appear in several diapers in a row.

If the stool is hard, this does signal constipation. This is unlikely to occur in an exclusively breastfed baby. However, if your baby seems to be in pain when she does move her bowels, there are several things you can do. One is for *you* to drink six ounces of prune juice or eight ounces of apple juice once or twice a day. Another is to eliminate cow's milk from your diet. If neither of these steps helps, call your baby's doctor.

To prevent infection in either you or your baby, wash your hands after diapering and before nursing him.

WHAT IS YOUR BABY LIKE?

All new babies have certain characteristics in common. They all have facial configurations particularly suited for nursing—the receding chin and flat nose that let them get their faces in the right position at the breast, and the well-developed cheek muscles they need for suckling. They all cry when they want something, they all eat often, and they all need to be taken care of. They're all tiny, dependent, defenseless, and incredibly appealing.

However, we now know scientifically what parents have always known—that each baby comes into this world with a unique personality. Studies that have followed children from birth into adulthood have found that individuals differ greatly right from the beginning in such characteristics as activity level; regularity in biological function (hunger, sleep, elimination); adaptability to change; acceptance of new situations; sensitivity to noise, light, and other sensory stimulation; mood (cheerfulness or crankiness); distractibility; intensity of feelings and responses; and persistence. From the time each of us draws our first breath, we have our own distinctive temperament.

How to Discourage Biting

A baby who is actively nursing cannot bite. Biting happens most often toward the end of a feeding, or when a baby is about to fall asleep. Babies are smart: Once they realize that every time they start to bite, they get taken off the breast, they learn that this kind of behavior isn't getting them what they really want, and they'll stop. The following suggestions work well:

• As soon as your baby starts to bite down on your breast, withdraw your breast. Break the suction by inserting your finger in the corner of his mouth.

• As you take your breast away, firmly say "No" every time your baby tries to bite.

• Do not smile when you say this; your baby may interpret this as a game you're playing. You might even look at your baby with a sad expression.

• One mother we know begins socializing her children by saying, "That hurts Mommy. We don't hurt other people," as she takes her baby off the breast for biting. She repeats this same litany over and over again as her children grow into toddlers, providing a continuing way to teach them not to kick, hit, or do other hurtful acts.

• If your baby is teething, give her a cold washcloth to bite down upon just before you nurse her. Also give her special teething toys and foods.

• Try putting him down, walking away for a moment, and then returning to put him back on the breast.

• If you can anticipate when the biting is likely to start, take your baby off your breast ahead of time.

• If your baby keeps biting, keep your finger close to her mouth and watch her carefully; as soon as she stops nursing actively or looks playful, remove your breast.

• Or quietly say your baby's name while drawing him close to you; this distracts him and gets him back to nursing.

Furthermore, children's temperaments influence the way we respond to them. A cheerful baby is treated differently from a fussy one, an active one from a docile one, and a predictable one from one with very irregular patterns.

Since you'll respond to your baby's personality, it's helpful try to figure out his temperament and to accept his uniqueness as an individual. You may recognize your child immediately in the following profiles, or decide he's a combination of several, or realize that his personality is different from

---

Cutting Down on Spitting Up

- If your baby seems to be gulping down milk at a fast and furious rate, try feeding him more often instead of waiting until he's desperately hungry.
- If you're engorged, your baby may be swallowing air as she latches on. To relieve engorgement before a feeding, express a little milk and apply a warm or cold compress to your breasts. Of course, if you're feeding your baby often enough, your breasts will not get the chance to become engorged.
- If your milk is coming too quickly at the beginning, express a little or let some flow into an absorbent cloth before nursing.
- If your baby seems to be eating more than he can handle, nurse on one breast only at each feeding.
- Prop your baby back at a 30-degree angle for twenty to thirty minutes after a nursing before you burp her. This helps the milk settle in her stomach and discourages it from coming up with the air bubble.
- When you do burp your baby, do it gently.
- Keep an ample supply of bibs and burping cloths at home and in your diaper bag, and stick to washable clothing yourself for the spit-up duration.

---

anything described here. Whichever way your baby is, the important thing for you to do is to accept and love him for the way he is, not for the way you would like him to be.

The Alarm Clock: She has an inner clock that wakes her regularly, about every two hours in the early weeks. She sleeps about the same time every day, tends to move her bowels at about the same time every day, is hungry at regular intervals, and in general has predictable patterns. She's easy to live with and easy to take care of.

The Nonconformist: This is the baby who tries parents' souls. He sleeps for two hours one morning, for fifteen minutes the next, and not at all the third. He's ravenously hungry Monday morning and totally uninterested in eating on Tuesday. He offers few clues to his wants. If left to set his own feeding schedule, he innocently runs his mother ragged.

This child benefits from parental guidance in helping to regularize his living patterns, but as one mother said, "Trying to schedule him is like walking up the down escalator." You may have to ride with his nonschedule for a while, and end up compromising somewhere between the regularity you would like and the irregularity that comes naturally to the baby.

You may actually find that there is more of a pattern to your baby's activities than you had thought. Try keeping a log of the times he nurses, the times he sleeps, and the times he moves his bowels. After a few days you may find a certain rhythm that was not apparent at first.

The Good Eater: She comes to the breast with a good appetite and an inborn knowledge of technique. She eats well, suckling so vigorously that she develops blisters on the middle of both upper and lower lips. These don't bother the baby; the skin falls off, another blister forms, and the cycle repeats itself till the baby's lips become used to her energetic nursing.

The Waiter: He doesn't become interested in nursing until about the fourth or fifth day. He may be sleepy from childbirth medication, or he may not feel like exerting himself until his mother's milk flows copiously. This baby needs to be seen by a lactation consultant or a doctor to be sure he isn't on the road to serious trouble.

The Dawdler: She's a slow eater who nurses for a few minutes, then rests a while. Other times she mouths the nipple, tastes the milk, and then sets to work. She takes the milk in her own good time and cannot be hurried.

The Dozer: He likes to sleep, especially at mealtimes. You may be able to rouse him by dabbing him on the forehead with a sponge dampened with cool water, expressing a little milk into his mouth, taking off some of his clothing, leaning him forward on your lap, walking your fingers up his spine, or massaging his legs and arms. Playing with him before a feeding may encourage him to stay awake, and changing diapers after the first breast may wake him up enough to take the second. (For other ways to wake a sleepy baby, refer to the box on page 111.)

The Overeager Beaver: She becomes so excited at feeding time that she moves her head quickly from side to side, grasps the breast, then loses it and ends up screaming in frustration. Handle her gently, speak to her softly, keep putting her back on your breast. Try to nurse her before she gets frantically hungry, even if you have to wake her sometimes to do it. Eventually she gets the idea and settles in.

The Biter: He comes down hard on your breast, chewing it as if he had been born with a mouthful of sharp teeth. However, even an infant can learn not to bite the breast that feeds him. For ways to discourage biting, see the box on page 207.

The Spitter: Fat and healthy, she spits up milk after practically every feeding. She may continue this until she's almost a year old and you're convinced that you, the baby, and the apartment will always smell like cheese. (The smell is a lot milder while she's on breast milk alone.) If the spit-up milk shoots out forcibly in what is known as "projectile vomiting," call your baby's doctor. Otherwise, don't worry. As one experienced family practitioner has said, "In a healthy baby, spitting up is a laundry problem, not a medical problem." For suggestions on how to cut down on spitting up, see the box on page 208.

The Lopsided Nurser: He develops a preference for one of your breasts. He's not lopsided, but you may soon get that way. What to do?

• If one breast is producing more milk than the other, offer the less full one first at every feeding: Your baby will drain it better and encourage it to produce more; when it does, you can go back to alternating if your baby is agreeable.

• Express or pump milk from the less favored breast and save it for a relief bottle.

• Switch nursing positions: Hold your baby more vertically or in the clutch (football) hold, or nurse lying down.

• Try the "slide-over" technique. Using the cradle hold, start your baby on the breast he prefers. When it is time to switch breasts, slide him over into a clutch hold at the other breast, not changing his lying position. A pillow on your lap makes it easier to do this smoothly without disturbing your baby.

• If you can't influence your baby to give both breasts equal treatment, forget about it and pad your bra on the smaller side when you go out. When you stop nursing, you'll regain your symmetry.

The Playboy/Playgirl: Practically every baby falls into this category at some time—usually about four or five months. By this time they're more aware of the world around them and eager to show how much they love you. He'll suddenly pull away in the middle of a feeding to flash you a bright toothless smile. Or she'll turn her head in response to a voice or footstep. He'll stroke your breast or face with his dimpled little hand. She'll play with the buttons on your blouse.

This is such a beautiful way to cement a loving relationship that you should make every effort to relax and enjoy these longer, more playful feedings. If you occasionally want the feeding to go more quickly, nurse in a dark, quiet room free from distractions.

WHAT WILL YOU CALL IT?

You may not be able to imagine a time when your baby will be talking and asking for "num num" or "nursy" or "titty," or some of the other words that sound so cute just between the two of you, but that might bring a blush to your cheeks if uttered, say, at your employer's family Christmas party.

So think ahead. You may be nursing long after your child has learned to talk. Use a word for nursing that won't embarrass you if your child says it at an inopportune time. Instead of using some of the more explicit words for nursing, one mother always asked her baby if he wanted to drink. When he started to talk, his word for nursing, "dra," was a code word between him and his mother. This mother's second child transformed "drink" into "gingky." Her third would ask for "mee" for "milk." The daughter of another mother, who would ask, "Do you want me to feed you?" came to call nursing "feed'ly," a code word that the outside world didn't know and didn't need to know.

LIFE AS PART OF A NURSING FAMILY

It takes a couple of months for you and your baby to become attuned to each other. The first few weeks you're both busy learning how to nurse and the next few, you're perfecting the art. During this time you come to know what to expect of your life together.

You learn that there are days when everything goes smoothly—and days when nothing does. You learn that there are days when your baby is cranky and days when you're cranky. You learn that you can cope with all these ups and downs because that's what life is all about. By the time these first couple of months have passed, the trial-and-error period is over. You don't have long lists of questions about breastfeeding. You know what to do—and you go about doing it. You and your baby are a nursing pair.

How long will you remain a nursing pair? This is up to you and your baby, a matter of personal preference, lifestyle, philosophy, personality, and individual needs. In Chapter 18 we'll talk about some of the choices you can make in deciding when to wean your baby. Till then we'll explore other facets of your life.

Your Other Life

When an actress takes off her clothes onscreen but a nursing mother is told to leave [the theater], what message do we send about the roles of women?

ANNA QUINDLEN, THE NEW YORK TIMES

While you're getting started at breastfeeding, you'll probably find that the only social life you're interested in for a while revolves around making friends with your baby and integrating the newcomer into your family. This is just as well, since you need your rest and the freedom from outside pressures. Still, the time will come when you'll want to see people and go places. There's no reason why you can't.

You'll also find that other concerns will assume more importance in your life as time goes on, concerns that will be affected by your status as a breastfeeding mother. We have already talked about some aspects of caring for yourself in Chapters 7 and 8, and we'll talk about other aspects of your life, like employment and your sexual relationship, in Chapters 12 and 13. In this chapter we'll raise some of the social and legal issues that may arise while you're nursing.

YOUR SOCIAL LIFE

Going Out with Your Baby

Once your baby is three or four weeks old, you can get out quite easily with him or her for visits with friends or a trip to a nearby restaurant. Babies this young are usually very agreeable to going out and bedding down for a while in carriage, sling, carrier, car seat—or your arms. Should your nursling want to be fed, you're right there. The only danger about this is that it seems so easy that you may tend to overdo it. If you find that you're going out so often and staying out so late that you or your baby is getting tired and irritable, cut back.

If your baby starts to cry while you're driving, remember that your first obligation is to keep both of you safe. To do this, you need to give your full attention to your driving. It won't hurt your baby to cry a little if you can't stop immediately. You can, of course, talk or sing to your baby, but you need to keep your eyes on the road and the traffic. Before doing anything more for your baby, get to a safe place where you can stop the car.

If your baby starts to cry while you're both passengers in a moving car, you may be tempted to take her out of her car seat to nurse her. Do not succumb to this temptation. The laws in every state require small children to be buckled into approved safety seats. (The state laws vary slightly regarding the age or size of the child.) The statistics paint a clear picture: Your baby's safety depends on being securely held in a car seat. Again, wait to nurse until the car is not moving.

For other suggestions about nursing your baby away from home, see the section "Nursing in Public," on page 214.

Going Out Without Your Baby

By the time your milk supply is well established and your baby has developed a regular enough schedule so that you can sometimes predict just when she'll want to be fed (this happens somewhere between six weeks and three months), you may want to go out from time to time without your baby.

You may miss an occasional afternoon or evening feeding, but it's best to miss as few as possible, preferably no more than one or two a week if you don't have to. You don't want your baby to develop a preference for the bottle, which will have a negative impact on your milk supply. Some mothers offer an occasional bottle from the age of six weeks on; some babies refuse to take a bottle if it isn't offered until later. Many babies, however, are quite willing to accept milk in a bottle or a cup from another person, whereas they won't take it from their mothers. (See the suggestions offered to working mothers in Chapter 12.)

If you need to be away from your baby often, you may want to express or pump your milk at those times. When you feel a let-down or at the time you would ordinarily nurse, find a private spot where you can express. You'll feel more comfortable, you'll be less likely to leak, and your breasts will get the regular stimulation they need to keep producing milk.

When you leave a relief bottle (which you should not do, if possible, before your baby is at least six weeks old), the best option is to leave your own breast milk, which you have previously expressed and refrigerated or frozen. (This is especially important if you have any concerns about allergies in your family.) Or if you have to, you can leave a bottle of ready-to-feed formula. Your baby should not be drinking plain homogenized cow's milk until at least one year of age. For information on expressing, storing, and freezing breast milk, see Chapter 17.

NURSING IN PUBLIC

Many women nurse their babies wherever they happen to be, with such skill that no one else is aware of what they're doing. Still, if you feel shy about nursing in front of other people, you don't have to. When feeding time comes, excuse yourself, go into another room, and feed your baby. Or start the baby nursing elsewhere and then rejoin the group. Usually the time your breast is most exposed is at the start of a feeding. Once your baby has latched on, it's easier to keep your breasts covered. See the suggestions that are discussed in the following section.

Most people will respect your privacy. In a public place where you can't be all alone, you can usually find a quiet nook where you'll be relatively unobserved. Or a companion may be able to shield you from public view.

However, if you feel comfortable about breastfeeding in front of others, there's no reason why you shouldn't. You need not feel apologetic or bashful about nurturing your baby the healthiest way possible. In fact, this right is legally protected, as discussed in the section "Breastfeeding and the Law" on page 217.

Nursing Comfortably in Public

Many women who never thought they could feel easy about nursing in public find that when they're out with their baby and the baby is hungry, they lose their reluctance very quickly. And the more you do it, the easier it gets. The basic ingredients for comfort are what you wear, where you go, how you act—and most of all, how confident you feel about your right to nurture your child wherever you happen to be.

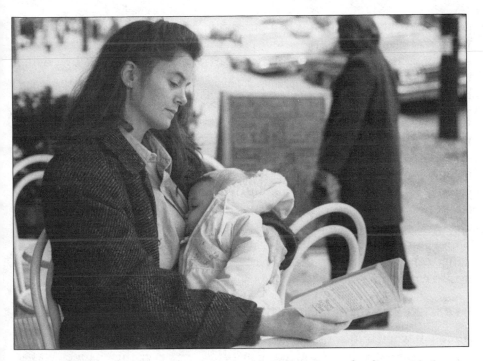

More modern women are nursing wherever their daily lives take them, with the confidence that they are doing the best they can for their babies.

What You Wear: With a little wardrobe planning, you can breastfeed modestly anywhere, so that no one can see your breasts. You can cover more of you by unbuttoning your blouse from the bottom up rather than from the top down. If you wear a knit pullover, you can easily pull it up so that your baby's body will cover your midriff and the pullover will cover your breast. Ponchos, loose-fitting cardigan sweaters and jackets, scarves, and shawls are all good cover-ups. So are the slings you carry your baby in, many of which will let you position your baby to nurse while you're carrying him. You may want to practice nursing at home in front of a mirror with different kinds of clothes until you feel comfortable about doing it in public. (Also see "Your Clothes" in Chapter 8.)

Where You Go: If you're out shopping at a department store, you can often find a comfortable chair in a well-equipped women's lounge, in the furniture department, in or near a women's fitting room, or in the store restaurant or children's department. In a restaurant, try to sit in a corner seat in a booth. In a bookstore, look for a comfortable area where people can sit and read—and you can sit and nurse.

When you drive, try to nurse your baby in your parked car before you get out at your destination. On a bus, train, or plane, try to sit next to the window. Be sure to observe safety precautions in any moving vehicle, by keeping your baby in an approved car seat or safety seat, and by staying belted yourself. It's hard to listen to your baby's cries when you can't reach her because of these restraints, but it's better than risking both your lives.

How You Act: You can position yourself for maximum privacy by turning your body away from the sight of passers-by. Some women discourage interaction with strangers by maintaining eye contact with their babies or a companion, while others openly meet other people's eyes and smile. Either way, your body language can show your own comfort with breastfeeding and will tend to discourage disparaging remarks and complaints. Note that almost all cases in which women have been asked to stop nursing (or to go somewhere else to nurse) have ended in apologies to them. But, most women would rather avoid the hassles in the first place. However, should you encounter difficulty, remember that the law is almost always on your side.

Pressures Against Nursing in Public

Although women in some of the most modest cultures in the world comfortably and naturally breastfeed their babies wherever they happen to be, many Western countries display a bizarre and contradictory set of values. In our society, women's uncovered breasts are displayed openly in movies and popular magazines and are barely covered on beaches from coast to coast. Yet our culture's insistence on defining the female breast as a symbol of eroticism has generated a taboo against showing it in public for its primary purpose. The sight of a mother suckling her infant—sanctified in paintings of the Madonna and Child and accepted in public areas of so-called less civilized countries around the world—is considered indecent in much of the Western world.

One reason for the low breastfeeding rates in the United States is our society's simultaneously lascivious and prudish attitude that sees breasts as sexual objects rather than as organs of nurturance. Newspaper columnist Ann Landers has told women not to nurse their babies in the presence of guests in their own homes. And nursing mothers continue to be humiliated at and even evicted from restaurants, hotels, and swimming pool areas. The vice president of one chain of retail stores, when contacted by a nursing mother who had been asked to move in one of the chain's stores, compared breastfeeding to the "streaking" fad of the 1970s, when college students would run nude through a public place, just for the shock value.

But why should a woman have to hide herself away from normal life and from other adults because she wants to do the best thing for her baby?

As we demonstrate in the following section, "Breastfeeding and the Law," more and more women are refusing to accept this taboo. They're nursing their babies in meetings, at parties, at concerts and ball games, on beaches, on airplanes, and in churches and synagogues. And they're getting support from other women.

As a result, more contemporary observers are becoming familiar with a sight that was once commonplace in Western society and is once again regaining its proper place as an acceptable practice. As women themselves accept the naturalness and the respectability of breastfeeding, cultural—and legal—acceptance of public nursing will keep apace.

BREASTFEEDING AND THE LAW

Legal issues intersect with a baby's right to be breastfed in a number of areas. We'll discuss public nursing, custody conflicts, jury duty, and extended breastfeeding here, and employment issues in Chapter 12.* Should you encounter problems in any of these areas, you may want to contact your local La Leche League leader, who should be able to offer some help in handling legal issues surrounding breastfeeding. To get the name of a local leader, first look under "La Leche League" in the white pages of your telephone directory. If you need further help, call the main office of the League (phone numbers are in the Resource Appendix). For further information about breastfeeding and the law, you can visit the La Leche League website (see the Resource Appendix) or consult a lactation specialist.

In some situations, as in the right to breastfeed in public, your local press and a local support group of other mothers may be even more helpful than an attorney. In other circumstances, an attorney is essential, as with custody conflicts, charges of abuse, or instances in which an employment situation may result in job loss or a need to file suit. Each case, of course, is unique and has to be dealt with on its own merits.

Your Right to Breastfeed Wherever You Are

In April 1997 in Cincinnati, Ohio, eighty nursing mothers, babies, and fathers marched outside a Wal-Mart store after a woman nursing her two-month-old on a bench just outside the women's dressing room had been

---

*Much of the following information is based on talks and papers by Elizabeth N. Baldwin, Esq., an attorney who specializes in legal issues involving breastfeeding. For information on reaching her or other lawyers knowledgeable in this area, see the Resource Appendix.

asked to move to the lavatory. The marchers were rallying to educate the public and to urge state legislators to pass a law ensuring women the right to breastfeed when and where it was necessary. As of this writing, the Ohio Civil Rights Commission has found probable cause of violation; a state senator has offered to sponsor a bill; and a great deal of support for breastfeeding has surfaced in the press and in the community.

And in July 1997 in Boulder, Colorado, a group of mothers held a "nurse-in" at a public pool to protest an incident in which a mother breastfeeding her six-month-old had been asked to leave the pool the week before. City officials apologized to the woman and agreed to support nursing mothers even if they should receive complaints from other patrons.

So far, as we go to press, seventeen states have enacted laws protecting the right to breastfeed.* Many of these statutes firmly assert that it is legal for a woman to nurse her baby anywhere it is legal for the two of them to be. The Florida law specifically states: "A mother may breastfeed her baby in any location, public or private, where the mother is otherwise authorized to be, irrespective of whether the nipple of the mother's breast is uncovered during or incidental to the breastfeeding." The New York law, the strongest legislation so far, protects breastfeeding as a mother's civil right and provides women with legal recourse if anyone tries to prevent them from nursing.

Why are laws to protect a woman's right to breastfeed necessary? Not because it is illegal *anywhere* to nurse in public, but because some people— fortunately, a minority—consider it indecent exposure and therefore criminal behavior. As we've said, this is ironic in a society like ours, which has seen women's clothes become more and more revealing over the past half century until little is left to the imagination.

Another major irony is that in many cases the harassed nursing mother's breasts are not even visible. People who complain about her are simply uncomfortable with the very idea of breastfeeding. As attorneys Elizabeth N. Baldwin and Kenneth A. Friedman write, "Most mothers who are harassed for breastfeeding are trying hard to be discreet. Although nothing shows, everyone knows what she is doing. These new mothers, breastfeeding for the first time in public, are often the ones who are picked on. [These mothers] are more likely to wean as a result of embarrassment and humiliation."

We need to protest every case of discrimination—after all, bottlefeeding mothers are not asked to feed their babies in private. We need to rally community support. And we need to make the point that breastfeed-

---

*California, Connecticut, Delaware, Florida, Illinois, Idaho, Iowa, Michigan, Minnesota, Nevada, New Jersey, New York, North Carolina, Texas, Utah, Virginia, and Wisconsin already have laws.

ing is never illegal. We also need to see mothers nursing in public more often, so that young people seeing them will accept this as the natural way to feed infants, an attitude that will serve the next generation of babies. If women are not made to feel as if they have to hide when they're doing the best they can for their babies, more women will do the best they can.

Protecting Your Nursling in a Custody Case

Unfortunately, many family breakups occur while small children are still being nursed, and sometimes the nursing becomes an issue between the parents. If you are involved in such an issue, you need to address it firmly and reasonably, and, whenever possible, by settling your disputes out of court.

Some judges pursue the laudable goal of promoting bonding between a child and a noncustodial father by mandating a certain number of hours or days of visitation with the father, away from the mother. All too often, however, the judge does not take into account a child's nursing status. There have been cases in which judges have ordered that breastfed infants spend the weekend, a week, or even longer with their fathers, ignoring the nursing relationship.

Judges who are not knowledgeable about breastfeeding often think that the milk is the issue, not the separation, not the loss of a cherished sense of comfort. Furthermore, they frequently think that an easy solution would be for the mother to express enough milk for the visit and send the required number of bottles with the baby. Neither of these beliefs takes into account the reality of breastfeeding and its significance in a child's life.

In other cases, a mother's decision to breastfeed her child beyond age one or, at the most, two years of age may give rise to an accusation that she is "enmeshed," or too entangled in her child's care, or is nursing for her own neurotic reasons, or is using breastfeeding to keep her child away from the father, or some other charge.

In either of these scenarios, you need to prepare well and you need to have good, competent legal advice. Many times it is essential to show not just the importance of breastfeeding, but the current recommendations regarding breastfeeding. For instance, the World Health Organization and UNICEF recommend that all babies be breastfed until age two or beyond, and the American Academy of Pediatrics (AAP) now recommends that all babies be breastfed for a minimum of twelve months, and then after that as long as it is mutually desirable. (This most recent AAP recommendation cites a study that discusses the normality of extended breastfeeding as late as age seven.)

Often it is helpful to show the judge in your case that you are your child's primary caretaker and primary attachment figure. Make sure to tell your attorney all the ways you care for and nurture your child so that she or he can help to prove this.

It is most important that you make the court understand that breast-feeding is not incompatible with your child's bond with her father. Unfortunately, many in the legal field mistakenly think that they have to pick one (breastfeeding) over the other (the child's bond with the father). Giving the court several alternatives as to how breastfeeding can continue at the same time that your child has significant contact with her father may help to dispel this myth.

It is well worth making the effort to work with your child's father with regard to breastfeeding. Even if he is uncooperative and unpleasant, you need to be reasonable, polite, and informative. You may want to do some or all of the following:

1. First, try to convince your child's father that you will encourage his bond with your child because you know that is best for the child. (It is, of course, with few exceptions.) You will help your case by refraining from angry words and name-calling.
2. Decide what you want and try to come to an agreement before you file any papers with the court. If you and the father can't agree, meet with a counselor or a mediator.
3. Develop a visitation plan that provides for frequent contact between your child and her father, while still respecting your child's breastfeeding needs.
4. If you absolutely cannot work it out yourselves, expert evidence may be essential to prove the importance of breastfeeding specifically regarding your child. Obtain testimony from your pediatrician, a psychologist, a lactation consultant, or some other authority.

If You're Called to Jury Duty

In some states, if you are breastfeeding your child (sometimes with an age restriction, like up to one year of age), are responsible for your child's daily care, and are not employed outside the home, you can be excused from jury duty. But what if you don't live in such a state?

If you're called to jury duty, take these steps:

1. Follow the directions in the printed summons you receive, and be sure to respond within the stated time limit. If you meet the criterion for any exemption, just check that box. For example, in Florida, you're automatically excused if you are not employed and are caring full-time for a child under six. Some states will excuse you for economic necessity if you cannot afford a baby-sitter.

2. Advise the authorities of your situation—that is, that you're a nursing mother of a baby for whose care you have full-time responsibility.

3. If your child has any medical condition that would make separation from you difficult, ask your pediatrician to write a letter, which you send in along with your own letter requesting a medical excuse.

4. If separation from your nursing child could result in a breast infection or other medical problem for you, ask your doctor to write you a medical excuse.

5. Consider asking for a hardship exemption. Write a polite, informative letter to the clerk of courts. Tailor the letter to your own situation. Include any facts that will bolster your case, including a medical condition in your family or the baby's father's family (like allergies) that makes it especially important for your baby to be breastfed.

6. If none of these exemptions apply, try to educate the court about the value of breastfeeding and the effect of separation on your baby and yourself. You may want to present information from Chapter 1 of this book, telling why breastfeeding is so important.

7. If none of the above exempt you and you do have to serve on jury duty, do not bring your baby with you into the courtroom. Many courts prohibit the presence of babies and can impose serious sanctions on anyone who brings one. It *is* outrageous that a governmental body would not see nursing a baby as a valid reason to postpone jury duty and would impose sanctions on a mother who brings her nursing child to the courtroom. However, if you don't want to challenge this rule, you can either ask someone to stay with your baby just outside the courthouse in the hope that your jury breaks will coincide with your baby's feeding schedule. Or you can leave bottles of your expressed milk with your baby-sitter.

Breastfeeding an Older Child

Over the past several years some rare instances have arisen in which social service agencies have questioned the propriety of extended breastfeeding. Although the issue is more likely to arise the older the child is, we know of no social service agency that has found extended breastfeeding to be considered abuse or neglect, regardless of the age of the nursing child. Says attorney Elizabeth Baldwin, "As more social service agencies become aware of the normalcy and frequency of extended breastfeeding, I have seen the issue resolved favorably even with six-, seven-, or eight-year-old breastfeeding children."

What should you do if you are reported for abuse because of extended breastfeeding—or any other unusual family practice? First, remember that every report of abuse must be investigated. Be polite and cooperative, without volunteering information or agreeing to anything. Remember that anything you say may be misinterpreted. Make a note of any accusations and if possible, ask the investigator if you can call back. Meanwhile, you may need to contact an attorney experienced in social service agency cases or a criminal lawyer if it looks as if the matter is not going to be resolved easily.* If you are contacted by the police, remember that your constitutional right to remain silent or to have an attorney present during questioning is for your protection. Volunteer as little as possible; let your attorney speak for you. She or he can do this most effectively if you empower your lawyer by educating him or her about the benefits and normality of extended breastfeeding. Good resources for educating anyone concerned about extended breastfeeding are the 1997 recommendations from the American Academy of Pediatrics and the books cited in the Bibliography.

The law is often no more than a reflection of society-wide values and customs. As our culture becomes increasingly more nursing-friendly, many of these conflicts will cease to pose problems.

YOUR OLDER CHILDREN

If you have other children, you may wonder about their reactions to your nursing their baby brother or sister. You may be afraid that your feeding your new baby in such an intimate way will make your other children especially jealous. Actually, your older children, especially the one closest in age to the new one, is likely to have ambivalent feelings toward the new baby— loving the baby and feeling jealous of him—no matter how you feed. This doesn't seem any worse when the baby is nursed. In fact, one study found that the older siblings of babies who were being bottle-fed misbehaved more at feeding time than did the siblings of babies being breastfed.

If you breastfed your older children, you can tell them that you fed them this way when they were babies and that now it's the new baby's turn. If you did not breastfeed them, there's no need to volunteer this information, but you don't want to be dishonest by implying that you did, either. Simply tell them that this is the healthiest way to feed a baby and that you want to be as good a mother as you can to the new baby, just as you want to be a good mother to all your children.

If they ask whether you nursed them as babies, you can explain that when they were little you didn't know how good breastfeeding was for the baby and the mother. Now that you do know, you want to do the best

---

*To find such an attorney, see the Resource Appendix.

thing. Most youngsters accept a simple explanation like this and are happy to hear that even adults keep learning new things.

You can expect your older ones to be on your lap or by your side as your baby nurses. (We're not talking here about toddlers whom you nursed throughout a subsequent pregnancy and are still "tandem" nursing, which we'll say more about in Chapter 16, but about those who were never nursed or were weaned some time back.) Accept this and make feeding times family times.

When you breastfeed, you have a free arm to draw your toddler close to you or to turn the pages of her favorite book. While the infant has your breast, your older child has your attention on his level. Show your other children in many ways that the new baby has not displaced them in your affection, but don't let them feel that they have the right to deprive the infant of the right to be nursed.

One way to keep your older child busy while you're nursing your baby is to set aside special toys or books that can be played with *only* while you're nursing, or to turn on a special video or audiocassette as a nursing-time-only treat.

Occasionally toddlers ask whether they can nurse, too. If you let your child try, he'll probably laugh and forget about it or may even put his mouth to your breast and then not know what to do about it. The suckling movements that come so naturally to a newborn seem to be easily forgotten. Many babies forget how to do it as soon as a month after they have been weaned. If your toddler is different, though, and does want to go back to nursing, you can point out to him that this is something that only little babies do—and you can follow this by giving him a treat that is only for "big" boys or girls. Or you can go ahead and "tandem nurse" both your baby and your toddler, a choice we discuss in Chapter 16.

Your older children can probably offer more help to you than you realize. Take advantage of their interest in being eager baby-amusers, willing fetch-and-carriers, and pleasant companions to you as they help you fold the laundry, set the table, or push the baby carriage. Some of the happiest family times occur in such everyday activities.

As a breastfeeding mother you have a lovely opportunity to provide some elementary sex education in an easy, natural way. The child who sees his little brother or sister at the breast learns some of the biological differences between men and women and gains a sense of the function and beauty of the human body. Your young daughter may be especially inspired by the thought that she will be able to care for her babies in this special way when she grows up. Your little boy may think he'll be able to do it, too—but will probably accept your explanation that he'll have other ways to love his babies.

The Working Nursing Mother

I see this as an opportunity to be a role model for some of the women in the firm who haven't had babies yet. I show them that breastfeeding and working full-time is doable—and that it's well worth the extra effort.

JESSICA, BOSTON, MASSACHUSETTS

Of course, *all* mothers are "working mothers." We change diapers, we do the laundry, we cook mashed potatoes, we clean up kitchens and bathrooms. We stay up all night with a sick baby or wrench ourselves out of a warm bed in the middle of the night to comfort a toddler scared by a nightmare. We play endless games of Candyland when we would rather curl up with a good book. In short, as parents we do all kinds of things that are described better as "work" than as "play."

But besides this often gratifying, often difficult family work, most parents take on other work, too. Across the world and throughout history, most parents of both sexes have always worked. Until relatively recent times, much of this work could be done without both parents having to leave their children in the care of others. Now, though, this is less often an option.

Over the past several decades we have seen two major changes in women's lives. The year 1969 marked a turning point in the history of American women: For the first time more mothers of school-age children were holding down jobs than were working as full-time homemakers. Since then the proportion of mothers in the workplace has continued a steady rise, with the biggest increase in recent years among mothers of children under the age of three. Now, more than half of all mothers of infants under one year of age are working for pay, full- or part-time, in or out of the home—the highest proportion in the history of the United States. When we use the term *working mother,* these are the mothers we refer to.

The year 1971 signaled a different kind of turning point: That year marked the nation's lowest breastfeeding rates in history. Since then the proportion of women choosing to nurse their babies has also risen steadily. As these two trends have come together, we see more and more women who are working outside the home and are also nursing their babies.

Yes, it can be done. Many women are doing it, and what's more, many women are enjoying combining these two activities. Working mothers often express a special appreciation of the joys of breastfeeding. Away from their babies for much of the day, they savor the special warmth and intimacy of the nursing relationship when they are home. They find that the intensity of the nursing experience helps to make up for the hours they are away from their families. Furthermore, many working mothers find that the ability to sit and nurse actually has a calming, relaxing effect on *them,* while reminding the baby who the real mother is!

Not that it's easy. Anyone who combines working for pay and caring for a family is bound to experience one conflict after another: You have only so much time and energy. Adding breastfeeding to your daily schedule imposes still another layer of activities and concerns. Yet more and more women are so convinced of the value of breastfeeding and are so committed to their work (for reasons of economic necessity, personal fulfillment, or both) that they are determined to carry out both activities. A few years back women were saying, "I'm going back to work. Can you help me wean my baby?" Now they say, "I'm going back to work. Can you help me keep on nursing?"

How do so many women manage to combine these areas of their lives so well? They line up the support they need—and they organize their lives for success.

FINDING SUPPORT

This is one time in your life when you need as much help as you can get. Your time to assist others will come, but for now you have to reach out for any aid that others can give to you. Help is where you find it.

If your partner takes over some of the household chores, cares for your baby in many important ways, and provides that all-important dollop of moral support that lets you know you're doing a good job, you're lucky. Of course this is only fair. If you're doing your part to win the bread, he should be doing his part to make the home.

If your partner provides verbal support for your efforts but not much more, you may be able to enlist his cooperation by letting him know how important his help is to your success at breastfeeding. (Ask him, for example, to read Chapter 14 in this book.) If he still does not do as much as you would like him to, look for help elsewhere.

You may be able to call upon your baby-sitter for help above and beyond the work she was hired for. Or you may be able to go to family members. (One mother told us of a time when she had to visit her husband in the hospital. She met her brother after work, he took her expressed milk, picked up the baby at the caregiver's home, and gave the baby the bottle.) Don't forget friends, neighbors, coworkers, employers, or local support groups like La Leche League, International Childbirth Education Association, or ASPO/Lamaze. It's especially important for single mothers to find people to help them through this gratifying, though demanding, period of their lives.

If your income permits extras or if anyone wants to give you a generous baby gift, there's no better use for money at this time than buying you some help. Hiring someone to do the cleaning, the cooking, the marketing, and the laundry is an investment that can pay off in your physical and psychological comfort, and ultimately in your entire family's well-being.

The special helper we talked about in Chapter 4 can be a lifesaver for the working mother. She (or he) can step in at times of emergency and lighten your load in many ways on a day-to-day basis. If you don't have someone in your life to serve this function, you may need to call upon some of the problem-solving abilities that serve you so well on the job to locate one or more people to share those all-important tasks.

PLANNING AHEAD: WHILE YOU'RE PREGNANT AND STILL ON THE JOB

The time to arrange for your maternity leave and to enlist your employer as your ally is during your pregnancy. If you have performed your work well and made yourself valuable to your employers, they will be eager to do whatever is necessary to bring you back and keep you happy. Highly valued employees can often obtain all sorts of concessions that company policy ordinarily prohibits, such as longer maternity leaves, temporary part-time schedules, and the opportunity to do some of your work at home.

If your position with your company is strong, ask for whatever you want. You may be pleasantly surprised at what you can get. One thing you might suggest to your personnel or human resource director would be contacting one of the organizations listed in the Resource Appendix under "Help in the Workplace." These organizations look at employee health and support programs from the employer's point of view, emphasizing how such services can increase productivity and profits by reducing employee absenteeism and turnover, and cutting child health costs. By meeting your needs now, your employer is likely to have a happier and more productive worker in the future.

Your Maternity Leave

It's your responsibility to tell your employer about your pregnancy before you show up in a well-filled-out maternity dress and before you tell your coworkers. Fairly early in your pregnancy, ask for an appointment with your supervisor to discuss your plans and your future with the company. Tell her how long you expect to continue working and how much maternity leave you plan to take. Before your meeting, familarize yourself with legal and company maternity provisions, so you'll get, at the very least, what you're entitled to.

The absolute minimum for your maternity leave should be four weeks; the federal Family and Medical Leave Act mandates twelve weeks of unpaid leave for companies with fifty or more workers. The more you can negotiate for (either paid or unpaid), the easier it will be for you. A good goal to shoot for is four to six months. With this amount of time, you'll be fairly well rested by the time you go back to work, your milk supply will be well established, and your baby may even be sleeping through the night and on a fairly predictable schedule.

Research shows that breastfeeding and employment are compatible—and that the longer a woman's maternity leave is, the longer she's likely to nurse. In one group of 567 working breastfeeding mothers, whose occupations covered a wide range (including mill and factory workers, police officers and postal carriers, secretaries, preschool through college-level teachers, business executives, attorneys, and physicians), the typical time of return to work was six to seven weeks after birth. Three-fourths of these women were back on the job before their babies were thirteen weeks old, and those who returned before the baby's fourth month were likely to wean earlier than those who stayed home longer.*

---

*This study, by Kathleen G. Auerbach, Ph.D., and Elizabeth Guss, specified only one cutoff point to differentiate early and late weaning—the first birthday. Most of these "early-weaning" mothers nursed until seven months or so, ages that in our society are not generally considered early weaning. See Chapter 18 for a discussion of different ages for weaning.

An Ideal Program for Working Breastfeeding Mothers*

In its 1997 policy statement on breastfeeding, the American Academy of Pediatrics urged employers to "provide appropriate facilities and adequate time in the workplace for breast-pumping." A number of corporate and public-sector firms that employ sizable numbers of women have already instituted full-scale lactation programs, and more and more are putting such programs in place. They are doing this not because of charity, but because it makes sense on the bottom line.

What does such a program involve? According to Rona Cohen, director of Sanvita Corporate Lactation Programs, the following components are important:

• A policy, agreed upon by department heads, senior administrators, and employees, which recognizes parents' responsibilities to both job and family.

• A maternity leave policy that is long enough to enable mothers to establish a breastfeeding routine and milk supply before returning to work.

• Providing breaks, flexible work hours, and part-time work so that women can pump their milk during the workday or nurse their babies, either at a nearby child-care site or at a place where someone brings their babies to them.

• Offering a clean, safe, and comfortable private area where mothers can go to pump their milk. This place should be easily accessible, should have lockable doors, should have access to electricity (so that an efficient electric pump can be used), and should be in a place where it will not disrupt work schedules.

*For information about organizations that help employers set up corporate lactation programs, see the Resource Appendix.

Furthermore, those mothers who didn't go back to work until their babies were four months old were less likely to feel that their employment affected their breastfeeding negatively. Still, 40 percent of those who returned before four months continued to nurse past their babies' first birthday.

Even if you have to go back to work earlier than you would like, you can still have a successful breastfeeding experience.

Your Breastfeeding Plans

It's not necessary to discuss your breastfeeding plans when you first speak to your employer. After all, that time is a long time away. Besides, your

• Renting or buying breast pumps: an electric one with a double pumping system to be kept at the worksite, available to workers on any shift; and portable pumps for travel and off-site use. Although the worksite pump can be shared, each woman needs her own attachable kit and tubing so that her milk will not come into contact with any surface touched by another mother's milk.

• Supplying a sink and a water source for washing equipment in or near the pumping room.

• Hiring a lactation professional who can counsel and support both female and male workers on combining parenthood and employment, who is available for consultation prenatally, during maternity leave, and after the return to work.

• Developing or coordinating with existing on-site or near-site child-care programs so that mothers can go to their babies during the day.

• Offering education to other personnel about the advantages to the company—and by extension, to them—of providing understanding and support for breastfeeding and other parenting needs.

A society like ours, which talks about how pro-family it is, should provide services that help parents give their children the best care possible. In this regard we are far behind many other countries. In Sweden, for example, new mothers receive 90 percent of their salary for nine months and may ask for nine more months of unpaid leave, with their jobs guaranteed. Of more than 100 countries surveyed as far back as 1975, 75 percent had laws requiring nursing breaks and child care in or near the mother's workplace. Our government could do much more to encourage employers to institute family-oriented policies. Providing tax incentives to businesses that institute lactation support programs, that provide day care assistance, and that help families in other ways is one goal we should work for.

employer may not be interested in discussing them with you. In fact, depending on the atmosphere at your workplace, you may decide never to discuss your nursing with anyone there, but instead to privately work out your own arrangements. Many women have found, however, that talking with their employers ahead of time was helpful in enlisting support and in reassuring the boss that the job was still important to them.

Good times to talk about these plans are just before you go on leave or just before you plan to return. If you do raise the issue of nursing, you will want to make the following points:

• Breastfeeding is not unduly time-consuming. You know other working women who have found it compatible with their work schedules, and you are organizing your life so that you will be able to handle it, too. At this time you might talk about how you plan to make up any time you might lose from work (by coming in early, staying late, or taking lunch at your desk).

• Breastfeeding mothers need not be restricted. With good organization, nursing women can be away from their babies if necessary for the complete workday (and sometimes even longer, although this is certainly a situation you don't want to encourage).

• In terms of your lifetime career, the period of time you'll be breastfeeding is really very short. You have shown your commitment to your work up till now, and that commitment will continue long after this important temporary interlude.

• The employer benefits economically from your breastfeeding. Since breastfed babies are usually healthier than bottle-fed babies (see Chapter 1 for specifics), you're likely to lose less time from work than you might otherwise. Research studies have borne this out: Women who continue to nurse after returning to work miss fewer days of work because of baby-related illnesses, and, when they do miss work, their absences are shorter. Your employer's health insurance plan also benefits: An internal study by Kaiser Permanente found that breastfeeding for only six months can decrease a family's health care claims by hundreds of dollars in the first year of life.

• If your employer's workforce includes a large number of young women, you might want to suggest that management consider adopting a lactation support program like the one described in the box on page 228. Such a program is inexpensive and easy to install. Yet it can go far toward attracting new workers, shortening the maternity leaves of the ones who are already there, increasing productivity by raising morale, and saving money. (John Hancock Mutual Life Insurance Company in Boston estimates that since its establishment in 1993 of a "mother's room" where nursing mothers can pump their milk, it has saved about $60,000 in time lost because of sick children.)

• You may or may not want to talk about your milk-pumping needs. If you do, make the point that you'll be able to do this on your coffee and lunch breaks, so you won't need to take time from your working day. Once you feel you have a sympathetic ear, you can ask for access to a private, comfortable place where you can pump your milk a couple of times a day.

PLANNING AHEAD: WHILE YOU'RE ON YOUR MATERNITY LEAVE

While most of your efforts during this brief time will probably involve getting used to caring for your new baby, establishing the breastfeeding relationship, and resting after the labor of childbirth, you will want to use these weeks at home to handle some important steps.

Finding Child Care

As a working mother, the most important person in your life after your husband and child is likely to be the person who takes care of your child. You need to find a caregiver who is both caring and capable. You also need to find someone who will support your breastfeeding plans, not sabotage them.

When you interview a potential caregiver, be sure to let her know that you plan to breastfeed your baby. Be alert to her responses: Does she seem to think this is a wonderful idea or a terrible one? Does she seem to feel that her domain is being invaded? Does she feel that it's a mistake for a working mother to nurse? If you get any clues to such feelings, you'll know that this person is not for you.

If she does seem responsive, however, you need to ask some more questions and to give her some information.

• Ask whether she has ever taken care of a breastfed baby.

• Tell her the kind of schedule you have in mind, how many feedings a day you want her to give your baby, how to store your expressed breast milk or formula, and how to thaw it if you'll be providing frozen breast milk.

• If she has never cared for a breastfed baby, you need to tell her about the differences in feeding schedules (breastfed babies eat more frequently), in bowel movements (looser and either more or less frequent, depending on your own baby's pattern), and in ways of soothing the baby (for example, avoiding bottles of water and pacifiers for at least the first few weeks).

• If your caregiver lives closer to your workplace than to your home, you may want to nurse your baby after you take her there in the morning and as soon as you pick her up at night. Be sure that this is acceptable.

• You may want to give or lend her a copy of this book, marking the pages she's most likely to refer to. Or you can write out the information she needs and put it in a convenient place.

While you may not be able to find a caregiver who has the same attitudes toward breastfeeding that you do, you do need to find one who will carry out your instructions. In other words, she can *think* the way *she* wants, as long as she *acts* the way *you* want.

Introducing Milk in a Bottle or Cup

Since the key to your success in combining working and breastfeeding will probably lie in your baby's having at least one or more feedings while you're at work, it's vital that you take special pains to help her like the bottle or cup, even if she doesn't love it. (She'll be saving her love for you.)

In our society we have generally assumed that babies who are not breast-fed need to get their milk in a bottle. But in many countries around the world, babies who cannot be nursed receive all their liquid nourishment in a cup, sometimes right from birth. United Nations agencies do not distribute feeding bottles at all, even to babies who cannot be breastfed.

Cup feeding has several advantages: There is no danger of nipple confusion; an open cup is easier to keep clean than either a bottle or a sipper cup; you cannot prop a baby alone with a cup the way you can with a bottle; and even premature babies can drink from a cup, since the swallowing reflex appears earlier than the sucking reflex. However, cup feeding may be more time-consuming, and, probably more important, it is an unfamiliar idea to most people—which may include the person who cares for your baby while you are at work.

If you can, get your baby used to a cup from an early age, and ask your caregiver to feed her this way. If this will not work for you, however, you do, of course, have access to bottles for the feedings while you are at work.

By and large, the earlier a baby is given milk in a bottle or cup, the more readily she will take it. Babies confronted with their first bottle at several months of age often refuse it absolutely and will sooner go hungry rather than drink from this strange, hard, unwelcome container so different from their mother's soft, warm breast. This usually happens only for a few feedings, however, until hunger takes over.

Yet there is a danger in introducing the bottle *too* early. Although some babies have no trouble taking a daily bottle along with their breast feedings right from birth, other babies who are offered bottles before they have fully mastered the skills of nursing at the breast develop "nipple confusion." They can't make the switch between sucking on the rubber nipple and suckling at the breast, and sometimes develop nursing problems.

It's important to strike a happy medium. Introducing a cup or bottle after six weeks of age may avoid both these problems. By this age, most babies are competent nursers and yet they're still flexible enough to try something new. Furthermore, the mother's milk supply is well established by now and flows easily enough to keep her baby happy.

If you must go back to work before this time, you'll have to introduce the cup or bottle earlier. If at all possible, try to hold off your return to work at least until two months postpartum, for both your sake and your baby's.

You may decide to introduce the cup or bottle gradually, about a week or two before you plan to go back to work, so that by the time you do go back, your baby is taking one cup or bottle feeding every day, at the same time every day. This time should coincide with at least one of the feedings when you'll be away, so that a pattern will be set. While your baby is nursing from one breast, express or pump from the other breast to keep up your milk supply. Your baby probably will drink less milk from the cup or bottle than she does from the breast, perhaps less than two ounces at a time. This is not a problem.

Some mothers hold off introducing a bottle or a cup until they actually return to work. Since some babies accept a bottle or a cup better from someone other than their mother, the baby-sitter can often manage this transition herself. Meanwhile, the mother remains totally associated with breastfeeding.

When you or another person (which is often more successful) first introduces milk in a cup or bottle, give it to your baby when he's not terribly hungry—maybe forty-five minutes after a feeding. This way, he'll be more receptive to something new and may be pleasantly surprised to find something good trickling out of it. Also, if you usually sit in a particular chair to nurse, have someone else, the baby's father, for instance, offer a bottle in some other chair, or some other room. For other suggestions on encouraging your baby to take a bottle, see the box on page 234.

Making the Transition from Home to Work

It will probably be easier for your baby to adjust to your going back to work than it will be for you. You can make it even easier for both of you.

If your caregiver will be coming to your home, ask her to come to work a week or two before *you* go back to work so that she can get to know your baby, as well as you and your routines. If you will be taking your baby to her home, plan to take him for a few increasingly longer visits before you go back to work.

- First, you and your baby should be with the caregiver for an hour or so just to get acquainted. Then your baby should be alone with the caregiver at a time when he won't need to be fed. Then he should be with the caregiver for a few longer sessions that include feeding times.

Offering Your Baby the Bottle

- Have someone else give the cup or bottle, right from the start. This is an ideal way for your baby's father to assume a larger role in his baby's care. The next best feeder is the person who will care for your baby when you go back to work.

- Introduce the cup or bottle when your baby is not frantically hungry.

- Some babies have definite preferences for one kind of nipple over another. Others don't care. Try a contoured nipple (like the Nuk or the Kip), but just buy one or two in case your baby doesn't like it. Be sure *not* to buy nipples especially made for premature infants if your baby is full-term; these nipples are made of thinner rubber, and some vigorous suckers have been known to bite pieces off and swallow them.

- Try to find "blind" nipples, which don't have holes in them; then you can make your own hole with a hot straight pin, to ensure that the milk won't come too quickly.

- To test the flow of milk, hold the bottle upside down. If milk pours out, the nipple opening is too big; if it doesn't squirt out when you squeeze the nipple with your fingers, it's too small. In the first case, there's nothing you can do other than throw the nipple out; in the second, you can make an additional hole or two with a hot straight pin.

WHAT IF YOUR BABY REFUSES THE BOTTLE?

Your baby may absolutely refuse to take any nourishment from a bottle. Some go on "hunger strikes" if they can't have the breast; no matter how ravenous they

- Take the time to show your caregiver how you want her to do things and encourage her to ask you about any problems or questions she may have.

- Be sure she knows how to reach you and your husband at work.

- If you take your baby to the caregiver, bring some familiar toys to carry the smells and thoughts of home and Mommy.

- Before your first day back on the job, hold a "dress rehearsal," a day when you'll be away from your baby for about the same length of time as on a typical workday, and when your caregiver will treat your baby the same way she will when you do return to work. This will let you iron out

get or how piteously they cry, they won't give in. Families cope with this in a number of different ways. One of the following may work for you:

• Nurse as much as possible while you're home, so even if your baby won't take a bottle while you're gone, she'll still be getting a good supply of milk.

• Brush your baby's mouth with the nipple and let him grasp it himself instead of pushing it forcefully into his mouth.

• Warm the bottle nipple and the milk to body temperature by running warm water over the nipple and the bottle.

• Ask someone else to pick up your baby while she's sleeping, but almost ready to wake, and feed her milk in a bottle. Do this for a while, and then try it when she's awake.

• If you have not already offered your baby milk or water from a cup, try offering him water first. Once he takes that readily, he'll probably also take milk this way. You don't need a special cup to do this. Any cup in your house will do, although the infant "sipper" cups with two handles and a lid are the least messy.

• Feed the milk through a large medicine dropper or a spoon—rubber-coated or plastic. Sometimes, once the baby has received a couple of ounces of milk this way and is not so desperately hungry, he'll be willing to tolerate the bottle for the rest of the feeding.

• Experiment with different kinds of milk. One mother discovered that her baby preferred fresh, refrigerated breast milk over thawed frozen milk. If you're feeding formula, try another brand, after consulting with your baby's doctor.

• Experiment with different feeding positions. Have your caregiver try propping your baby against her raised legs, or holding him facing out, so he can't see her. (We don't know why this works, but some babies feed better this way.)

any kinks in your scheduling—and will reassure you that you can handle both home and work.

• Whether you nurse at the caregiver's house or at your home, be sure that she will not feed your baby for a couple of hours before you come to pick him up so that he'll be hungry enough to nurse vigorously. It may take a few days to work out this scheduling; it is extremely important for your baby's satisfaction at the breast, for your milk supply, for your comfort, and for the success of the breastfeeding relationship.

Learning How to Pump or Express Milk

If you plan to leave your own milk with your baby-sitter to give to your baby for the feedings you'll miss, the need for pumping or expressing milk is obvious. With this technique you'll be able to get milk from your breasts while you're at work, bring it home, and give it to the caregiver to give to your baby the next day. You'll also be able to make extra milk that you can store in the freezer for emergencies or unexpected feedings.

Even if you plan to use formula for missed feedings, however, pumping or expressing is an important skill to have. It can help you relieve the pressure of overfull breasts so that you feel more comfortable, it will diminish leaking, it will keep up your milk supply, and it will help to prevent the breast infections that often result from engorgement. In the Auerbach and Guss survey mentioned earlier, 86 percent of those 567 working mothers either hand-expressed or pumped milk at missed feedings, and the women who did this tended to nurse longer.

Learning these techniques is a perfect activity for "What I Did on My Maternity Leave." You can't expect to do your learning when you're back on the job, pressured by time, dressed for success, and in an environment that probably provides less than ideal levels of comfort and privacy. If you start doing it at least three weeks before you go back to work, you'll have time to practice and you should be fairly proficient by the time you need to be.

One technique that's especially valuable is expressing from one breast while you're nursing your baby on the other breast. This method enlists your baby as your partner, since you'll be getting the benefit of the let-down triggered by your baby's sucking, and your work will be easier. You'll need help from another person the first time you try this, even if you're extremely dextrous. Or you can express from the non-nursed breast immediately after nursing from the other one.

If you have trouble mastering this (as many women do), try instead to pump or express some milk about an hour after a nursing while your baby is otherwise engaged. The amount you produce doesn't matter, especially in these early sessions. The point is to learn the technique.

Expressing while you're still at home will let you stockpile milk in your freezer. If you plan to feed your baby breast milk alone, you'll have a backup supply for emergencies and days when your supply may be low. If you plan to supplement with formula, a few extra bottles of breast milk are a happy bonus for your baby.

For step-by-step directions on both hand-expression and pumping and for a comparison of the different techniques and the different kinds of pumps, see Chapter 17. You'll also find directions for storing and then using the milk that you have expressed.

BACK AT WORK

Your Work Schedule

Try to make your first day back at work a Thursday or Friday. This will give you the weekend to rest up, to analyze the way your workday went, and to see how you can help it go more smoothly. Try to take off the first few Wednesdays: a mid-week break will also make the transition easier.

If you can go back to work part-time for a while, this will be ideal. Survey after survey shows that mothers who work part-time seem the happiest

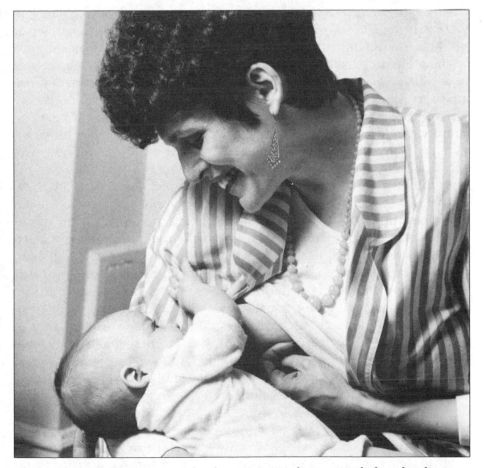

Working mothers often treasure that last nursing in the morning before they leave the baby and the first one after they return home at the end of the working day. The babies love them, too.

with their lives, compared to full-time employees and full-time homemakers. This is especially helpful, of course, for the breastfeeding mother, especially if you go back to work before your baby is four months old. Research has also shown that mothers who work no more than twenty hours a week are likely to continue to nurse as long as homemaker mothers.

If you have the option of working part-time and can plan your schedule, fewer hours per day work out better for breastfeeding than fewer days per week. In other words, if you plan to work about twenty-four hours per week, you'll do better putting in five hours a day for five days instead of eight hours for three days. You'll have to balance this advantage for breastfeeding with such disadvantages as a higher expense of child care or a long commute to work and make the decision that's best for you.

The possibilities for alternative scheduling are limitless. On some jobs you can bring some of your work home. On others you can take advantage of flexible scheduling or of sharing your job with another worker. At some workplaces you can take your baby to work with you. Or you may be able to combine two coffee breaks into a single longer break, which you can then attach to your lunch hour so you can go to your baby. (One mother we know meets her caregiver, her older son, and her nursing baby in a park on sunny days and in a coffee shop on cold or rainy days.) Explore the possibility of these options with your employer. Even if they never thought of such arrangements in the past, they may be willing to give it a try.

You may decide, after adding up the costs of child care, commuting, clothes, lunches out, and so forth, that the only way for you to come out ahead is to find work that you can do at home. Or you may be in a position to postpone your return to paid employment until your child is older.

Years ago the mother who worked outside the home was criticized for leaving her children. Today the climate has changed so far in the other direction that criticism is often directed at women who have the financial option of staying home for a few years and who enjoy caring for small children and running a household. It would be a shame if women came to accept the judgment that a person is only as interesting and valuable as her job and her income—a way of thinking far too common among men. Bringing up children is important work, and our society needs to recognize that *every* mother is a working mother. You're the only one who can decide whether this is the sole work you want to do in these years and whether it's financially feasible for you.

Whatever your decision, if you're happy with it, your children are likely to thrive. According to research, the more satisfied a woman is with her life, the more effective she is as a parent, and the better adjusted her children will be.

Your Nursing Schedule

While there are many different ways to arrange your breastfeeding schedule, a fairly typical one for a full-time mother of a small baby with fairly regular habits may go something like this:

1. Wake up in the morning one hour before you need to begin to get ready for work. Take your baby back to bed with you for a quiet, leisurely feeding.
2. Nurse your baby again just before you leave him at the caregiver's home or at the day care center. This one is optional, depending on how much time has elapsed since the first morning feeding, and on you and your baby. If you do have time, it's a nice way to say "Good-bye, I'll see you soon."
3. If you're leaving your own milk for your baby's feedings, express or pump two to three times during the workday (on morning and/or afternoon coffee breaks and/or at lunchtime).
4. If feasible, nurse your baby at noon, either by going to her or having her brought to you.
5. Nurse your baby right after work, at the child-care site if you have a long ride home or, preferably, at home. Ask the caregiver not to feed your baby for a couple of hours before you're expected.)
6. Nurse just before you go to sleep.
7. Nurse one or more times during the night. (This is optional, depending on your baby's schedule. Many women find that getting up once during the night is not exhausting, especially if they and the baby go right back to sleep afterward, which is easier if they are sleeping in the same bed.)

No one is typical, and every woman has to learn what works for her. One flight attendant, for example, went back to work after three months, making three trips a week. She chose night flights so that she would miss only one or two feedings, used a breast pump every three or four hours, put her breast milk in bottles that she packed in ice till she got home, and then froze the milk for use during her next flight.

Another mother nursed full-time for her baby's first six weeks, then substituted formula for two daytime feedings a day for the next two weeks, and went back to work after two months. She continued to nurse only three times a day—morning, evening, and bedtime.

Some working nursing mothers schedule "reverse cycle feeding," by which they feed their babies frequently during the evenings and at night

(continued on page 242)

A Day in the Life of One Working Nursing Family

The following schedule represents a fairly typical weekday in the life of Charlotte Lee-Carrihill and Brian Carrihill, when their son, Colin, was three years old, and their daughter, Laura, was three months:

Charlotte is an executive at a Wall Street investment banking firm; Brian is a computer graphics specialist. This family's extraordinary success in handling two careers and two children, one of whom has been and the other of whom is being breastfed, rests on their willingness to work together toward common goals, support from family members who live nearby, good organization, and Charlotte's vast reserves of energy, which let her keep an almost unbelievably active schedule.

Each family needs to find its own way of doing things. This is how life works out in one household, but it might not work well in yours. You need to recognize your own and your family's unique personal needs and to plan your schedule accordingly. You may, for example, be able to sleep a little later in the morning, get to your place of work a little bit later or leave a little bit earlier, and your partner may be able to shoulder more or less of the child-care duties.

Once you have your schedule worked out, you need to keep it flexible. Life has a way of interfering with the most careful plans, requiring quick changes and an acceptance that even the most ideal schedule has to be written in pencil, not ink.

6:00 A.M.   Charlotte nurses Laura, who usually sleeps in the same bed with her parents for the first few months of her life. If Laura doesn't wake up by herself, Charlotte wakes her for the nursing. Brian is already awake and getting dressed.

6:15   Charlotte showers, washes her hair, dresses.

6:30   Brian leaves for work.
            Charlotte dresses Colin, who sleeps through the entire process. She then dresses Laura, who has also fallen back to sleep.

7:00   Charlotte takes Colin and his lunchbox (packed the night before) out to the car. She puts him in his carseat and covers him with a blanket, which she leaves in the car all the time, so the children have an easier awakening. She goes back into the house to get Laura, Laura's bag (containing diapers, an extra outfit, a bib, toys—all packed the night before—plus the day's supply of expressed milk put in at the last minute), and her own briefcase (containing a cylinder-type breast pump, a thermos, a washcloth, a brush to clean the pump, paper towels, and nursing pads, in addition to papers she needs for work, also packed the night before).

7:10	Charlotte drops Laura off at the caregiver's home. (She leaves some equipment there all week, including a stroller, a walker, a quilt, a blanket, and one bottle of frozen breast milk for emergencies.)
7:25	Charlotte drops Colin off at his nursery school/day care center.
7:30	Charlotte parks her car near the subway, takes the train into work.
8–8:30	Charlotte arrives at her office. She eats breakfast either in the cafeteria with coworkers, at a breakfast meeting with clients, or alone at her desk.
10:00	Coffee break — Charlotte goes into the ladies' room where she pumps her milk and pours it into a thermos, which she'll carry home in her briefcase. She can now do both breasts in about ten minutes.
12–1:00 P.M.	Lunch, usually at her desk, usually followed by a short trip outside to do errands and get some fresh air.
1:00	Trip to the women's bathroom to pump milk.
4:00	Trip to the women's bathroom to pump milk.
5:00	Charlotte leaves her office.
5:40	Charlotte picks up Colin at school.
6:00	Brian picks up Laura at the caregiver's. Charlotte arrives home and gives Colin a snack to tide him over till dinner, which she starts to prepare. Over the weekend she plans the week's meals. If she gets home late or for some other reason can't hold to the original plan, she takes something out of the freezer that can be prepared quickly.
6:30	Brian and Laura arrive home. Charlotte nurses Laura. Brian brings Charlotte something to eat while she's nursing—a banana or a mini peanut butter sandwich. She also sips on a glass of ice water (which she does during most nursings). Brian takes over dinner preparations.
7:00	Brian, Charlotte, and Colin sit down to dinner. Laura is nearby in her swing or playing on a quilt on the floor.
7:30	Brian washes the dinner dishes while Charlotte bathes Colin and Laura. Brian dries Laura and dresses her; Charlotte does the same for Colin.
8:00	Charlotte nurses Laura. She nurses her on cue all evening, every hour or two, whenever Laura seems to want to nurse. Usually this averages five or six nursings between 6:00 P.M. and 6:00 A.M.

(continued on next page)

(continued from page 241)

	Charlotte finds this relaxing, as well as a good way to keep up her milk supply. She also nurses on cue over the weekend.
8:00	While Charlotte is nursing, Brian is building with blocks or coloring with Colin. During the nursing, Charlotte may join in to play games, read, or watch TV with the two of them. (TV is limited to one hour a day on weekdays.) Weather permitting, the four of them may go out for a walk. (Occasionally the family goes out to dinner with family or friends. It's very rare for Charlotte and Brian to go out on weeknights without the children.)
8:30–10:00	Sometimes Charlotte throws a load of clothes into the washing machine and dryer; sometimes she does hand laundry. She always does next-day preparation: She lays out the next day's clothing for the children and herself; she makes Colin's lunch; she packs Laura's bag (except for the milk); she packs her own briefcase.
10:00	Brian gets Colin ready for bed, and Charlotte reads to him. Because Colin takes a long nap in nursery school, he is not ready to go to sleep early. His parents are content with his schedule, since this gives them more time with him.
10:00–10:30	Charlotte nurses Laura and puts her to bed. She sometimes goes for a short run with a friend.
10:30–11:00	Brian and Charlotte find quiet time together.
11:00	Charlotte and Brian go to sleep. They sometimes move Laura, already asleep in their bed, to her bassinet beside them.
3:00 A.M.	Charlotte nurses Laura.

so the babies won't be hungry during the day. Some babies seem to save their "up" time for these nighttime nursings, which are easier when mothers bring the baby into bed with them to nurse rather than awakening completely. If you can concentrate on the bonus of together time instead of the lost sleep, these snuggled-together sessions can be highlights of the nursing experience.*

Clearly, there's no single "right way." For the way one remarkable family manages, see the box on page 240.

---

*This schedule was described by Marilyn Grams, M.D., who used it while nursing her babies, in her very personal book, *Breastfeeding Success for Working Mothers.*

Travel

If your job requires travel, this poses especially difficult challenges. Ideally, you'll be able to postpone any trips until your baby is weaned. The next best thing is to keep trips brief, no more than overnight. If you can't do either, you still don't necessarily have to wean because of the trip. The ingenuity of mothers and the adaptability of babies can be astonishing. You may be able to take your baby and caregiver with you. If so, you might be able to maintain the same basic schedule as at home. If not, you can arrange for feedings in your absence.

If you know about your trip ahead of time, you can express milk and build up a frozen supply. Or your baby can take formula while you're away. In either case, you'll want to express milk during the separation to keep up your supply and to feel comfortable. Try to rent an electric pump if you'll be staying at one place for several days.

While it's sometimes possible to work out such arrangements, it's far from simple; it's to both your advantages (yours and your baby's) to make every effort to avoid this kind of separation while you're nursing.

Your Coworkers

Some nursing mothers find that their fellow workers, both male and female, take an interest in them and help them in ways both large and small. One woman, for example, pumped her milk under a stairwell while a male colleague stood guard to protect her privacy. Others report that their coworkers answer their phones for them while they're on their "pump breaks." Unfortunately, other mothers are targets of resentment from colleagues, who may complain about a woman's expressing milk in an employees' lounge or bathroom or about her "getting away with" something that other workers are not.

Women handle their on-the-job relationships in various ways. Some don't tell their fellow workers what they're doing. Others go out of their way to let people know—and to show them that they are indeed doing their jobs as well as ever. One stock analyst (known in her firm as the "Dairy Queen") is able to deal with the hostility she sometimes senses from women in her office by understanding where it comes from.

"I realize," she says, "that some of these women's resentment comes from their own pain or regrets that they didn't do this for their babies, or that they're not able to be with their children as much as they would like, and I don't let their remarks bother me. I know I'm doing this because it's important for my baby, and I can't be ruled by other people's derogatory attitudes and comments. "

Wardrobe Tips for the Working Breastfeeding Mother

Appearance is especially important for women who face an audience of adults each day. Since you're apt to feel better about yourself and what you're doing if you're happy with how you look, you'll want to look as good as you can, even while you're dressing for breastfeeding. These suggestions, plus the ones in Chapter 8, may help:

• Wear breast pads in your bra, at least for the first few weeks. They'll prevent leaking milk from coming through and showing. Be sure to change them when they get wet, to prevent sore nipples and to avoid the possibility of moisture showing through.

• Wear bright or dark print blouses or tops. They won't show any leaking that does occur as readily as solids and they won't show the outlines of your nipples or your breast pads. Stay away from whites and pale colors; they reveal to everyone what you may want just your baby and your partner to see.

• Cottons and synthetic fabrics stand up best in case of leaking. Silks and linens may become stained. Clinging materials will show the outlines of nipples and breast pads.

• Everything you wear should be washable. Nothing should need more than touch-up ironing.

• If you're self-conscious about your more bosomy figure, wear a lightweight blazer or loose jacket during your workday.

• Don't try to squeeze into too-tight prepregnancy clothes. Chances are that you're a few pounds heavier than you were then, and clothes that strain are unbecoming to even the slimmest women. Try wearing what you wore to work early in your pregnancy before you put on maternity clothes.

FEEDING YOUR BABY WHILE YOU'RE AT WORK

You need to decide long before you go back to work what your baby will drink in the feedings she receives from her caregiver. You have two choices—your own milk that you have expressed and pumped earlier, or formula. Straight cow's milk is not an option, since babies should be twelve months old before they are fed plain cow's milk.

- Tight blouses and shirts are especially treacherous: They rub against your nipples and might trigger a let-down at inconvenient times, like on the subway or in an important meeting. More important, they can cause a clogged duct or breast infection.

- Keep a spare blouse at work (one that can be worn with most outfits) in case you leak or spill milk on the one you're wearing.

For ease in expressing milk or nursing your baby during the workday:

- Wear two-piece outfits or dresses that button in the front.

- Wear blouses or tops that button down the front or pull up easily.

- Don't wear cotton sweaters; they tend to lose their shape during the day after being pulled up two or three times.

- Wear a nursing bra to work. It's more convenient to be able to undo one side at a time instead of having to take off your entire bra. You'll also welcome its good support.

DEALING WITH LEAKING

- This is most common in the first month or two of nursing, when your breasts are full or it's nearly time to nurse or express, and when you're thinking about your baby.
- If you can hold off going back to work for two months, leaking is less likely to occur at work.
- You can often prevent it by anticipating when it's likely to occur and expressing milk to reduce breast fullness.
- If you do feel tingling, cross your arms across your chest for about ten seconds. As one mother told us, "I like the elbow pressure against my breast as I 'fiddle with an earring.' Only another nursing mother will know what I'm *really* doing."

Breast milk is superior in many ways to formula, for the reasons spelled out in Chapter 1. Modern formula, however, is a viable alternative, and many babies thrive on it. The one caution in introducing formula at an early age is the possibility of a baby's showing an allergic reaction to it either now or in the future.

If you do feel that you can, as many women do, undertake and follow through on a program to express or pump milk for your baby, he can enjoy the benefits of breast milk for the entire time that you're nursing. Given your work conditions, your schedule, and your own inclinations, however, if you decide not to do this, you can substitute formula for the feedings you'll be missing. If neither you nor your baby's father has a family history of allergy, this is quite safe.

If you find that you're not able to express enough milk to meet your baby's needs, you can combine formula and breast milk. Or you may want to switch entirely to formula for feedings while you're at work. Remember that it's better to give some breast milk than none, that worrying about the possibility of your baby's going hungry will decrease your milk output even more, and that the value of the nursing experience does not rely only on the volume of milk you produce.

If you're anxious about the amount of milk you're producing, leave some formula with your caregiver. It's better to do this and to be able to enjoy the emotional closeness when you do nurse than to be so worried about the quantity of milk you're providing that neither you nor your baby will enjoy the nursing experience.

Whichever you decide, you'll want to learn how to pump or express milk, either to provide your baby's sustenance or to relieve your own discomfort. Basic instructions for expressing, pumping, storing, and giving breast milk are in Chapter 17. We'll deal here with some special considerations for the working woman.

Equipment You'll Need for Pumping Your Breast Milk

• A pump that's easy to carry and store, since you'll either be taking it to work with you every day or storing it at work. If you keep it at work, you need another pump to keep at home. You'll also want one that's easy to clean, especially since the washing facilities at work may not be up to the standards you have at home. The most efficient kind is an electric pump with a double pumping kit.*

• Either a thermos or a cooler to use with the bottles or milk storage bags. If you use a thermos, get the kind used for fluids, not solid foods, of the best quality you can find. Before you leave home in the morning fill it with ice cubes to keep it cold. When you express, dump out the ice, dry the inside of the thermos, and fill the thermos with your milk. If you use a cooler, put ice packs in it when you leave home.

Instead of pumping into a thermos, some women pump into a wide-

---

*One model comes in a shoulder bag that stores the double pumping kit, the pump itself, collection bottles, and cooling elements. You can also buy a unit to run it from the cigarette lighter in your car, or a rechargeable battery to use when electricity is not available. For information, contact the companies listed in the Resource Appendix.

mouthed jar and then pour the milk into a bottle or milk storage bag. They then store it among ice cubes or ice packs in a thermos jug or small cooler. The method works fine. The disadvantage is that it involves carrying bulkier equipment. Some women like the disposable bags that fit into nursing bottles because they lie flat in a freezer, are easy to stack, and thaw quickly. Others find them hard to handle and easy to puncture. Some of the bags made specifically for storing breast milk are sturdier, but more expensive. You have to find out what works best for you.

- A photo of your baby, to prop in front of you while you express. Seeing your baby's adorable face can help trigger your let-down.

- A brush for cleaning the pump after each use.

- A washcloth for patting your breasts dry after expressing. (Do not wipe. Wiping removes natural oil secretions and can cause chapping and soreness.)

- Cloth or paper towels for wiping the rim of the thermos and the pump.

- An extra set of nursing pads.

- A bag or briefcase, in which you can carry your equipment between work and home in separate plastic bags.

Where to Express

Find a clean, quiet, private place. Ideally, a quiet office with a door you can lock, either your own office or another that you can arrange to use, is best. A vacant meeting or conference room may be available. Some women go out and sit in their cars (some electric pumps can be plugged into the cigarette lighter). Others use a women's lounge or bathroom. One confessed to a special fondness for the stall in her bathroom designed for women with disabilities, since it's roomier and has a convenient shelf for placing her paraphernalia. If you're using an office, check for windows so that you can maintain your privacy.

When to Express

If you are hand-expressing or using a manual pump, at first it may take you up to thirty minutes each session to drain both breasts. Eventually you may be able to get it down to eight minutes each time; some women continue to need fifteen to twenty minutes. Electric pumps are much faster and take no more than about ten or fifteen minutes total right from the start. The more you practice at home, the better you'll do.

You should be able to find enough time between your coffee breaks and your lunch hour. Some women eat while they pump or at their desks. In your eagerness to make the most of your time, however, don't neglect your diet. You need to keep up your strength. If you can't get enough pumping time during your breaks, you may be able to make arrangements to come into work earlier, stay later, or take work home. Or you may be so efficient that you can do your job in less time.

How Much to Express

At first you may not get more than an ounce at a time, but eventually you can probably count on expressing three to five ounces of milk at each session. However, different women produce different amounts, all of which may be normal. You'll most likely produce more milk early in the day and early in the week. If you can't get enough for your baby's next-day feedings, try some of the hints given in Chapter 17. It's still worth pumping even if you get just one ounce from each side, since you can mix your milk with formula.

When you're at home, evenings and weekends, nurse your baby on cue, or even more frequently than the baby "requests." This will help you increase your milk supply. Don't give any bottles or cups at all when you're home.

How to Handle Expressed Milk

If your worksite temperature is higher than 72°F and you cannot refrigerate the milk, store it in a clean container and put the container in a cooler with ice or ice packs. Cap the container tightly, keep it out of the sun and away from heating units, and refrigerate it as soon as you get home. It will be ready to take to your caregiver the next day, packed in a cooler. Refrigerated milk will keep well for up to 48 hours. If you have more milk than you'll use within this time, freeze it immediately. As soon as you get home, pour your expressed milk into clean four-ounce plastic bottles. The bottles don't need to be sterilized if the milk has been kept cold, but they do need to be washed thoroughly to be sure that no milk particles are left. Rinse them out, swish a bottle brush around the inside, including the rim, and then wash in hot, soapy water. Rinse well. If you have a dishwasher, wash them in there.

In the first six to ten hours after expression, human milk kept in a capped clean container does not grow bacteria, even at room temperature (66° to 72°F). One of the qualities of human milk is its ability to slow the growth of bacteria. So even if you are not able to keep your milk refrigerated or on ice until you get home, you can still collect it.

You can freeze your milk directly in the plastic bottle. The four-ounce size is best so that you can defrost small amounts. You may even want to freeze milk in one- and two-ounce quantities for "snacks." Try to keep an extra emergency stock in the freezer so you won't get nervous about running out. You can build up your stockpile at home by expressing from one breast while you are nursing your baby from the other.

Breast milk will stay well for two weeks in your refrigerator freezer compartment; it will keep for three to four months in a separate door freezer that you open fairly often. If you have a deep-freeze unit that is not opened often and that maintains a consistent temperature of 0°F (check with a freezer thermometer), your milk will keep for six months.

Be prepared for the unexpected, which will always happen. One mother dropped and broke her thermos of the day's expressed milk—and saved the next day by expressing while she nursed that evening and the next morning. Her baby was already sleeping through the night, so the mother set her alarm to wake herself up every three hours all night long to express enough milk for the following day. Thanks to the law of supply and demand, her breasts responded to the frequent stimulation.

Negotiating with Your Employer

If your employer is not supportive of your pumping or breastfeeding on your breaks, find out what her concerns are, and then see how the two of you can work out a solution. For example, if your employer feels that you are taking too much time from your work, you may be able to reassure her that you will be taking less time within a couple of weeks, once you get your routine under way, and that you will make up any lost hours. Or you may find that you can do your pumping or nursing in a shorter time right away. If coworkers object, ask for the basis of their complaints and see how you can meet their concerns. Also, explain, calmly and reasonably, why the health benefits of nursing are so important to your baby.

One woman asked the lactation consultant at her local hospital to write her employer, explaining the benefits of breastfeeding for mother, child, and employer. Another called her coworkers together to describe these benefits. And another went out of her way to have her company's nursing-friendly atmosphere recognized during World Breastfeeding Week.*

---

*World Breastfeeding Week (WBW), observed August 1 through 7 every year since 1992, aims to generate public awareness and support for breastfeeding. The week's activities around a specific theme are coordinated by the World Alliance for Breastfeeding Action (WABA). For more information about WABA and WBW, see the Resource Appendix.

Employers are not legally bound to accommodate nursing mothers. The only way you could approach the problem legally would be to charge discrimination—if, for example, other employees are given smoking breaks equal in time to what you would need to pump. However, it's always better to resolve a problem amicably, through education and discussion, rather than calling in the law. But if your earlier efforts do not bear fruit, you may benefit from speaking to an attorney. (See the section "Breastfeeding and the Law" in Chapter 11 and the Resource Appendix for suggestions on finding legal help.)

Formula

If you plan to offer formula to your baby at one or more feedings, this change must be done gradually, to avoid engorgement and the risk of breast infection. For each feeding that you want to eliminate, you'll need to allow between four and seven days. If you plan to switch to formula exclusively, the weaning process should take at least a couple of weeks. (Remember that pumping alone produces some nipple stimulation and therefore some milk.) As you begin to substitute formula for your own milk, you may need to express manually to relieve your discomfort. If so, save your milk. You can use it for your baby, occasionally substituting breast milk for formula.

On weekends and holidays, you can maintain your weekday schedule, except for one additional breastfeeding. This keeps your milk supply at a fairly constant, comfortable level. Again, you may want someone else to give those feedings, since your baby may not accept them from you.

Working mothers, like other breastfeeding mothers, cite fatigue as their biggest problem. Since it's especially hard for you to get the rest you need, you have to be ruthless in cutting out everything in your life that is not essential or enjoyable. Doing your work, taking care of your family, and taking some time to care for yourself should be the only things you have to worry about for the time you're nursing.

This is the time to cut back on the extraneous and enjoy this precious time of your life, so that you can look back in later years to many happy memories of this special shared experience. As one breastfeeding working mother says, "It lasts for such a tiny part of the children's lives that it needs to be cherished."

Breastfeeding: A Sexual Passage

Of course I didn't always feel sexy when I was nursing the baby—which is a good thing while I was feeding her ten times a day! But sometimes the combination of nursing her and seeing my husband in bed next to me made me want to rush through the feeding so that Bob and I could make love.

KATE, BRADFORD, NEW HAMPSHIRE

I'm sure that nursing had something to do with my lack of interest in sex. My body was in use all day long. I felt as if somebody was constantly sucking on me and holding me and being held by me, and by the time night came around I just wanted to draw an invisible circle around my body and say, "No trespassing."

LILY, SARASOTA, FLORIDA

Nursing mothers seem to fall about equally into two distinct camps. Some, like Kate, experience increased sexual appetites and enjoy a much less sexually inhibited relationship with their partners. Other women, like Lily, find that they are not nearly as interested in sex for the first six months after childbirth as they had been before or will be again.

Nursing is a sensual experience. But this sensuality most often translates into a sense of satisfaction similar to the euphoria that follows orgasm rather than the intensity and excitement of orgasm. Nursing mothers most often talk about a calm feeling of completion that combines physical and emotional fulfillment. In her book *Free and Female*, Barbara Seaman describes breastfeeding as "a sensual and sensuous experience unlike any other, somewhat related to and yet different from good sex."*

A number of studies have found that, in general, breastfeeding women resume sexual activity sooner after childbirth than do bottle-feeding mothers,

---

*Barbara Seaman, a noted activist in the women's health movement, first became involved in women's health issues in the 1950s after she had her first child. Only after her baby son became sick did she find out that the pills hospital personnel had given her were laxatives, which she was unknowingly passing on in her milk. Nursing was so rare in those days that no one even thought to ask this mother whether she was breastfeeding.

and that nursing and sexuality are positively related. Among more than one thousand nursing mothers polled by New York psychologist Dr. Alice K. Ladas, 30 percent of the women reported that their sexual relationships with their husbands had improved after nursing, while only 2.5 percent reported worsened relationships. Most of the women who said they now had a better sex life had considered their sexual relationship excellent before nursing, while all the women in the other category said they had had a poor sexual adjustment to begin with.

Women who feel sexier while nursing might be particularly sensuous and comfortable with their bodies. They may have fewer feelings of embarrassment about handling or exposing their breasts than other women do. They may even welcome the opportunity to breastfeed as a chance to experience a new kind of bodily sensation. They may be more sensitive to physical sensations and more accepting of body secretions. They may have especially erogenous breasts that respond to the constant stimulation of the baby's suckling. Or they may have especially high stores of the hormone oxytocin in their system. While this potent chemical is contributing to their success in nursing, it may also produce increased levels of eroticism.

On the other hand, many factors can diminish a nursing woman's interest in sex. You may yearn for the intimacy that you and your husband enjoyed before your baby was born.* And you may want very much to resume your sexual relationship, but be distressed to find problems that you hadn't expected suddenly getting in the way. Both you and your partner may be puzzled and concerned about what is happening—or has, in fact, already happened—to your sex life. What you need to remember is that you can—and almost certainly will—overcome any obstacles. But it may take a little time.

One condition that affects almost all new mothers, and their sex lives, whether they nurse or not, is fatigue. Taking care of an infant is hard work. Furthermore, as a new mother, you never get a good night's sleep. Add to this the first-time mother's concern about her ability to care for her new baby and her all-too-common sense of herself as less attractive, and it's easy to understand many new mothers' temporarily lower interest in lovemaking.

The "touched-out" feeling expressed by Lily is also common. Many nursing mothers immerse themselves so deeply into their babies' care and derive so much pleasure from the physical as well as the emotional closeness they experience from breastfeeding that they don't need this kind of closeness with

---

*If you are in a nonmarital adult relationship, simply substitute the word *partner* for *husband* in this discussion. In almost all cases, what applies to a husband-and-wife relationship also applies to other committed bonds.

Pelvic Floor (Kegel) Exercises

You may have been doing these exercises to strengthen your pelvic floor while you were pregnant. Actually, it's a good idea for every woman to do them, whether or not she is expecting or has just had a child and whether she is young or old, to keep her pelvic floor muscles (also known as the pubococcygeal or the perineal muscles) well toned. These muscles are the ones that support the uterus, the bladder, and the rectum—everything inside the pelvic cavity—and the ones that contract spontaneously during orgasm.

Named after Arnold Kegel, M.D., the gynecologist who first developed them in the 1940s, principally to control urinary leakage, these exercises speed healing from childbirth, minimize pain and swelling, and strengthen the perineal muscles. Well-toned pelvic floor muscles enhance the experience of sexual intercourse for both you and your partner and also help resolve any problems of minor incontinence.

To do them, contract and relax the group of muscles directly between your legs that involve the urethra, the vagina, and to a lesser extent, the anus. Hold the contraction for five to ten seconds, as if you were holding back the flow of urine; then slowly release the tension and relax the muscles for a few seconds. When you first begin, you may have trouble holding the contractions, but with practice your muscles will become stronger. Right after delivery, these muscles may be numb and you may not feel the contractions, but the sensations will return. Do the repetitions from twenty-five to thirty times a day.

You can do them sitting (in a chair or while driving), standing (while brushing your teeth or in line at the bank), or lying down (while nursing or watching TV), and no one else will be able to tell what you're doing. You can evaluate your progress if you do them while you're urinating; you'll see how much better you get at holding back and then releasing urine. You can also do the exercises during sexual intercourse, to the enhancement of both partners' pleasure. And you can continue doing them for the rest of your life, to maintain muscle tone and strength.

their partners. In fact, they sometimes need the exact opposite—a time when they can pull into themselves like turtles in a shell, and "reclaim" their bodies for themselves.

Furthermore, female physiology almost seems to discourage sexual activity in the nursing mother. Because of her lower levels of estrogen (caused by the higher levels of prolactin in her body during lactation), her vaginal wall becomes thinner and more sensitive, and there is less vaginal lubrication. Many women find that their nipples and breasts are less sensitive to touch while they're lactating. Some women also find that their nipples lose their ability to become erect on stimulation, even though they still become elongated in the baby's mouth. (These responses may be nature's way of discouraging another pregnancy too soon.)

No matter which camp you fall into, whether you're eager to resume sexual relations as soon as possible or just willing to go along in the beginning for your partner's sake, you probably have many questions about lovemaking. You wonder how soon you should go back to enjoying regular sexual relations—and whether you should restrict your activities in any way, for your own sake or for your baby's.

RESUMING SEXUAL ACTIVITY

Men and women generally have different attitudes toward sex, especially during pregnancy and after childbirth. While sometimes the woman is more sexually eager than the man, the more common situation is for the man to press for a resumption of sexual relations, especially intercourse, while the woman is content to go without it for a while. Some researchers suggest that women can accept disruptions in their sexual relationships more easily than men do and that they're more apt to dismiss the impact of child rearing as a temporary sexual inconvenience, while men seem more likely to feel that children interfere with sex. How much of this is physical and how much cultural? This is a hard question to answer, but there are some obvious physical reasons.

A man's body does not, of course, undergo the changes that a woman's does. His shape does not change; he is not uncomfortable in various positions; he is not exhausted and sore after childbirth. Nor do the hormones in his body change radically during pregnancy, after childbirth, and during lactation. All of these physiological differences affect women in various ways, one of which is often a reduced desire for sex. Furthermore, men often find emotional comfort in the sex act itself, while women are more likely to be comforted by being held and caressed. Still, women who may not be hungry for sex themselves will often be ready to resume relations because they want to give of themselves to their partners.

When to Begin

Most doctors advise women not to engage in sexual intercourse until after their postpartum examination. This is to prevent the two biggest postpartum risks, infection and hemorrhage. Either one can result from the introduction of an object—any object—into the vagina before it is fully healed from childbirth. Before you are ready for intercourse, you want to be sure that any vaginal tears or episiotomy incisions have mended, that the tenderness in your perineal area is less severe, that the placental site (the place on your uterus where the placenta had been attached until it was sheared away during childbirth) has healed, and that your vaginal canal has again developed the microorganisms that protect it from infection. Generally, once soreness has gone, stitches have been absorbed, and bleeding has stopped, intercourse is safe.

This postpartum exam usually takes place at about six weeks after delivery, but may occur sooner, depending on your doctor's policy and on your desires. If you want an earlier postpartum exam than your doctor customarily schedules, ask whether this is possible. It's also a good idea to ask your doctor to explain to both you and your partner together the reasons for abstinence before this exam. Men who understand these reasons are less likely to pressure women to resume intercourse before the women are ready. In fact, even if your doctor says you're ready, this doesn't mean that *you* feel you're ready.

How to Begin

Sexuality is not, of course, restricted to intercourse, and there are many other ways by which a couple can keep their sexual relationship alive. You can enjoy physical, sensual closeness by many other paths. You can, for example, bathe together and be nude in bed together. You can caress and fondle and stroke and massage each other. You can pleasure each other through oral or manual alternatives to intercourse.

The first time you resume sexual intercourse, you will probably find that you're still quite tender in the perineal area. Intercourse may well be painful, and you may worry that it will always feel this way. Fortunately, this is only temporary: Life—and sex—do get better. If you had a cesarean birth, you may experience abdominal discomfort. You may have both abdominal and vaginal pain if you had an unexpected cesarean after a difficult labor. This is common and, again, is almost always only temporary.

Talk to your partner ahead of time, so that he understands how your body feels and how he can help you to make this first time a good time. He needs to know that he can alleviate your discomfort by going slowly, and by allowing manual or oral stimulation first until you are ready for penile penetration. It will also be helpful to use a vaginal lubricant (like K-Y jelly, AstroGlide, or contraceptive jelly or cream) and a position that allows you to control the depth of penetration, such as the female-superior or side-by-side positions. Any discomfort should go away soon after intercourse. If pain persists for seven to ten days afterward or after the first half-dozen times postdelivery, call your doctor. You should feel good (even if tired) after having had a baby; if you don't, your pain may signal a medical problem.

If you began doing Kegel exercises soon after delivery (see the box on page 253), you are likely to enjoy intercourse more when you do resume.

If any activities or positions are painful for you now, let your partner know. Being a martyr won't feel good for you—or for him. He'll sense your lack of enthusiasm for sex and may attribute it to problems in your feelings for him rather than in your physical feelings. Meanwhile, as you let him know what does not feel good, be sure to show or tell him what *does* feel good.

Many nursing mothers wonder whether their breasts belong to their baby during lactation and should therefore be off-limits to the baby's father. They need not be. You can be a sexual partner during the time you are nursing your baby, and you can share your breasts with both your baby and your partner. Your breasts do not have to stop performing their erotic function just because they are now performing their biological function.

There is no reason why your partner cannot stimulate your breasts both manually and orally during the time you are nursing, if you enjoy this. Furthermore, your child's father won't be stealing candy from his baby if he gets an occasional swallow of your good milk. (Some couples regularly include this in their lovemaking.) There is plenty more where that came from, and as we've said before, the more milk that is removed from your breasts, the more they will produce.

You may find, particularly in the first couple of months, that your breasts become hard and tender an hour or two after a feeding. At these times, intercourse in the male-superior position is apt to be uncomfortable. You would probably be more comfortable in such positions as the female-superior, side-by-side, or rear-entry. This might be the perfect time to experiment with lovemaking positions that you have never tried. You may even discover something you like better than your former favorites. In any case, the tenderness of the newly lactating breast goes away soon. After a couple of months, it will not be a factor in how you do what you do.

Spurting of milk during and immediately after orgasm is fairly common among nursing women, with the milk usually flowing more slowly from the breast that has been suckled more recently. While many women feel happy about this show of excitement, those who want to avoid spots on the sheet find that making love right after a feeding helps. It's also possible to wear a bra during sex. (There are some very appealing lacy nursing bras.)

One woman told us, "When Joe and I first realized that every time I experienced orgasm my breasts would spurt milk, it was a big source of satisfaction for both of us. There was no doubt in his mind that I had reached a climax, and I loved being able to show it in one more way."

YOU AND YOUR MARRIAGE

The months following the birth of a first child constitute a major transition in a marriage. As with any other new experience, you are likely to welcome parenthood with mixed emotions. The birth of your first baby brings home to you and your husband more dramatically than any other event in your lives the realization that you are no longer children but are now adults, newly responsible for another human being.

Eager as you may be to grow into this phase of life, it's only natural that you feel anxious about what it will mean and what will be expected of you. If you and your mate have been able to communicate well before the arrival of your baby, you will have a good base to help you adjust to parenthood. If not, it's especially important for you to make extra efforts now to let each other know exactly how you feel.

Like every other woman in the world, you have to learn to be a mother. It does not happen magically via labor and delivery. You need time and practice to feel at home in your new role. Meanwhile, while you are worrying about your ability to be a good mother, your partner has his own conflicts to struggle with as he faces up to the responsibility of parenthood. Yet all too often, both husband and wife assume that their partners know how they feel, and neither one expresses his or her real concerns.

The experience of breastfeeding introduces other elements into this period of your life, since as a lactating woman, you are experiencing a powerful phase in the female cycle of sexuality. The physiological changes that occur in your body in connection with pregnancy, childbirth, and lactation are likely to affect your emotions, your sexual desires, and your adult relationship. Breastfeeding dramatizes the physical and emotional ties in the new pairing (you and your child) that overlap with those in the preexisting couple (you and your husband). Furthermore, both you and he are bound to respond in some way to those cultural signals in our society that accentuate the sexual symbolism of the breasts.

Different women respond differently to this aspect of their reproductive and sexual functioning. Like the women quoted at the beginning of the chapter, some find that breastfeeding enhances their sense of themselves as sexual beings and others feel that it relegates their sexuality to the "back burner." Let's look at some of the ways in which breastfeeding serves as a sexual passage.

The Five Phases of
Female Sexuality

HOW OUTSIDE PRESSURES AND EMOTIONS
CAN INFLUENCE ALL FIVE PHASES

- *The menstrual cycle:* The most regular cycle can be disrupted by excitement or anxiety. Many a bride, for example, has carefully set the date for her marriage—and yet still menstruated on her wedding day. And the tension of a job or family crisis often brings on or suspends a woman's menses.
- *Orgasm from sexual stimulation:* The tremendous impact of outside influences on sexual interaction is obvious to anyone (male *or* female) who can't get in the mood for sex because of the distractions of financial, family, job, or health problems. A woman (or man) at the brink of orgasm may be abruptly "turned off" by a piercing yell from the nursery, by the ringing of the telephone, or by a fear that their privacy is about to be invaded.
- *Pregnancy:* Conception itself may be affected by emotional influences. Studies in animal and human reproduction suggest that stress may affect hormone production in a way that interferes with ovulation.
- *Childbirth:* Outside events also influence childbirth. An emotional or physical shock can bring on premature labor, and the mother's anticipation of childbirth often seems related to the ease and duration of labor and delivery. A woman who is frightened of giving birth is apt to have a more difficult delivery than one who understands the physiology of childbirth.

FEMALE SEXUALITY

Historically, sexuality has been discussed mostly in terms of male-female genital intercourse. People have been considered fulfilled sexual beings if they have been able to reach orgasm through intercourse. This definition has tended to focus on men, either ignoring women's needs for sexual gratification or assuming that they should achieve gratification in the same way men do.

Today, though, we recognize the distinctly female sexual experience. With this awareness, we have developed a more global definition of sexuality, keying it more into sensuality and to the many pleasurable sensations that can be reached through a wide range of activities, which may include, but are not limited to, intercourse. By thinking of sexuality in this way, we expand the possibility of sexual fulfillment to include the later years of life, as well as

• *Lactation:* Mothers and midwives have long known that a woman's ability to give milk to her baby is influenced by pain, embarrassment, and emotional conflict. Drs. Michael and Niles Newton confirmed this observation in the laboratory, when they showed that a nursing mother will give significantly less milk when she is distracted during feedings by feelings of discomfort and various annoying conditions.

PHENOMENA COMMON TO MORE THAN ONE PHASE OF FEMALE SEXUALITY

• *The breasts enlarge* just before menstruation, during pregnancy, just before orgasm, and during lactation.
• *The nipples become erect* upon sexual stimulation, during childbirth, and during lactation.
• *The uterus contracts* during orgasm, childbirth, and lactation.
• *Body temperature rises* during ovulation, childbirth, orgasm, and lactation.
• *A woman usually feels an urge to take care of her loved one* (the baby) during pregnancy, after childbirth, during lactation, and (her partner) in a fulfilling sexual relationship.
• The hormone *oxytocin* surges through a woman's body during orgasm, during childbirth, and during lactation. This hormone causes the uterus to contract and the nipples to become erect. Oxytocin is also the stimulus for the milk-ejection reflex and probably the reason why milk sometimes spurts from the breasts of a woman in orgasm.

those times in earlier years when intercourse may not be possible, advisable, or desirable, such as the weeks just before and just after the birth of a baby.

Both men and women can and do derive great pleasure from such noncoital activities as kissing, stroking, touching, cuddling, massage, and oral and manual genital stimulation. In addition, women's sexuality is even more wide-ranging, closely tied in as it is to the five phases in female reproductive capacity: the menstrual cycle, orgasm, pregnancy, childbirth, and lactation.

All five of these phases are controlled to a large measure by the interaction of hormones released inside a woman's body. Estrogen, progesterone, testosterone, follicle-stimulating hormone (FSH), luteinizing hormone (LH), oxytocin, and prolactin are among the hormones that help to make a woman a sexual being. Some of these substances manage the course of the menstrual cycle, causing ovulation and fertility. Some dominate during pregnancy. Others signal the onset of labor, the production and release of milk, and the climax of orgasm. Most of these hormones have more than one function. While some are more active during one phase of the female cycle than are others, the interaction among them is responsible for some remarkable similarities in the various sexual phases, as shown in the box on page 258.

Female sexuality, then, involves a complex series of responses that carry over from a woman's reproductive capacity to her maternal functions. Yet in our society, woman's interest in sexual intercourse—in achieving her own orgasm and in helping her man to achieve his—has been stressed, while those elements of sexuality related to childbirth and lactation have been virtually ignored.

Dr. Alice Rossi, a sociology professor at the University of Massachusetts, has suggested that our "male dominant family and political systems have imposed a wedge between maternalism on the one hand, and female sexuality on the other. We define maternity in culturally narrow ways, clearly differentiate it from sexuality, and require that women deny the evidence of their senses by repressing the component of sexuality in the maternal role."

Fortunately, this attitude is being overcome, partly due to the women's movement and partly due to greater acceptance of sexuality in general. The work of sex researchers William H. Masters and Virginia E. Johnson had an enormous influence on the ways in which people think about sex. In the past several decades we have learned a great deal about the actual physiological mechanisms related to sexual activities and responses. We have felt freer to communicate with our sexual partners about how we feel and what we like, and many couples have found that their sexual rapport flourishes in such an open climate. The same can happen when we are open and understanding about aspects of sexuality in the maternal role.

THE SENSUOUS NATURE OF BREASTFEEDING

Nursing is supposed to be enjoyable for both mother and baby. If it were not, our species could never have survived the thousands of years when no substitute for human milk was available. Some researchers have concluded that when women are encouraged to accept and enjoy the sexual pleasure breastfeeding can offer, they give more milk. This makes sense, since the letdown reflex is highly subject to emotional influences. Indeed, the good feelings associated with breastfeeding may be built into our natures to strengthen the bond between mother and baby in the early months of life.

In *Human Sexual Response,* the 1966 book that reported on their pioneering research, Masters and Johnson included the results of interviews with 111 women during and after their pregnancies. These women talked about their sexual behavior, feelings, and responses during pregnancy and immediately following childbirth. Of this group, only twenty-four women nursed their babies (a reflection of the low popularity of breastfeeding when this research was done).

Some of these nursing mothers reported experiencing sexual arousal while suckling their babies. Several said they felt guilty about this and worried that they were "perverted." Some women did not breastfeed because, they said, they were afraid that they might be sexually stimulated from the suckling. (Only three of the women in the Masters and Johnson study reported incidents of orgasm while nursing, which bears out the rarity of this among the general population.)

It shouldn't be surprising that breastfeeding has its sensual components. For many women, their breasts are highly erogenous zones, sensitive to the slightest touch and capable of sending messages of excitation throughout the body. In fact, some women reach orgasm from having their breasts fondled. The nerve pathways from the nipple to the brain are the same, no matter what the stimulation is. During lactation, of course, the breasts are constantly stimulated both by the mother's own handling and by the baby's extensive suckling and sometimes frequent stroking.

As one mother told us, "There is something very earthy about nursing a child that can pleasantly affect the husband-wife relationship. And I also feel that a good breastfeeding experience makes you more open and womanly. Because of nursing I was able to have orgasms, which I had never had before."

Furthermore, since our society has eroticized the breast even beyond its own intrinsic nature, most nursing mothers are very conscious of their breasts as sexual symbols as well as sources of nutrition and comfort for their babies. (This, of course, is why so many women are reluctant to breastfeed in public. Even if they don't see the act as sexually provocative, they know that there are others who will.)

Unfortunately, many women who experience the normal, albeit relatively rare, sexual arousal while nursing their babies are apt to feel guilty—so guilty that they may wean their babies early and refuse to nurse future children. In our society sexual feelings are supposed to stay in their place—to come out of hiding only when a culturally determined suitable partner is present. Yet we are sexual beings, and our sexual feelings spin a thread that runs through the fabric of our entire lives.

Most women do not experience sexual sensations from breastfeeding;

those who don't needn't feel that they are repressed or inhibited. They simply have a different, just as normal, experience. In his landmark book *Sexual Behavior in the Human Female*, Dr. Alfred E. Kinsey stated that only half of all women seem to derive any satisfaction from having their breasts fondled—and that both oral and manual stimulation of the female breasts are often more exciting to the man who touches than to the woman who is touched. A woman whose breasts are not normally erogenous is not likely to become erotically stimulated by the suckling of her infant. And even a woman whose breasts ordinarily respond to her partner's loving touch or kiss may find that during lactation, they become almost insensitive to touch—his as well as his baby's.

Also, it's been said many times that the most powerful sex organ in the human body is the brain. Situations that we think about as sexual are more arousing than those that we don't imbue with sexual connotations. Thus, a woman may be concentrating so fully on feeding and interacting with her baby that she is not even aware of physical sensations that in other circumstances might be very erotic.

In sum, there is no right or wrong way for you to respond sexually to the nursing experience. You can be a successful nursing mother if you do become erotically aroused by breastfeeding—or if such feelings are the farthest thing from your mind.

BIRTH CONTROL

As a nursing mother, you are less likely to become pregnant than women who are not fully breastfeeding. If you are giving your baby nothing but breast milk, you are less likely to become pregnant than are women who feed their babies formula, or a combination of human milk and formula or other foods. Based on records in societies where long-term nursing is the rule, and on studies of exclusively nursing, partially nursing, and bottle-feeding mothers in this country, we can point to considerable evidence that breastfeeding postpones pregnancy. However, lactation is not a foolproof method of contraception, especially as your baby grows.

If your baby is being fully nursed, that is, is receiving no supplemental bottles or solid food and is being breastfed at least two or three times during the night as well as every four hours or oftener during the day, the hormonal balance in your body will prevent ovulation and therefore pregnancy for three to six months, or even longer. This is because the hormonal changes in your body during lactation delay the return of ovulation and of your menstrual periods.

Generally, if you are fully breastfeeding, you may have one "sterile" menstrual period before you begin to ovulate. But you cannot depend on it. Women have become pregnant while fully lactating or before their menses have resumed. If you do not want to conceive right away, you will want to use some form of contraception.

What Kind of Contraception Should You Use

The Lactational Amenorrhea Method (LAM): One of the most dramatic research findings in recent years has been the proven effectiveness of exclusive or nearly exclusive breastfeeding coupled with the absence of menstrual periods as a means of delaying pregnancy for up to six months. Even though folk wisdom and society-wide statistics have for many years attested that women were less likely to conceive while they were breastfeeding, only during the past decade have scientific investigations confirmed this. LAM, the Lactational Amenorrhea Method, draws on these studies, which have been conducted in several different countries.

LAM is effective if you can answer "yes" to the following three questions:

1. Are you still not menstruating, not even spotting? (Bleeding before day 56 postpartum is not considered a period.)
2. Are you nursing your baby at least two to three times during the night, as well as every four hours or more often during the day, and giving him nothing but breast milk?
3. Is your baby less than six months old?

If you meet all three of these conditions, your chance of conceiving is less than 2 percent, a rate that compares very favorably with most forms of birth control.* When any one of these circumstances no longer exists, it is time to begin an alternative method of family planning if you wish to be sure of healthy spacing between your pregnancies.

The big advantage of LAM is that, as an introductory method effective in the first few months after childbirth, it gives you some time to decide on the method of contraception you'll use on a regular basis. Meanwhile, you're not ingesting any hormones and you don't have to buy any special paraphernalia. You are just relying on your own body's ability to prevent pregnancy.

---

*This rate is based on clinical trials with nursing women in Chile, Ecuador, and Rwanda.

Contraception for the Nursing Mother*

RECOMMENDED DURING LACTATION

METHOD	COMMENTS
Lactational Amenorrhea Method (LAM)	Supports breastfeeding and baby health. Should begin right after birth. About 98% effective for up to six months, and maybe longer if woman continues to breastfeed often, day and night, and is still not menstruating. Requires frequent breastfeeding; not effective if mother and baby are regularly separated for more than four to six hours.
Male Condom	No effect on lactation or baby. About 85% to 97% effective;* effectiveness is enhanced when used with a spermicide. Can be begun anytime after delivery. New polyurethane condoms have several advantages over latex ones: For one, they seem to allow more sensation during sex because they conduct heat well.
Diaphragm	No effect on lactation or baby. Can be begun four to six weeks after delivery. Woman needs to be fitted after each birth. About 80% to 95% effective. Used with spermicide, which provides lubrication. Must be inserted no more than six hours before intercourse and left in place for 6 hours afterward. May be irritating to nursing mother if her lower estrogen levels cause vaginal dryness, and may be dislodged in certain positions if vagina is relaxed after childbirth.
Female Condom	No effect on lactation or baby. Can be used anytime after delivery and inserted up to eight hours before intercourse. About 80% to 95% effective.
Spermicide (foam, jelly, cream, film, tablet, or suppository)	No effect on lactation; virtually none is transmitted through milk, and no reports of absorption or ill effects on baby. Can be begun anytime after delivery. Must be applied within five to ten minutes of each act of intercourse. About 75% to 95% effective, with relatively high accidental pregnancy rates; less of a problem during lactation; may complement LAM and condoms. Some people are allergic.

*The first number given is the effectiveness rate for the method as commonly used; the second number is for correct and consistent use.

Cervical Cap	No effect on lactation or baby. Must be fitted after birth. Can be begun four to six weeks after delivery. About 60% to 85% effective for women who have had children.
Intrauterine Device (IUD)	No effect on lactation or baby. Can be begun immediately or six weeks after delivery. About 99% effective. Nursing women report fewer complaints of pain, bleeding, and insertion problems than do other women. Problems of uterine perforation can be minimized by careful assessment of uterine size; uterus may be smaller during lactation.
Sterilization	If you are absolutely sure that you do not want any more children, either you or your partner can choose surgical sterilization. Female sterilization can often be performed at time of delivery. Doing it right away is best for nursing mothers, since one study found that women sterilized four to six days postpartum produced less milk for as long as two weeks. Other studies, however, found little difference. Immediate sterilization had no effect on lactation. Male sterilization (vasectomy) can be performed at any time. Both are about 99% effective, and both should be considered irreversible.

NOT RECOMMENDED DURING LACTATION

Birth Control Pill (combination of estrogen and progestin)	Reduces amount of breast milk and may affect composition; requires more supplementary feedings for baby. Baby may gain weight more slowly. Some steroid in breast milk may be passed on to baby; however, no long-term effects reported on children up to age eight; no effect on growth up to age seventeen. Should not be begun for at least three months, preferably not until six months, and ideally not at all while nursing. If used, should be taken at beginning of longest interval between feedings. Mother should offer extra suckling time and nurse more frequently to rebuild milk supply. About 93% to 99% effective in preventing conception.
"Mini-pill" (progestin-only contraceptive pill)	No effect on lactation or baby reported in the research literature, but some mothers have reported diminished milk supplies if they started to take the minipill before their milk supply was fully established. Preferable to combined birth control pill, but still better to wait until

(continued on next page)

(continued from page 265)

	after weaning, or at least until baby is eating a mixed diet. Can be begun at time of first menstrual period, or at least six weeks after delivery. Should be taken same time every day. About 97% effective.
Injectable Contraceptive (Depo-Provera®, others)	May produce slight difference in milk composition (more protein, less fat). Steroid in breast milk can be transmitted to baby. No reported effect on children up to ten years. About 98% to 99% effective. Preferable not to use during lactation, but may begin six weeks after delivery. If begun before this time, milk supply may diminish. Injection required every three months. Return of fertility delayed four to nine months after last dose.
Norplant® Implant	No effect on lactation. Some steroid in breast milk. No reported effects on baby. Preferable not to use during lactation, but may begin six weeks after delivery. If used before this time, milk supply may diminish. About 99% effective.
Natural Family Planning (Rhythm Method)	These methods may require long periods of abstinence, but most have rules that can be applied during lactation. They may be harder to use efficaciously during breastfeeding, since they depend on regularity of menses, of body temperature, and of mucus patterns, all of which are irregular in nursing women and cannot predict ovulation. However, the natural protection of nursing may compensate somewhat, and the use of such less effective methods remains a personal choice.
Coitus Interruptus (withdrawal)	Very unreliable in preventing pregnancy. Usually sexually unfulfilling for both partners.
Emergency Contraception (the "day-after" pill)	The use of birth control pills in higher doses of hormones than usual, to be taken within forty-eight hours after unprotected intercourse, has not been studied in lactating women.

When LAM No Longer Applies: For up to six months after delivery, you are safe using LAM, which is not a device or a technique, but simply the consequence of your frequent and almost exclusive breastfeeding. But then you need to adopt another method of birth control if you do not want to conceive right away. You have to weigh the pros and cons of each choice and decide upon the method that best suits your own physiology, personality, and lifestyle—as well as those of your partner.

The best kind of contraceptive when LAM no longer applies, or when you wish to start another method, is the nonhormonal kind. If you took birth control pills or wore an IUD before getting pregnant, it may be hard to adjust to one of the preferred barrier methods (diaphragm, cervical cap, condom, and/or spermicide), the use of which is closely tied to the specific time of intercourse. While these methods may at first seem intrusive and a nuisance, many couples make inserting the diaphragm or putting on the condom a part of their sexual foreplay and consider doing it together an act of shared love and responsibility. For a comparison of various birth control methods, see the box on page 264.

YOUR HUSBAND IS STILL YOUR LOVER

Yes, this can be a trying time in the life of a marriage. You may suddenly find, as you struggle in the morass of diapers and colic and nursing, that you would like to be a little girl again and have someone else care for both you and your baby. Meanwhile, your partner, who is awed by the competent way you feed, bathe, and diaper your baby, sees only your outer shell of self-assurance. You may seem so capable in carrying out your maternal responsibilities that he underestimates your need for him. He may feel left out of the tight little circle around you and your baby.*

At the same time, this new responsibility of caring for a baby often reawakens a new father's own dependency needs. One study found that expectant fathers' heightened needs for mothering showed up in an increased frequency of phone calls and letters to their own parents and requests for stories about their own birth and infancy.

At this time your partner needs your reassurance that he has not slipped to last place in your life. While he recognizes intellectually that your baby requires a great deal of your time and energy, he may not be able to help resenting all the attention lavished on the newborn—attention that was formerly his alone. In addition, he sees you sharing with your baby not only your time, energy, attention, and affection, but also the breasts that were formerly revealed only to him. Is it any wonder that he should be a little jealous of his own child?

Such feelings are natural, but many men are ashamed of feeling this

---

*Besides making special efforts to invite your husband into the parenting picture, you may want to suggest that he read the next chapter, "Especially for the Father."

way and will not admit them. Others express them quite openly. This is one of those times when clear communication is essential.

Meanwhile, you need to explore your own feelings. Are you sensing some conflict between your role as a mother and your role as a sexual partner? You may want to think about the attitudes you grew up with—whether you had the sense that your mother enjoyed sex, whether you absorbed a feeling that once a woman became a mother, she wasn't sexy anymore, whether the changes in a woman's body in pregnancy and childbirth signal the end of her attractiveness.

If you can talk about these feelings with other women or with your partner—or both—you may find that you are more responsive to the idea of making love again. It's most important to let your partner in on how you feel emotionally and physically.

The birth of a first baby often signals a low point in a couple's sexual relationship. As one husband told us, "My wife and I had had a very good sex life, but when our two children were small, both the quality and the quantity of sex went way down. We were both tired most of the time, we couldn't be spontaneous, and we never felt as if we had any privacy. We thought we had been prepared for this—but we were prepared in our minds, not in our hearts—or elsewhere in our bodies. But we never gave up—and finally it got better." The key is—never to give up.

Talk, Talk, Talk

It's often difficult to talk about sex, but since neither of you can read the other's mind, you need to share your feelings. You might tell your partner how much you value the intimacy between you—but that right now you're often too tired to act on it. Let him know that your lack of interest in making love is not a lack of love for him.

Suppose you love the back rubs he gives you—but he considers them a prelude to intercourse, which you're not always ready for. You need to tell him—in a loving way—how you feel. And you need to ask him what you can do to help him feel valued and loved.

Suppose that your baby is a few months old now, and your partner says, "You never want to make love anymore! How long is this going to last?" You may want to give it a try just to be agreeable. And you may be agreeably surprised to find that once things get started, you find your own interest rising.

St. Louis sex therapist Beverly Hotchner uses an analogy with food when one partner is more interested in sex than the other: "Let's assume that your partner is really enormously hungry and you're not hungry at all. Wouldn't you be willing to sit down and have a cup of coffee just to be sociable? Sometimes when you do this, the food starts to look pretty good and you take a little nibble and your saliva starts flowing, and suddenly you think, 'Hey, I think I'm going to have some.' You don't have to have a whole course—you can have just dessert.

"It's the same with sex. If you're tired and don't feel aroused, you can masturbate your partner or hold him tenderly while he masturbates. Or you can take a bath together, which is very sensual. What people really hunger for is affection and closeness and warmth and relaxing and fun together. And they have thousands of ways to get that. They don't have to limit themselves to intercourse."

You can show your partner in many ways that he is still very important to you and that your love for him has not diminished because of your love for his baby. It's hard to have to think of one more thing at a time when you're facing so many new demands, but it's important to make extra efforts to preserve and enhance your connection with your partner. You can adjust to being a mother without forgetting that you are still in a committed adult relationship. The suggestions in the next section might help you both over some rough spots.

Keeping Romance Center Stage

• Make at-home dates ahead of time with your partner. These are evenings when you're not available for company, when you take your phone off the hook or let your answering machine pick up, when you set aside time just for each other. You need this relaxed time together, whether you use it for talking, for a relaxing massage or hot bath, or for an evening of watching a special TV show or maybe an erotic videocassette.

These evenings at home can, of course, be wonderful times for making love. While planning ahead for lovemaking may seem unromantic at first, it's worth noting that in our society marriage is the only structure that demands spontaneous sex. Dating couples and extramarital lovers know they have to plan ahead to see each other—and they usually find the planning itself erotic. Married couples can have an "affair" with each other, too. You may be able to phone or e-mail each other during the day, or leave romantic notes where your partner will see them.

• Invite your partner to enjoy the sensuousness of parenting by bringing him into bed, bare-chested, while you are nursing the baby, and following feeding sessions with three-way cuddling, or by taking family baths together. This brings the father into the family circle and enables you as sensitive parents to transmit a warm, comforting sensuality without being inappropriately seductive.

• Bc flexible. If before the baby arrived, you usually made love at bedtime, planning your day differently now may help you get together more happily. Some couples like to make love in the early morning after the baby's first nursing of the day. Some partners are able to get home for lunch at a time when their babies conveniently take a nap.

One husband who had felt ignored because his wife was always asleep by the time he got into bed with her after the 11 o'clock news finally realized that he could get into bed with her at about 8:30, snuggle for a while, and make love. Then, after she went to sleep, he would get out of bed to watch the news.

• Even though you are nursing, you can still leave your baby for short periods of time. Once the course of breastfeeding has been established, many couples plan an evening out once a week so that they can enjoy each other's company in a more carefree way. This need not be anything more elaborate than a trip to a movie or a nearby ice cream shop—but can, if you're feeling extravagant, include a few hours at a local motel.

It's best if you can plan to go out at a time when your baby usually sleeps, but if there is no "usually," you can nurse your baby just before you leave and then leave him or her with a competent sitter—possibly a student nurse, an older woman, or a college student, if no grandparent is available. Once your milk supply is well established (usually by the end of the second month), you should be able to be away from your baby during feeding time by leaving a bottle that contains your own milk, which you've either hand-expressed or pumped earlier in the day.

While you and your partner are renewing your relationship, your baby can be learning to trust other people besides the two of you. As Margaret Mead told me (Sally Olds), babies are most likely to develop into well-adjusted human beings when they are cared for "by many warm, friendly people"—as long as most of these loved people remain in the infants' lives.

• Disruptions of the dinner hour seem to hit some men harder than anything else. You can minimize these by waiting to prepare dinner until right after a feeding. Then if you and your partner pitch in together, you might be able to cook and eat dinner before your baby needs you again. Or Dad may take over dinner preparations for a while, even if his "taking over" means taking out.

No matter how much of a gourmet you may have been before the birth of your baby, be prepared for drastic changes in your eating habits, at least for the first few months, when your baby's schedule is apt to be irregular. The best kind of meal for now is one that involves a minimum amount of preparation—a casserole that can be put together whenever one of you has the time, fish that can be broiled quickly, or a salad or stew that won't mind waiting. If you have access to good, nutritious take-out food and can afford the extra expense (along with paper plates), this is the time to splurge.

• The simplest meal can take on a romantic aura if you eat by candlelight on your good china (which is no harder to wash than your everyday ware).

• If you're used to having an occasional drink before or with dinner with your partner, you don't need to give it up. It's probably best to time your cocktail hour to come soon *after* a feeding. You can enjoy a quiet interlude for the two of you over a glass of wine while you're catching up with each other on the events of both your days.

• If your baby sleeps in the same bed with you, you need to show a little ingenuity. Bed is not the only place where lovemaking can take place. Why else was the rug in front of the fireplace invented? Or you might slip quietly out to a guest bed, a living room couch, or any other welcoming surface while your baby is asleep.

One couple whose two-year-old daughter continued to fall asleep every night in their bed would wait until she was sleeping and then tiptoe out to her room and make love in *her* bed. They would sometimes put on music before their daughter went to sleep and let it continue to play to drown out any sounds they might make. In these child-rearing years some parents who work hard at finding the time and the place to make love get an added excitement from the illicit feeling that reminds them of their teenage years, when they would "make out" out of their parents' sight.

• Pay attention to yourself. Your baby will think you're beautiful no matter what, but you'll feel better about yourself and show your partner that you care about his opinion if you can do some minimal grooming feats shortly before you expect him home. You might expend the energy to run a comb through your hair and put on a shirt that doesn't carry that unmistakable perfume of spit-up milk.

If you're ordinarily small-breasted, you might enjoy dressing seductively during the time you're nursing, when you're more bosomy than you have ever been before. If you're less thrilled about your added pounds and curves, you'll feel and look more attractive if you buy one or two flattering outfits to fit your current figure (see Chapter 8).

- If you're eager to resume sexual relations, don't be shy about letting your partner know. He may be waiting for a signal from you. If you couldn't care less, you may want to go along to please him. Reaching orgasm is often less important than the physical closeness of sex. While women more often seem to be comforted by being held lovingly, men tend to find genitally oriented sexual activity comforting and life-enhancing.

One of the most important things you can do for your husband—and your children—is to bring him into the family circle as early as possible. This decision can help your children forge a close relationship with both parents and can help them feel good about themselves throughout their lives. If your partner is interested in doing things for his baby, don't limit him to fetching and carrying. Encourage him to hold, play with, and bathe the baby. Remember: You are not the only person who can do the right thing for your child. Also remember: The stronger your child bonds with both her parents, the better off she will be. However, if your partner is not terribly interested in doing a great deal with your young infant, it's better not to push him but to wait for his attitude to change—as it probably will the first time his baby smiles at him.

If you are with a person you love, you are lucky, indeed. You have the opportunity to give of yourself and to be physically close to your baby—and to your partner. You have fulfilled your birthright—that cycle of sexuality that only a woman can know.

Especially for the Father

I had been breastfed myself, and I was happy that my wife wanted to nurse our children. I found it really attractive in a humanistic, caring sort of way. I also think it's important to be physically close to your children—you wouldn't dream of taking a baby animal away from its mother. Touching and giving pleasure is a lot of what breastfeeding is all about.

JOHN, RENO, NEVADA

Why, you may wonder, should we have a chapter for fathers in a book about breastfeeding? The answer is easy: Because you, as a father, are a vital part of the nursing experience; because it will enrich your life as well as those of your wife* and baby; and because your support and help are needed as much now as they will ever be in your family's life. As a father, you are in the unique position of providing a source of strength and balance for your entire family—and to grow through the challenges and opportunities your new role as father affords you.

As a new father, you have embarked upon a new adventure. Like most adventures, it will have its times of exhilaration—and its times of anxiety. Both are normal.

Throughout history most men have hungered to father children and have taken their parenting seriously. Today, however, men in our society seem to have an even deeper involvement in bringing up their children than many did in times past. Our new society-wide appreciation of the father's role in his children's lives acknowledges that his participation in their care is at least as—or even more—important than his traditional responsibility as family breadwinner.

There are some interesting signs of this new appreciation. In public

---

*If you are not married to the mother of your baby, you can just mentally substitute the word *partner* wherever we have written *wife* or *husband*.

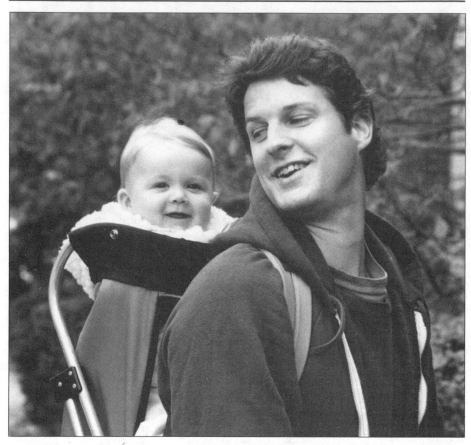

The father who plays with and cares for his baby develops a very special attachment that will enrich both their lives.

places we see men out alone with their small children. In baby supply stores we see strollers with longer handles and diaper bags with fewer frills. In television commercials we see fathers diapering and bathing their children. In airports we see diapering tables in the men's restroom. This growth of fathering is bound to enrich the lives of the men doing it, as well as those of their families.

BREASTFEEDING'S BENEFITS FOR YOU, THE FATHER

As the father of a breastfed child, you can appreciate the advantages that nursing confers on your wife and your baby (described in Chapter 1). You can also find benefits for yourself, such as the following:

- You don't have to worry about running out of formula at an inopportune time and dashing around trying to find an open store.

- When you go places with your baby, you have less to lug—no bottles or cans of formula, no sterilizing equipment. Since the father is usually the one who carries all the paraphernalia required by a new baby, you'll appreciate this lightening of your load when you go on vacation, visiting, or on family errands.

- Breastfeeding puts less of a load on the family budget.

- You can get to know and appreciate a new aspect of your wife's womanliness.

BECOMING A FATHER

Before a baby is born, we have a warm fuzzy feeling about the delights of parenthood. And yes, parenthood *is* wonderful and no one who has never been a parent can truly appreciate that special depth of feeling you can have for a child.

But—being the father of a new baby is not unalloyed bliss. There will be mornings when your adorable baby will not look at all adorable to your bleary-eyed gaze, after you have been up with him all night. The very helplessness of an infant means that your wife will need to be more attuned to your baby's needs than yours. But even though you know intellectually that you are an adult who can wait for gratification, while your baby cannot—you may not feel so adult, emotionally.

Listen to what one new father has said about what he calls, with some embarrassment, "spousling rivalry": "I feel like a big baby, jealous of my own son. I love the baby, sure, but I miss having a wife who cares about me. She goes on and on about him, which I can understand, but occasionally it would be nice if I got the feeling that she cared how I am."

Most new fathers are apt to feel somewhat shut out of the family circle, no matter how their babies are fed. Some men can accept these feelings more easily than others—but virtually *every* new father has them to some degree. You're not abnormal; you're not a selfish brute; you're not immature for experiencing twinges of jealousy and hurt after the birth of your baby.

Remember that this is a time of transition. Your familiar household routines are completely disrupted. You and your wife have to learn how to carry out your roles as parents. You have to take into account the needs and wants of a very noisy addition to your family. You have new responsibilities toward your wife as she recuperates from the physical demands of pregnancy and childbirth and copes with the hormonal changes accompanying these events. You may feel sexually frustrated, since lovemaking has already taken a moratorium for a while, and even when it resumes it will probably take some time to get back to the level you enjoyed prebaby. Your older children are especially needy now. Your social life is disrupted, and you may worry that you'll never again have the freedom and the fun you and your wife used to have together. In addition, you have new financial strains, especially if your wife had been making a substantial contribution to the family income and is now taking an extended maternity leave. You not only have to cut back to living on one income—you have all the added expenses brought by the baby.

But you need to remember that these early days hold excitement and thrills, as well as concerns, and that you and your wife are embarked on an inspiring adventure. The more involved you get, the more gratifying it will be.

THE FATHER'S IMPORTANCE IN THE FAMILY

A common refrain of many happy breastfeeding mothers is: "I couldn't have done it without my husband's help." While some expectant fathers are afraid they'll feel like a fifth wheel in the family after a baby is born—especially if the baby is breastfed—the reality is far different. You are needed.

Your emotional support and encouragement are even more important to your breastfeeding partner than they would be if she had chosen to bottle-feed. This is because a woman's ability to give milk is so strongly influenced by her emotional state. If she is feeling your love and support, her let-down reflex is more likely to function well. As a result, your baby feels satisfied, your wife feels gratified, and you can bask in both of their happy states of mind and body.

You have a vital role to play in the lives of your wife, your new baby, and your other children. A strong, supportive, helpful husband can often make the difference between breastfeeding success and failure and between family harmony and discord. Let's talk about the different ways—both emotional and practical—by which you can show this support.

Encouraging Your Partner to Breastfeed

Your opinions on breastfeeding are important to your wife, and your encouragement is vital to her success in this endeavor. Study after study has found that a father's favorable attitude toward breastfeeding is the most important factor in a mother's decision to begin. You are more important in this regard than a doctor, a nurse, or a lactation consultant.

Before you can encourage your wife to breastfeed your child, however, you have to be convinced of the value of nursing for both mother and baby. You may have some worries about your wife's becoming a nursing mother—worries that you can allay by learning more. It's important to read Chapter 1, which discusses the benefits of breastfeeding; Chapter 2, which answers such common concerns as a woman's fear of losing her figure and her fear of being tied down; and Chapter 13, which talks about a nursing woman's sexuality. You may also want to browse in some of the other chapters in this book, like those that talk about the social and work lives of the breastfeeding mother.

If your baby has not yet arrived, you can learn a great deal about breastfeeding and other issues related to the arrival of your baby by attending prenatal classes for expectant parents. If you want to be present during your baby's birth, you'll probably have to have some prenatal education before you can obtain permission to stay with your partner during labor and delivery. Even if you're not going to be in the delivery room, it will still help you to learn about childbirth. Prenatal courses usually discuss breastfeeding and the postpartum period, as well. Another advantage to enrolling in one of these classes is the opportunity to see that you are not alone, that other men share your concerns and possible confusion.

After your baby is on the scene, you might enjoy attending a special meeting for fathers held by a local chapter of such organizations as the International Childbirth Education Association, La Leche League, or ASPO/Lamaze, where you can air your questions and receive authoritative answers. Or you may want to take your questions to your doctor or midwife, to your parents, to your brother or sister, or perhaps to a friend whose own wife breastfed her children.

Being Your Wife's Strongest Ally

Even today, when most people accept—or at least give lip service to—the benefits of breastfeeding, your wife may encounter discouragement from relatives, neighbors, her employer, or even her doctor. If *you* wholeheartedly support her desire to breastfeed, she will be better able to handle any out-side opposition.

You can support your wife most effectively if you are really convinced that breastfeeding is best for baby and mother. But even if you are not 100 percent convinced, you can appreciate the fact that *she* is and you can show your love by helping her as much as possible. What can you do?

• Let her know that you are happy with her choice.

• Let everyone else know that you stand behind her decision.

• Speak to the doctors—your wife's and your baby's—to tell them you'll help her in any way you can.

• Arrange to take one or two weeks off from work after your baby's birth, so that you can be on hand to help your wife and bond with your baby.

• Answer the phone and doorbell to let your wife rest or breastfeed with-out distraction.

• Fix her a snack or bring her a drink while she's nursing.

• Speak to well-meaning friends and relatives who may be showing their disapproval of breastfeeding or doubting your wife's ability to nurse. Be her buffer and defend her against their subtle (and not-so-subtle) disparaging remarks. If you make it plain that she is not to be discouraged from nurs-ing, people will probably take their cues from your attitude and will keep any negative opinions to themselves.

• Remember that your wife is probably busier and more wrapped up in her daily schedule (especially if this is her first baby) than she ever has been be-fore and ever will be again; that the hectic pace of these first few weeks does abate; and that with a little time she will become more calm and less anx-ious about her new responsibilities.

• In a good relationship, you need to feel free to express your worries as well as your joys, your anger as well as your happiness. But because of the great effect the emotions have on the course of breastfeeding, if you can de-fer expressing your more negative feelings at least for the first few weeks af-ter your baby's birth, you will be making a great gift to your baby, as well as to your wife. Try to understand why she may be more irritable than usual, why she forgets to do things, and why she sometimes seems distracted when you're talking to her.

As important as your role is in your baby's nursing, you should not sti-fle all your feelings. But do try to deal with them in as adult a way as possible so you can spare the new mother, at least in the first few weeks after your baby's birth, as much emotional upset as possible. The calmer and more relaxed a woman is, the better able she is to produce and give milk.

In the especially sensitive early days after childbirth, a woman flourishes from being lovingly cared for. Even the simplest gestures—like bringing her a glass of juice while she's nursing, bringing home a small gift, or offering to go to the store—can go far to make her feel appreciated and to alleviate the down-in-the-dumps feeling that often follows childbirth.

Learning How to Cope

What do other fathers do? How do they deal with the challenges of parenting the breastfed baby, supporting the breastfeeding mother, and meeting their own needs as well? According to one study, fathers of happily breastfed babies developed five coping techniques:

1. They were realistic about the sometimes inconvenient ways breastfeeding affected their lives as well as those of their wives.
2. They accepted the situation, often by reminding themselves that breastfeeding was best for their children, and that it would not last forever.
3. They focused on the benefits breastfeeding held for them—like not having to get up at night. (Many, whose babies did not sleep in the family bed, did get up to bring the baby to their wives, but then they rolled over and went back to sleep until it was time to take the baby back to her own bed.)
4. They did other things for their babies—bathed them, diapered them, held them, walked with them, put them to sleep.
5. By playing an active role in their children's lives, both during the nursing days and after weaning, they forged close attachments with their children that were comparable to their wives' bonds.

YOUR BABY'S MOTHER IS STILL YOUR LOVER

One of the most important ways you can boost your wife's morale is to keep showing your interest in her as a woman. You are still her man and she is still your woman. You have a relationship that includes more than shared parenthood. She needs to know that you still consider her interesting and attractive, that you still value her opinions as much as ever, and that you still share interests besides the baby.

As we point out in Chapter 13, some women find that the sensuality of lactation makes them more interested in sex, while others find this a time of diminished sexual interest. Even if your wife is in the latter group and is not interested in resuming sexual relations as soon as you are (which is no reflection of her feelings for you), she still needs to be reassured of your love. This reassurance can take such physical form as cuddling and kissing even when it does not include sexual intercourse. Your patience now is likely to be rewarded when your wife once again becomes interested in sex.

One study of 194 couples found that the first sexual experience after childbirth was considered satisfying by more than two-thirds of the new fathers, but by fewer than half of the mothers. Pain and fatigue are major factors in many new mothers' more negative experience of sex.

Another major factor in the less satisfying sexual experiences of some women is their feeling about their own attractiveness. Women who don't like the way they look—because they're heavier than usual, because they have stretch marks, or because they feel "top-heavy"—don't feel like desirable sexual partners. As a result, they may withdraw from sex.

It's clear, then, that there are things that you can do with regard to all these factors. In the previous chapter we talked about ways to lessen the discomfort of renewed sexual activity. It's important to realize the problems that pain causes for some women and to be patient as well as flexible in your sexual techniques.

One happily married father of adolescents recalls the period just after their births as a time of "less sex and lower-quality sex." His advice to other men: "After childbirth and breastfeeding, you go back to square zero. You're almost starting out all over again. You don't know how you and your wife will relate to each other. You don't know what you'll be doing in bed. You may not do some things you used to do, but you may be doing some new things. And then the hardest thing: Try not to be anxious. And when you are anxious, just accept your anxiety as something you'll both get beyond. Just relax and concentrate on having pleasure."

You can help your wife feel better about her desirability by letting her know that you like the way she looks. If you can accept the fact that she may be heavier than usual throughout lactation and if you value those curves as symbolic of her fertility and her ability to nurture, you will be helping her to accept herself, too. One way to show her that you think she's beautiful is to tell her so; another is to take photographs of her, especially while she's nursing the baby. Other ways are to surprise her with an occasional appearance-related gift, such as a piece of jewelry or a pretty item of clothing that she can wear right now. You might even go shopping together, enjoying the outing as well as the gift.

It's also important to talk. Sharing thoughts and feelings is the cornerstone of a close relationship, and the timing and manner in which you talk to each other go far in determining the quality of your communication.

As Susan, a mother of three small children, told us, "We didn't do a lot of talking, of sharing our gut feelings until this past year. I never said to Bill right after our first child was born, 'I really love you but I need some space now for me.'" Her husband added, "And I never said anything to her about how deprived and left out I was feeling. What we did do was fight. I found a lot to criticize in Susan—the house was a mess; the kids were dirty; I didn't have any clean socks."

Now, after they've begun talking more, Susan says, "Now I realize that it wasn't the socks—it was the sex. Or rather, the lack of it. Now I can let the house go and I don't get those complaints. In fact, he pitches in and does more himself. As hard as it is, we manage to find time and energy for each other—for talking *and* for sex."

ROLLING UP YOUR SLEEVES

While the kind of emotional support we've just been talking about can be enormously helpful to your wife, she's sure to appreciate more practical kinds of help, too. Fortunately, these days there is a much less sharp distinction between work that's appropriate for either sex. There's no longer any stigma attached to a man's cooking or cleaning, just as there's no onus attached to a woman's painting a wall or putting up storm windows.

Every woman benefits from as much rest as she can get after giving birth. Her body has to recover its strength, even while her sleep is constantly being disturbed. Although a run-down nursing mother can produce milk, the effort will take its toll in her own health and in the quality of care she can give to her baby and to the rest of her family. The more rest she gets, the better off everyone in the family (including you) will be.

One of the most important things that you can do as the father of a breastfed baby is to be available to your wife and baby in those crucial early days after your baby's birth. The success of breastfeeding often hinges on what happens in the first week or two. If you can take a week or two off from work, you can help your wife and you can bond with your baby.

One valuable gift you can give your wife is to help her get the rest she needs at night. This helps you become closer to your baby, too. When he awakens during the night, you become the one on call. If your baby is sleeping in a separate bed, you become the one who gets up out of bed, gets the baby, brings him to your wife, and helps her get into a comfortable nursing

How a "Breastfeeding" Father Can Nurture a Baby

- Take your baby out of the crib at any time of the day or night to carry her to her mother for feedings.

- If you're home during the first week after your baby's birth, learn how to care for your baby's umbilical cord, and take over this responsibility.

- Change diapers, either before, after, or during the mid-feeding break.

- Walk around with your baby, carrying him in a baby carrier to feel his soft warmth next to you and to let him enjoy your presence.

- Rock or walk her when she's unhappy or soothe her in some other way (as suggested in the box on page 200).

- Enjoy one of the most fun-filled parenting activities for anyone who likes to play in water—giving your baby a bath.

- In a warm room or under a blanket, hold your baby, clad only in a diaper, against your bare chest, where he's able to hear your heartbeat and feel your warm (and maybe fuzzy) skin. Even though you can't breastfeed, you can bond through that wonderful skin-to-skin contact, and you can provide your baby with a different tactile experience from the one he has with his mother.

- Hold and stroke your baby and show how gentle and loving your touch can be.

- Give your baby a soothing massage (see the box on page 200).

- Work through some baby exercises with her.

- Sing to him.

- Talk to her.

With these last two activities, you'll not only be establishing a relationship—you'll also be furthering your baby's language development, an important contribution to your child's overall cognitive growth.

position. After the feeding, you diaper the baby and put him back to bed. Or you can welcome your baby into your bed; he will cry less often and wake you less often, since his mother will be able to nurse him at his first stirrings.

By being on night duty this way, you'll be performing the vital function of conserving your wife's energy so that she'll be better able to breastfeed—and better able to get through the day. There's no way to overestimate the psychological as well as the practical benefits of this help.

Another way to help the new mother conserve her energy is to hire someone to come in to help with the housework for a while if your budget permits. Your investment will pay off in everyone's good spirits and in time both you and your mate can devote to each other. If this is out of the question, pitch in yourself. You can market, cook, vacuum, do laundry, bring home take-out food, and take care of the baby and any older children.

One father told us, "The more I do in the house the better our relationship gets—especially our sex life. My wife isn't so tired, she feels good about herself, and she feels good about me. Besides, it's satisfying to know that I can do things I'd never done before, like whip up a pretty good meal."

YOU CAN BE A COMPLETE FATHER

One common worry among partners of women who plan to breastfeed is that there will be no way in which they can help to care for the baby. While this fear is very real to men who want to be actively involved in their babies' lives, it has to bring a smile to the face of any experienced parent. There is so much more to taking care of new infants besides feeding them!

You and Your Baby

If you want to be close to your baby, you can be. Just because your baby's mother went through nine months of pregnancy, bore your child, and is now nursing, this does not mean that she is the only person who can care for your baby. You can be just as tender with your baby as any woman might be—with no loss to your masculinity.

It is sometimes difficult for today's fathers, who may not have felt a nurturing bond from their own fathers in a time when male and female roles in our society were more stereotyped, to know how to become close to their children. But many men are finding the nurturant sides of themselves and are forging close attachments with their children, right from infancy.

What can you do to become close to your baby? A lot, as shown in the box on page 282.

You'll want to have time alone with your baby. This isn't "babysitting," which by definition involves taking care of someone else's baby. This is parenting. This is taking care of your own child. This is an activity that knows no gender limitations.

You can do your one-on-one parenting between feedings at first, giving your wife a chance to rest or go out while you and your baby enjoy your tête-à-tête. Or you can take the baby out in carrier or carriage. As your wife's milk supply becomes well enough established to miss a feeding (after the first six to eight weeks), you may be giving your baby an occasional bottle or cup, either of expressed breast milk or of formula. For tips on bottle- and cup-feeding, see Chapter 12.

At home with your family, you can take off that protective shell you may wear all day at work. You can free yourself to express those warm, tender emotions that are yours to give. A man who can freely give and take loving feelings can know completion as a human being.

You and Your Older Children

If you have older children, one of the most meaningful things you can do for them, for your partner, and for yourself is to lavish extra time and attention on them after your wife comes home with the new baby. If *you* as an adult feel pushed to one side, imagine how *they* feel.

Plan outings with them when they can have your undivided attention. Offer special treats to show them how important they are to you. The extra time you spend with your older children will mean as much to your wife as to the children themselves, since her mind will be more at ease, knowing that they are happy while she is taking care of the new baby. They'll also provide extra benefits to you as you get to know your children better and reap more of the rewards of parenthood.

As David Stewart, Ph.D., has written in his wise little pamphlet *Fathering and Career: A Healthy Balance,* "Careers are fickle, but parenthood is forever." As this father points out, while many things in life can wait, the growth of a child is not one of them. "To enjoy a two-year-old," he says, "you must do it when he or she is two."

You can create extra time for your children (which will be meaningful both to them and to you) by waking up earlier or by setting aside time when you come home in the evening. You can declare a temporary moratorium on overtime, travel, and weekend work. It's a question of priorities: If you consider time with your children a necessity, you'll find time for it.

GETTING SUPPORT FOR YOURSELF

It sounds as if a great deal is being asked of you at this time. You're right. A great deal is. That's why you'll benefit by having someone that *you* can turn to for comfort. New fathers need special helpers, too—caregivers who, as described in Chapter 4, can offer friendship, reassurance, and both practical and emotional support.

At a time when you have to be more giving to both your wife and your baby, you may feel like being taken care of yourself. Both you and your wife are likely to have mixed-up feelings, and each of you needs a lot of moral and practical support.

Many men consider their wives their best friends. This may work at most times in their lives, but when they have an issue they cannot talk to their wives about, these men have no one to go to. Often, men are unable to talk to another man about their most deeply felt feelings for fear of showing their vulnerability. Yet as most women have learned, sharing ourselves, including the selves we usually don't show to the outside world, is often a bridge to intimacy with another person, who can then share something of himself.

This may be an ideal time in your life to seek out a man you feel you can trust (if you don't already have such a friend in your life). Some good candidates include your father, brother, brother-in-law, clergyman. Or you might approach a coworker or tennis partner with whom you are friendly. You'll probably get the best kind of understanding and possibly even practical advice from someone who's already been through this stage in his life, but if you can't find someone like that, you can at least find someone who can turn a sympathetic ear your way and just listen.

The role of fathers in their babies' lives has become a major research interest for contemporary psychologists. They have found that attachments and close ties form between fathers and their children during the first year of the children's lives and that the fathers then go on to exert a strong influence over all aspects of their offspring's development. Anyone who plays a large part in a baby's day-to-day life will have an important influence on that life. After the birth of your new baby, then, you can justifiably feel proud of the major contribution you are making to the lives of your wife and your children.

Preventing and Treating Nursing-Related Problems

Help! I have a nursing problem that I seem unable to solve, and I don't know if I can continue to breastfeed. Nobody I know had anything like this, and I'm worried.

MARIANNE, UNIVERSITY CITY, MISSOURI

You probably will not encounter problems while breastfeeding your baby, but if you should run into any, this chapter can help you resolve a number of possible situations. If your questions are not answered here, call your doctor, nurse, midwife, childbirth educator, lactation consultant, or local La Leche League leader.

If you ran into a breastfeeding problem with a previous baby, don't assume that it will occur again. Breastfeeding history does not necessarily repeat itself. Each nursing situation is unique, and now that you're more experienced, breastfeeding is likely to go more smoothly the second time around. On the other hand, this is a different baby, and each baby brings his or her own personality, habits, and feeding patterns to the table, sometimes with problems as a result. Don't blame yourself or your baby if something goes wrong. Just look at the situation as it is and see what you can do about it.

When you come across the lists of suggestions in this chapter, you need to be aware that you don't need to follow every suggestion listed for a particular problem. Try one or two remedies and see what happens. If the condition does not clear up, try one of the other ideas. If nothing works, call one of the practitioners mentioned above. This chapter represents the most current thinking about the issues covered here, but your practitioner may advise you to do something differently. If that happens and you agree, fine. But what should you do if you don't agree?

DISAGREEMENT WITH YOUR DOCTOR

Suppose the physician taking care of you or your baby gives you advice that contradicts other information you've received. You may be advised to stop or suspend nursing, you may be told to feed your baby formula or solid foods when you want to offer only breast milk, or you may be told to nurse your baby less frequently than you think necessary. What do you do?

First, you want to find out why the doctor is giving you this advice:

• Is it a consequence of a specific problem that has arisen with either you or your baby?

• Are you having a problem, perhaps with painful or infected breasts or nipples?

• Is your baby jaundiced?

• Is your baby not gaining weight at the rate the doctor feels is appropriate?

In this chapter we discuss some of these and other problems that may give rise to conflicting advice, and we present the most current remedies for them. Some of these solutions may be at odds with the advice you are receiving. Because each case is unique, however, your own physician is in the best position to evaluate your situation and make recommendations. *If your baby is sick or not thriving or has any special problem, it can be dangerous to disregard medical advice. If you don't have confidence in what your doctor says, find another competent doctor and get a second opinion* (see Chapter 4).

But if your baby is healthy and you're well informed, try discussing your differences with your doctor. Some doctors routinely recommend supplemental bottles of formula, early weaning, or early feeding of solids for all their patients, either because of long-established practice or because of their own opinions about desirable lifestyles, which may be different from your own. You need to separate medical advice from personal opinion.

One mother approaches such situations by saying, "I'm not comfortable with that. Can you suggest something else?" Another has found this way effective: "I use the words 'I feel' when I disagree with my doctor. If you 'think' or 'insist,' he won't like it. But if you 'feel' you would like to do or not do something, this is a gentle way to open the discussion, because nobody wants to step on your feelings."

Another mother who ran into a disagreement with her doctor over breastfeeding her jaundiced baby took him professional literature supporting her position and said, "I don't know whether you saw this recent research recommending that mothers of jaundiced babies continue to nurse them. Can you read this and tell me what you think of it?"

You may want to suggest that your doctor consult the books for professionals cited in the bibliography. You might also want to check with La Leche League International to see whether the League or any members of its Health Advisory Council have published materials on the topic or can suggest other sources you might consult.

Still another mother, who bolstered her argument with her knowledge about breastfeeding, found that her doctor was won over not only by the information she presented, but by her strong commitment to nursing her baby.

How you approach this situation depends on your personality and your sense of your doctor, as well as the specific issue under discussion.

ENGORGEMENT (HARD, SWOLLEN BREASTS)

Your breasts will normally become larger, heavier, and somewhat tender about two to five days after childbirth. The combination of the swelling of the tissues, the increased circulation of blood in the breasts, and the pressure of the newly produced milk can sometimes make them feel hard, tight, and uncomfortable. The skin on your breasts may be shiny and your nipples flat and distended; these are signs of engorgement. Although this is common for the first few days, it is not inevitable and can usually be avoided.

The best way to relieve, minimize, or even prevent engorgement is to feed your baby as soon after birth as possible and frequently from then on. Instead of waiting for your baby to cry, which is a late sign of hunger, feed him whenever he shows such early signs as sucking his fist, making sucking motions with his mouth, moving around, looking more alert, and so forth. Women whose babies nurse vigorously and often right from the start rarely suffer from engorgement. If you should become engorged, however, the procedures listed in the box on page 289 should help relieve the engorgement in a couple of days.

Ways to Relieve Engorgement

• Feed your baby frequently, eight to twelve times in a twenty-four-hour period in the first few days after birth, even if you have to wake her to nurse.

• Express or pump a little bit of milk before feeding to soften your breasts and make them easier for your baby to grasp.

• If your breasts are severely engorged, massage them once or twice a day before feeding, starting gently at the outer edges with your fingertips and going toward the nipple area. A mild cream may make the process easier, but don't get any on the areola, because that would make it harder for you to express any milk. It may help to do the massage in the shower.

• Apply warm, moist compresses about ten or fifteen minutes before a feeding (and before a massage). Between feedings, apply cold compresses. The warm compresses aid the let-down reflex, and the cold packs relieve swelling and pain. You can apply cold in an ice pack or a blue freezer pack wrapped in a thin towel. You can apply heat in a moist-heat pad, a small hot water bottle wrapped in a towel, a towel soaked in hot water, or in a hot shower. If you use a heating pad, be very careful not to burn your skin.

• Wear a firm bra for support. Be sure it's not too tight, since this can make you more uncomfortable and also cause other problems. Try taking off your bra while you're nursing, to be sure it is not constricting your milk ducts.

• Apply fresh cabbage leaves to your breasts. This simple home remedy seems to help some women. Pull two outer leaves from an ordinary head of cabbage, strip out the large vein in each leaf, cut a hole for your nipple, and rinse the leaf. Then lay the leaves on your breasts. We don't know why they work, but they're convenient, cheap, not injurious, and disposable, and some women report that they relieve pain. You might try it if you don't mind staining your bra—and smelling like dinner.

• Do *not* use a nipple shield.

• If you cannot breastfeed immediately but will resume nursing, express or pump your milk. An electric pump is the easiest and most efficient (see Chapter 17).

• Take a pain reliever—either one of the over-the-counter agents listed in the box on page 174, or something your doctor can prescribe that will not affect your baby or your milk.

• If only one breast is engorged because your baby is consistently not suckling from it, this may be a sign of a possibly serious medical problem. To rule this out, see your obstetrician.

When the engorgement goes away—and it will—be assured that you still have plenty of milk. Once your milk supply is well established, your breasts become softer and stay that way most of the time.

Sudden Weaning

If for any reason you have to wean your baby abruptly, you run a high risk of engorgement. In this situation, your approach will be different from the procedures given in the box on page 289, which you would follow if you were continuing to nurse. For suggestions on relieving the discomfort of abrupt weaning, see Chapter 18.

SORE NIPPLES

Many women experience mild, temporary tenderness the first few days after giving birth, and sometimes through the first week or two. If you're not in real pain and if your discomfort is relieved when your milk comes in and lets down for your baby, you don't need to do anything special. This mild to moderate initial tenderness usually goes away in a few days, as your milk begins to let down. But if your nipples look red and chapped or cracked or if you feel severe pain during or after nursing, do something right away. Don't wait until the pain becomes unbearable, because that will make the problem much harder to clear up.

Not all women experience nipple discomfort during early nursing. If you have positioned your baby properly from the start, and if he has latched on well, you can usually prevent sore nipples. Some infants, though, have more trouble than others learning how to latch on and to suckle; as a result, their mothers' nipples begin to hurt.

Proper positioning techniques almost always alleviate or completely eliminate sore nipples. So check the way you're holding the baby. Is she in a position so she can get enough of your breast in her mouth without straining? If not, take another look at the pictures and text in Chapter 6 and try repositioning.

Sometimes you may be doing everything right, but your baby may have a suckling problem. Some babies, for example, suck their tongues instead of the breast, or suck their lower lips along with the breast. Others thrust their tongues forward or because of a tight frenulum (the membrane that attaches the tongue to the floor of the mouth) cannot grasp the nipple properly (see page 307). If your nipple soreness persists beyond the first two or three days of nursing, ask someone knowledgeable in lactation to observe you and your baby while you're nursing. They may be able to pick up any problems in suckling and give you advice.

Dermatologist Donald A. Sharp, M.D., likens cracked nipples to chapped lips. If your lips get dry, you put on a cream to restore their internal moisture and you avoid surface wetness by not licking your lips. The same principle applies to nipples.

If your nipple cracks (develops a fissure), the current dermatological recommendation is "moist wound healing." This method of healing accelerates the healing process, eliminates scab formation, and provides pain relief. It involves restoring internal moisture by increasing the moisture content of the skin. To create the moist healing environment for sore, cracked nipples, apply pure, medical-grade, anhydrous lanolin, which is soothing and will also lubricate the skin and help it retain its internal moisture. Pure lanolin does not need to be wiped off before feedings because it will not harm your baby.

You can also express a little bit of your breast milk and apply it to the affected areas. You will thus be taking advantage of the healing and antibacterial properties of human milk, as well as its moisturizing benefits. And of course, you don't need to wipe it off your nipple before your baby nurses.

Even if some blood appears in cracks in your nipple, you can continue to nurse; your blood will not harm your baby. But if you are bleeding, you should take immediate measures to heal your nipples.

Treating Sore Nipples

• Be sure your baby is properly positioned for nursing, with her chest facing yours, her face and nose facing your breast, and her mouth covering all or part of your areola, as described in Chapter 6. Be sure that your nipple is well into your baby's mouth and that your baby's gums are compressing the milk ducts under the areola. If she is not properly positioned, take her off the breast carefully (breaking the suction with your finger) and bring her back to it. If you are in any doubt about your nursing technique, consult a lactation specialist.

• Do not let your baby chew on your nipple. If you feel this happening, carefully take him off the breast as above and bring him back. If he keeps doing it, end this feeding session.

• Express a little milk manually before putting your baby to the breast; this will start your milk flowing, help your let-down reflex operate more quickly, and lubricate your nipple.

• Practice a relaxation technique just before nursing (see the box on page 192).

• Nurse your baby more frequently, but perhaps for shorter periods of time. Your breasts are less likely to overfill and your baby is more likely to suckle gently.

• Offer the less sore breast first most of the time. This will give your milk a chance to let down from the sore nipple, and your baby won't be suckling as hard by the time he gets around to his second course.

• Change your position at each feeding. Lie down, sit up, hold your baby in different positions so that you can change the position of your baby's jaws on your breast. If you have a crack in your nipple, it's especially important to position your baby so his mouth clamps down elsewhere.

• If a scab forms on your nipple during early nursing, leave it alone.

• Avoid all irritating and drying substances. Do not use soap, alcohol, tincture of benzoin, or witch hazel on your nipples.

• Do not wipe away milk left on your breast after a nursing. In fact, you can express a few drops of your milk and rub that gently onto your nipples. As we said earlier, mothers around the world treat their children's irritations and infections with human milk. Your milk's curative powers can help you, too.

• Soothe the soreness with a cream prescribed by your doctor or with pure lanolin. Lansinoh for Breastfeeding Mothers® can be purchased from your local pharmacy or through Ameda/Egnell (see the Resource Appendix). It is hypoallergenic and thus safe even for people who are allergic to wool, and it does not need to be wiped off before your baby nurses.

• If only one breast has a sore nipple, breastfeed only on the other one and pump (with an electric pump) from the sore breast. If the nipples on both breasts are sore, consult with your lactation specialist on the best course of action. You may need to stop nursing completely for a couple of days, during which time you can pump or express your milk. (Using an electric pump is usually less irritating than your baby's suckling might be.)

• Keep your nipples free of surface wetness:

If you wear breast pads to catch leaking milk, change them when they get wet. Do not use the kind with plastic liners.

Wear an all-cotton bra, not one made of a synthetic fabric.

If you wear breast shells (milk cups) to bring out inverted nipples, empty them often.

Walk around the house with your nipples uncovered when you can. If the air in your home is very dry (as in an overheated apartment), use a humidifier or keep a pan of water on the radiator.

If it is too painful to have clothing touch your nipples, apply a light coating of modified lanolin and insert in your bra small mesh tea strainers from the hardware store, from which you have removed the handles; or plastic breast shields (described in Chapter 4).

• If your nipples are tender after showering, apply a coating of lanolin before you take your shower.

• Occasionally take an ibuprofen or a glass of beer or wine to ease your discomfort.

• Occasionally sore nipples are caused by thrush, a fungus infection, which may be affecting both you and your baby. See the section on page 294 for treatment suggestions.

• Do *not* wear the rubber or soft plastic nipple shields that are sometimes recommendeded to insulate your sore nipples from your baby's suckling. These shields consist of a cone attached to a rubber nipple. The cone fits closely over the breast and the baby sucks from the rubber nipple. They don't provide the stimulation your breasts need to keep making milk, they rarely relieve the soreness, and they cause some babies to develop nipple confusion, as explained in Chapter 5.

• If you have been pumping your breasts with a hand pump, you may have been doing it too vigorously or improperly. Switch to an electric pump, which has a gentle motion.

• If, as happens in rare cases, your soreness continues to worsen until your nipple cracks and bleeds and is absolutely too painful to nurse from, take your baby off the affected nipple for twenty-four to forty-eight hours. Nurse him often on the other breast. If necessary, give him expressed milk or formula in a bottle or cup. Express or pump your milk from the affected breast every three hours, or every time you would ordinarily be nursing.

Gradually resume nursing on the breast with the sore nipple, starting twice a day. Continue to express milk from the sore breast at other feeding times until your nipple is healed enough to work up to the full nursing schedule. Apply pure lanolin to heal the nipple fissures.

• If you have a persistent rash around your nipples that does not clear up, see your doctor to rule out any underlying problem.

THRUSH

Thrush, a yeast infection caused by the fungus *Candida albicans,* loves milk and places where milk goes. It isn't serious, but it can be quite painful. If your baby has it in her mouth, it may hurt her to nurse. If you have it on your nipples, it may hurt you to breastfeed. If one of you has it, you may be passing it to the other.

To check your baby, look inside her mouth for milky white spots or a coating on her tongue, gums, or on the insides of her cheeks. She may also have a diaper rash. Or she may have no symptoms at all. You may have pink, flaky, crusty, itchy, or burning nipples; a burning pain inside your breasts during or soon after feedings (which signals an infection in the milk ducts), and you may also have a vaginal yeast infection. Thrush sometimes develops after antibiotic treatment in mother or baby; also, women with diabetes are more prone to develop thrush. If you suspect thrush, see the suggestions below.

• Continue to breastfeed your baby.

• Call your doctor, who will probably prescribe liquid nystatin for the baby's mouth and a nystatin cream for your nipples. Other prescription and over-the-counter drugs (like gentian violet) are sometimes recommended.

• Follow the treatment for both of you for two weeks, even though your symptoms may clear up in a couple of days.

• While your baby's infection is clearing up, wash your nipples after every nursing in a solution of one teaspoon of baking soda or one tablespoon of vinegar to one cup of boiled warm water. Dry your nipples gently and apply the same medication your doctor has prescribed for your baby. You don't have to wipe it off. This way you're both getting the benefits of the treatment.

• Try dietary measures, such as yogurt with active cultures or supplements of lactobacillus acidophilus. If you are especially susceptible to this kind of infection because you are diabetic or have an immune system dysfunction, you should also limit your intake of sugars. Do this in conjunction with the treatment your doctor ordered. Over-the-counter or alternative remedies sometimes do nothing for a yeast infection and can even make it worse. You should treat yourself *only* if you have previously been diagnosed and treated by a professional for a yeast infection, and then only if you're absolutely certain about your symptoms.

• To prevent reinfection, wash your hands and your baby's hands often, and dry them with soft paper towels that you discard after one use.

• Do not give your baby any milk expressed and frozen during the thrush outbreak.

• Thoroughly wash anything that goes into your baby's mouth. Boil rubber nipples, pacifiers, teethers, and toys for twenty minutes once a day and discard them after a week. Boil breast pump parts. Wash nonboilable toys and breast pump parts thoroughly with warm soapy water.

• Change your nursing pads after each feeding.

• If thrush recurs after two courses of treatment, include your husband in the treatment plan, since thrush can be transmitted during sexual relations.

CLOGGED DUCT (PLUGGED DUCT, "CAKED" BREASTS)

In this condition, which can occur any time during nursing, one or more of the milk ducts are blocked so that the milk cannot pass through them. If you develop a clogged duct, you're likely to find a small reddened lump on your breast that's painful to touch. If not treated, this condition can lead to a breast infection, so you should take immediate measures, as suggested below.

• Be sure your bra (or other clothing, like a T-shirt or sweater) is not so tight that it is pressing on the milk ducts. You may want to get a bra in the next larger size. Or try going without one, at least while you're nursing. Also check other items that may be putting too much pressure on your breasts, like a baby carrier or a shoulder bag.

• Breastfeed more often and for a longer period of time, so that your baby can help you empty the breast.

• Change your position with every feeding, so that the pressure of your baby's suckling will hit different places on your breast, exerting pressure on different ducts.

• Express or pump milk from the affected breast after each feeding if your baby has not nursed long and vigorously, to get out as much milk as possible.

• If dried secretions seem to be covering your nipple openings, wash them off very gently after each nursing with a piece of cotton saturated with warm water.

• Offer your sore breast first, so that your baby will drain it more thoroughly.

• Apply moist heat several times a day (with a moist-heating pad, a hot water bottle, hot wet towel or washcloth, or tub bath or shower). Follow this with gentle massage on the area of the clogged duct.

• Get extra rest.

• Do not wear a nipple shield, which will make it even harder for your baby to drain your breast adequately.

• Do not sleep on your stomach, which puts pressure on your breast.

• Continue to nurse. If you stop suddenly, your breast is likely to get too full, the condition will worsen, and infection may result.

• If your baby refuses to nurse on the breast with the clogged duct, see your obstetrician. There may be a changed taste in the milk from that breast, which may be a sign of an infection or other problem.

• If a lump remains for more than three days, see your obstetrician. While the lump is most probably related to breastfeeding, it may not be and must be looked at promptly.

• If you repeatedly suffer from clogged ducts, consult a lactation specialist to reevaluate the way you're holding your baby or the way your baby is suckling.

BREAST INFECTION (MASTITIS)

When breast infections occur, they usually show up between two and six weeks after birth, but they may appear earlier or much later. A breast infection may be a complication of a clogged duct or the result of an infection carried from the baby to the mother or picked up elsewhere. Symptoms tend to appear suddenly and may include some of the following: headache, an intense localized pain, a lump that may or may not feel sore, engorgement with the breast hot and tender to the touch, redness, fever, a cracked nipple that looks infected, red streaks on the breast, and a generally sick, achy, flulike feeling. If you see any of these symptoms, begin treatment right away. If you still have fever after twenty-four hours of treatment, call your doctor.

Mothers with breast infections used to be told to stop nursing immediately. We now know that breast infections clear up more quickly and with fewer complications when the mother continues to nurse, and nurses frequently, from the affected breast. There is no danger of the baby's becoming ill from nursing at an infected breast; he probably harbors the same germs in his mouth and nose that may have caused the problem in his mother's breast. Occasionally a baby may not nurse well at an infected breast because the milk tastes salty. If this happens, express or pump from the infected breast and nurse from the uninfected one.

It is important to treat a breast infection right away, as suggested below. With treatment, the fever should drop within thirty-six to forty-eight hours, and the soreness and hardness will go away soon afterward. If symptoms do not disappear within three days of treatment, call your doctor.

• Call your doctor immediately upon development of symptoms of mastitis. The usual treatment for mastitis is the administration of an antibiotic for a course of from ten to fourteen days, in addition to other treatment, as indicated below. This will be safe to take while you continue to nurse. Once prescribed, the antibiotic should be taken for its full course, even if your symptoms have gone away before then.

• Go to bed immediately and stay there as much as you can. If you can't stay in bed, rest as much as possible.

• Apply moist heat to the infected breast with one or more of the following: moist-heating pad, hot water bottle, hot wet towel, soaking in a basin of warm water, warm shower, or warm bath. Nurse soon after application of heat.

• Do *not* apply an ice pack.

• Nurse frequently, as often as every two hours around the clock. This will keep your milk flowing, will avoid engorgement, and will drain the infected area of the breast. Be sure your baby is well positioned, and change positions so your baby is not always putting pressure at the same spot on your breast.

- Offer the sore breast first at each nursing so that it can be drained more completely.

- Be sure your bra is not too tight. You may want to get one in the next larger size. Or try going without one, at least while you're nursing. Also check other items that may be putting too much pressure on your breasts, like a baby carrier or a shoulder bag.

- Drink plenty of fluids.

- Do not wean suddenly if you can help it, since this can contribute to an abscess, a serious and painful infection that may require surgery.

- If you suffer repeatedly from breast infection, see your family physician, your obstetrician, or a breast surgeon, especially if a lump is not reduced in size after three days of treatment, if the mastitis keeps reappearing at the same place on your breast, and/or if you have dimpling on the breast. Breast cancer is extremely rare in lactating women, but it does occasionally occur and you must have it ruled out.

- If you have been checked out for repeated breast infection and reassured that it is not caused by a malignancy, check for other factors that may be causing the mastitis—allowing your breasts to become too full, not alternating them, improper positioning of your baby, inadequate washing of your hands before nursing, using an unclean breast pump, or not getting enough rest. Change what you can and seek medical help at the first sign of infection.

GALACTOCELE (MILK-RETENTION CYST)

Occasionally a nursing mother develops a non-tender lump in her breast. If you find a lump in your breast and if it does not change or go away within three days, you should see a gynecologist who is knowledgeable about lactating breasts.

The lump may be a galactocele, a benign milk-retention cyst, which is caused by blockage of a milk duct and which does not become infected. Galactoceles can be diagnosed in two ways, either by performing an ultrasound test or by aspiration to determine whether the cystlike structure contains milk. If you have a galactocele, you probably will not need surgery, and you do not need to wean your baby. These cysts rarely need to be removed surgically.

SUDDEN INCREASE IN BABY'S DEMAND

Your baby may have seemed happy with a nursing schedule that the two of you have worked out, but then just as soon as you think you've settled into a routine, he begins to ask for more. You wonder what has happened, and you worry that you don't have enough milk. This is a fairly common occurrence and nothing to worry about. It can occur for a number of reasons and is usually easy to resolve. All you have to do in most cases is nurse more frequently for several days. This will build up your milk supply and get your baby over the transition.

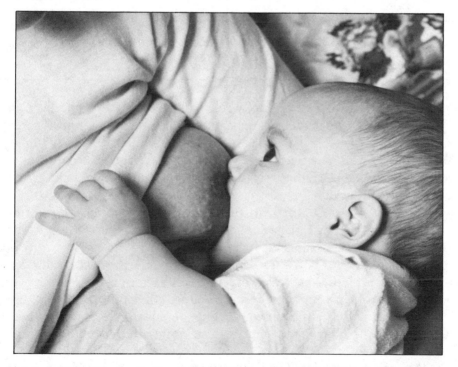

This baby is suckling well, directly facing her mother, taking enough of the breast into her mouth, and obviously enjoying the experience.

One reason why this sometimes happens lies with the baby's growth. Babies grow irregularly. During periods of particularly fast growth, sometimes called "growth spurts," they need more fuel. The most common times for this apparent increase in a baby's need for nourishment are three weeks, six weeks, three months, and six months of age. While you're nursing more frequently, you may also be able to increase your milk supply in other ways (see Chapter 10). After your baby reaches six months of age and still seems hungry no matter how often you nurse him, he may be ready to start eating solid foods. This readiness usually occurs sometime between six and eight months of age (see Chapter 18).

Another reason for what seems like a sudden increase in your baby's appetite may lie with you. Nursing and motherhood may have become so easy and manageable that you forgot to mother yourself. You work more, you go out more, you do more, and you forget about resting enough and eating right. As a result, your milk supply may diminish. This is easy to remedy. Take a look at your life and cut back on outside involvements while you take better care of yourself.

THE BABY WHO GAINS TOO SLOWLY

Occasionally a baby of two or three weeks will have gained practically nothing since birth. Or a baby may have begun to gain and then for no apparent reason hit a plateau. The baby may be crying constantly, obviously hungry all the time. Or he may sleep for several hours at a stretch, seem to nurse well, and seem happy. Either way, it's worrisome. Is the baby sick? Or not getting enough to eat?

Any baby who doesn't gain or seems unhappy much of the time should be examined by a physician. See the box on page 125 for signs that your baby should be evaluated right away. A baby who is sick won't do well at either breast or bottle until her condition is dealt with. If your doctor does not find any medical problem, see a lactation consultant, who may be able to help your baby become a more efficient nurser. Also, take a look at your own health. Are you feeling good, eating enough, and getting enough rest? Are you taking drugs that could interfere with your milk production?

If, as is usually the case, no physical problem is found with either you or your baby, you can take a number of steps to encourage weight gain and normal growth, as suggested in the boxes on pages 301 and 303.

Helping the Slow-Gaining Infant

Look at Your Breastfeeding Patterns

• Is your baby nursing no oftener than every three or four hours, either because she sleeps for several hours at a stretch and doesn't "ask" to nurse, or because you've been encouraging her to go longer between feedings? If so, nurse every hour or two, even if it means waking your baby up every couple of hours during the day.

Helping the Older Baby Who Isn't Gaining

Sometimes there's a sudden loss of weight or a failure to gain weight in a baby several months old, who has been doing fine up until now. If this happens, look for the following:

• *Is your baby teething?* If she's drooling a lot and trying to put everything into her mouth, she may be teething and finding nursing uncomfortable. Whenever you see her sucking her fist or fingers, pick her up and nurse her. More frequent short nursings will provide her with the nutrients she needs, while lessening the discomfort. After nursings you can give her ice-chilled teething rings until she seems more comfortable. If she seems extremely uncomfortable, ask your doctor for suggestions.

• *Has he become so efficient at nursing that he zips through his feedings and is ready to stop after five minutes?* If so, he may not be getting enough milk. Try burping and switching breasts several times during a session; the new surge of milk after a second let-down may interest him in staying at the breast.

• *Are you doing too much?* Cut back as much as possible on your activities for a while. Rest more, eat and drink more, and take better care of yourself to increase your supply of milk.

• *Is she easily distracted?* Does she break away from the breast to look around and see what's going on about her? Breastfeed in a quiet, dimly lit room.

• *Does he spend many happy hours with a pacifier, or sitting in a swing?* Devices like these can be wonderful helpers for a busy mother, but if your baby is losing weight or not gaining as fast as he should, put them aside for a while. Pacify and amuse your baby more with your breast; when he is once again gaining well, you can reintroduce the other pleasures.

• *Does your baby begin to nurse, then reject the breast?* If so, see the section "Temporary Rejection of the Breast."

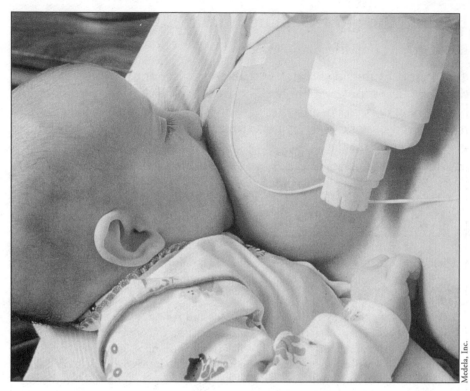

Medela, Inc.

A nursing supplementer delivers milk to a baby while the baby is suckling at the mother's breast. It's helpful to babies whose mothers don't seem to have enough milk to foster normal weight gain and those who need help mastering efficient suckling techniques.

• Has your baby been sleeping more than six hours at night before eight to twelve weeks of age? If so, wake him every four hours at night.

• Have you been timing feeding sessions, removing your baby when *you* think it's time, allowing only twenty or thirty minutes? If the baby is swallowing frequently (no more than two sucks to a swallow), let sessions run for at least forty-five minutes.

• Has your baby been taking only one breast at a feeding? If so, nurse from both. If she falls asleep after one, burp her and change her and then nurse on the other side. Switch breasts more than once during a feeding. This encourages multiple let-downs and, as a result, more milk.

• Is your baby getting milk or water from bottles? If so, your breasts may not be getting enough stimulation, and your baby may be experiencing nipple confusion. Eliminate the water. If your baby needs supplemental formula, feed it through a nursing supplementer (see the box on page 303), an

Nursing Supplementers

These devices deliver milk to a baby while the baby is suckling at the mother's breast. The two most commonly used methods are the Supplemental Nursing System (SNS)™ made by Medela, Inc., and the Lact-Aid Nursing Trainer™ System.* Whichever one you choose should be used only under the supervision of an experienced lactation specialist, and your baby should be closely monitored for healthy weight gain.

With the SNS a thin plastic tube runs from a plastic bottle hung upside down (to take advantage of gravity) from a strap around the mother's neck. The end of the tube is placed next to the mother's nipple and held there with surgical tape. As the baby nurses at his mother's breast, he simultaneously suckles the tip of the nursing tube and the mother's nipple, and his efforts are rewarded by the flow of milk via the tube. The bottles come in different sizes to accommodate premature babies and those with cleft palate or other feeding problems.

The Lact-Aid consists of a soft, presterilized plastic bag that contains the milk. The bag is attached to a plug that in turn is attached to a slender nursing tube. The filled and assembled supplementer is worn on an adjustable neck strap in the mother's nursing bra between her breasts.

In both these systems, the baby suckles the breast and the tube simultaneously, receiving milk as soon as he starts to nurse. Because of the way the system delivers fluid to the baby, it provides a type of oral patterning that helps to improve or train the baby's suckling skill and coordination. Meanwhile, the device helps to increase the mother's milk supply, since the baby is stimulating her breasts more effectively. Throughout, the baby is getting the nourishment he needs, and both mother and baby are able to enjoy the experience of nursing at the breast, with all the warmth and intimacy that are such a rewarding part of breastfeeding.

---

*For information on obtaining nursing supplementers, see the Resource Appendix.

---

eyedropper, a teaspoon, or a cup. Even some premature babies have been able to drink from a cup.

Remember, though, that this last suggestion does not help the baby to learn how to suckle correctly. Furthermore, you need to be very careful if you use an eyedropper approach or a cup, since there is the risk of putting more fluid into the baby's mouth than he is able to swallow easily, possibly causing him to aspirate it into his lungs.

• Is your baby using a pacifier to fill her sucking needs? If so, take away the pacifier and present your breast; this way she will get nutrition along with suckling.

Look at Your Baby

• Does your baby arch his back during nursing? If so, he may not get enough of your breast in his mouth. Hold him in the clutch (football) hold with his feet up behind you so that he can't push against anything.

• Is your baby so excitable that she keeps losing the breast? Try swaddling her in a blanket.

• Some babies become frustrated if the milk does not flow freely. It may help if you express a little bit before you begin to nurse.

What to Do Now

• Suppose you're already doing everything suggested above. If so, the first thing to do now is to make *extra* efforts to build up your production of milk. The best way is to nurse more frequently, as often as every hour or two. Other suggestions, as given in Chapter 10, may also help.

• If, after one or two days of this frequent-feeding regimen, your baby is still not gaining, seek the advice of a lactation specialist who may help you and your baby to overcome whatever obstacles have been keeping your baby from gaining.

• The lactation consultant will look closely at your baby's suckling technique, as explained in the the following section.

• The consultant may suggest that you supplement breastfeeding with formula or expressed breast milk delivered through a nursing supplementer.

Checking Your Baby's Suckling Technique

In some cases, babies fail to gain weight because they have a suckling problem. The quality of a baby's suck is at least as important as the frequency and duration of feeding sessions. Some of the same problems of suckling technique that we talked about in connection with sore nipples in the mother can also cause poor weight gain in the baby. Fortunately, these problems can often be overcome by changes in positioning or other management of breastfeeding.

Lactation consultants are specially trained to evaluate suckling technique as part of their expertise in breastfeeding management. Others who are sometimes able to help you identify and solve your baby's problem are physicians, childbirth educators, or La Leche League leaders. For proper assessment, it will probably be necessary for the consultant to observe a nursing session.

Before you consult a specialist, however, you can do a little detective work on your own. Ask an observer to help you check the following:

• Does your baby seem to be sucking her lower lip along with your breast? If so, take her off the breast, start her over again, and pull out her lip after she's attached.

• If your nipple tends to point down, point it straight into your baby's mouth by pressing down on the top of your breast with your thumb.

• If your baby seems to clench his jaws and clamp the end of your nipple, pull down on his jaw with your index finger; when he begins to suck properly, release the pressure.

• Pull down your baby's lower lip while he's nursing. Either you or a helper can use a small mirror and see whether his tongue can be seen between his lower gum and your breast. If not, he may be sucking his tongue. If you cannot see your baby's tongue:

Remove him from your breast.

Put your index finger on your baby's chin, pressing it down a little, and let him use his rooting reflex to find your nipple and take it in his mouth.

Or put your finger in his mouth, flatten his tongue, and insert your nipple on top. You'll need a helper for this. Repeat until he's doing it right.

If neither of these techniques works, ask your baby's doctor or a lactation consultant to look at your baby's tongue; occasionally the membrane attaching it to the floor of the mouth (the frenulum) is too short and needs to be clipped (see page 307).

• Test your baby's sucking technique by the Marmet Suck Assessment: Trim the fingernail on your index finger, wash and rinse your hands, stroke your baby's cheek toward the lips, and when her mouth opens, insert your finger with the nail down. If your baby is sucking correctly, the following will occur:

The sides of her tongue will curve around your finger

Her tongue will cover her lower gum ridge

You'll feel a sucking motion starting at the tip of her tongue and rolling back with a wavelike motion

She'll suck your finger far back into her mouth

Your finger pad will touch her soft palate

She won't gag

She'll suck rhythmically, occasionally resting without breaking suction

If your baby's suckling does not feel like this, she may have a suckling problem that a trained lactation 'specialist may help you correct.

THE BABY WHO GAINS TOO FAST

While we used to think it was impossible to overfeed a breastfed baby, an occasional totally breastfed baby seems to be very heavy. This is a baby who is gaining so much weight that he is in the top five percent of weight for a baby of his length. Although it was once thought that a fat baby is a healthy baby, we now know that too much fat is no good. It's not healthy now, and it may lead to obesity later in life.

However, "overweight" is quite rare among nursing babies who benefit from a system (breastfeeding) that is basically self-regulating. Most heavy breastfed babies slim down when they begin to crawl and move around more.

This is *not* an issue during the first couple of months of life. A very young infant should be fed frequently, with no concern about overfeeding. By the time a baby is four to six months old, however, the mother of an extremely plump baby might be wondering if her baby is getting too fat. Mothers who have a great deal of milk sometimes offer the breast every time the baby opens his mouth, and some babies are agreeable about taking the breast even when they're not hungry.

As we've noted before, babies cry for all sorts of reasons, many of them entirely unrelated to hunger. Just as it's inappropriate to offer an older child a cookie every time she's unhappy, you don't want to program an infant to satisfy her every want by putting the breast into her mouth.

If your baby seems to be gaining too quickly, try offering only one breast at each feeding (expressing milk from the other breast if you're uncomfortable). Meanwhile, try to meet your baby's needs in a variety of ways that don't involve feeding him.

TEMPORARY REJECTION OF THE BREAST ("NURSING STRIKE")

There are two kinds of breast refusal—that by a newborn who does not even begin to nurse, and that by a baby who has been nursing well and then decides to go on strike and refuses to take the breast. In either case, you can almost always figure out why this is happening and help your baby nurse happily.

If Your Baby Has Not Nursed at All

If your baby rejects the breast almost from birth, check the following possibilities:

• She may be having a problem latching on. Check the way you're holding her and experiment with other positions. If you are engorged, relieving that condition (see the box on page 289) may make it easier for her to take your breast.

• Your baby may be "tongue-tied." Some infants have a tight frenulum. This is the stringy fibrous membrane that connects the lower part of the tongue to the floor of the mouth. If it's too tight, the baby cannot extend his tongue far enough to take hold of the nipple. A lactation consultant can usually diagnose a short frenulum. Then you can ask your doctor to clip the frenulum, a procedure that is quick and painless and can be performed in the doctor's office. There may be a small amount of bleeding for a minute or so; as soon as this stops, your baby can and should be put to your breast.

• Some infants, right from birth, fight being held and fight being nursed. You're not doing anything wrong; you just have a baby whose personality makes it hard for him to settle into your arms and onto your breast. You need to experiment with ways to calm your baby and to find a position that he will accept. You also need to remember that your baby is not rejecting you and that you are not to blame. You may need to express your milk for a while and feed it to your baby by cup, dropper, or nursing supplementer, until he feels comfortable in the nursing situation. One mother finally got her baby to nurse by leaning over him and dangling her breast into his mouth.

The Older Nursing Baby

Sometimes in the first few weeks after birth, but more often between four and ten months of age, a baby will nurse a couple of minutes, then arch his back and cry. Nothing the mother can do will induce him to go back, and

When an Older Baby Refuses the Breast

• *Has your baby turned against the taste of your milk?* It may have changed be-cause of a cream you're using on your breasts, a new food you're eating, a new medicine you're taking, a new strenuous exercise program you've begun, a de-veloping infection in your breast, or because you are pregnant. Explore these possibilities, one by one. Keep a log of what you eat and what your baby's reac-tion is, so that you can identify and eliminate an offending food. Schedule nurs-ing sessions before exercise sessions, as suggested in Chapter 7. If you feel a lump in your breast, first treat it as a clogged duct; if it has not healed in three days, see your obstetrician.

• *Is she teething?* If her gums are tender from the pressure of new teeth coming in, it may hurt her to nurse. If she bit you, she may have been startled by your cry of pain and be afraid to nurse again.

• *Is he wildly hungry?* If he can't seem to wait for the milk to let down, try pick-ing him up about fifteen minutes before you would ordinarily feed him, or ex-press a little milk first to give your let-down a chance to work.

• *Does she have a cold?* She may be having trouble breathing through her nose. Use a vaporizer in the room where she sleeps or ask your doctor whether nose drops would help.

• *Does he have thrush?* This mouth infection, described earlier, can make nurs-ing painful. If you suspect it, treat it immediately, first to relieve your baby and also since the infection can spread to you.

• *Does she have an earache?* If so, she may find nursing painful.

• *Is your baby consistently refusing only one breast?* If so, see your own doctor, since this may signal a medical problem that should be explored.

• *Are you under tension?* If you're going through a particularly difficult time emotionally, your feelings may be coming across to your baby, who in turn becomes too upset to nurse. Make a conscious effort to forget about your cares, at least while you're nursing. You'll enjoy these oases in your life and your baby may be calmer, too. See the suggestions to help you relax in the box on page 192.

---

yet it's obvious that he wants something. What's wrong? And what can you do about it? As with so many other child-rearing issues, you have to look closely at your own baby and see what is going on in his life. The following suggestions have worked in some situations, and the box above lists several possible causes, along with some specific solutions.

• If you want to continue nursing, don't substitute bottle-feeding for the times you would ordinarily nurse. Doing that may make the problem worse. Chances are that this "nursing strike" may last only a day or two, and your baby will then go back to being an eager nurser.

• If your baby has begun to eat solid foods, increase her portions of these for a few days to tide her over. If she has been eating large amounts of solids, however, this may be causing the problem. She may be too full of food to be interested in nursing.

• Express or pump your milk and give it to him in an eyedropper, a teaspoon, or a cup until he resumes taking the breast.

• Keep offering your breast. The most effective time to do this is to pick him up while he's asleep or very sleepy; he won't remember to reject the breast, and once he's back in the routine of nursing, he may decide it's pretty good, after all.

• Vary your nursing positions. Your baby might prefer one you haven't used yet.

• Nurse in motion—in a rocking chair or walking around.

If none of the possible reasons listed in the box on page 308 to explain why your baby might be refusing your breast seem to apply to your situation, if none of the suggested remedies work, if after a week she's still refusing to nurse, and if she's more than six months old, she may be signaling her readiness to be weaned. While some children want to nurse long after their mothers had thought they would, others surprise and disappoint a mother by wanting to give up the breast earlier than she wants to herself. For suggestions on making the weaning process as comfortable as possible, with the least amount of emotional upset for mother and baby, see Chapter 18.

Special Situations

I was so worried about my tiny baby, but when I pumped my milk to give to her, I knew I was doing something for her that no one else in the world could possibly do. Then when I was finally able to put her to my breast, it made up for all the time we had been separated from each other.

NORMA, GLENCOE, ILLINOIS

There are a number of situations involving a mother or baby—or both—that can affect the course of breastfeeding. For example, what if your baby is born early? What if you or your baby gets sick? What if you have had breast surgery? What if you have more than one baby and want to nurse both, or all, of them? And what if you began to feed your baby with bottles, and then decided to initiate breastfeeding?

These are the sorts of circumstances discussed in this chapter. Most women do not encounter them. But if you do, you will have special questions that require special answers. You will want to know how your situation is related to your ability to nurse your baby. One thing you need to know is that in many such instances, you and your baby will both benefit from breastfeeding.

If you need more information about any of the topics discussed in this chapter, you can call your doctor, nurse, midwife, childbirth educator, lactation consultant, or local La Leche League leader. Or you may find answers to your questions in a more specialized book.

BREASTFEEDING YOUR PRETERM (PREMATURE) INFANT

A birth that comes before the end of the normal gestation period is often a frightening event, especially if a baby is born very early and/or very small.

However, medical technology has advanced so dramatically that, with modern care, even the tiniest babies have an excellent chance of growing up healthy and normal.

In your desire to do as much as possible for your baby, you are likely to feel disappointed if you cannot breastfeed him right away, as you had intended. However, you can express your milk for him immediately after his birth and either supply it to hospital staff or freeze it for later use. Then, as soon as your baby is able to suckle at your breast, you will have the milk to offer him.

Whether your baby gets your own breast milk right from the beginning or not until he has achieved a certain size and strength, you *will* be able to breastfeed him. Remember that prematurity is a temporary condition, but that breastfeeding can continue for many months.

Many women have expressed or pumped their milk for the first several weeks of their babies' lives. This milk has been fed to the baby either by tube or by bottle, helping to assure a good start in life. After the baby has become stronger, mother and baby have gone on to forge a fulfilling, satisfying nursing relationship. As one mother said, "Breastfeeding a premature baby means a few weeks of uncertainty and inconvenience, followed by many months of blissful happiness, contentment, and satisfaction."

This route is eminently doable—but it does take time, effort, patience, persistence, and most of all, determination. It's much easier if you can marshal support from your family, your friends, hospital personnel, and breastfeeding consultants. Many women are grateful that they persisted through the early difficult times until they were able to establish a normal breastfeeding relationship. Other women, who found it too difficult to maintain the kind of schedule required early on and switched to formula, feel that the breast milk their babies received in their first days or weeks of life gave them a better start than they would have had without it. Some women who decided against breastfeeding at the beginning changed their minds later and were able to relactate, a process described in this chapter.

How and What Will Your Preterm Baby Eat?

Procedures for feeding a baby born before term vary, depending on the infant's size, strength, and special needs. Your baby may be technically classified as preterm, but be well formed and strong and lack only a few ounces to be considered of normal weight. In this case, you can probably start to nurse immediately. Very tiny infants, however, are often not able to suck at all; they may have to be fed by *gavage* (via a tube that goes from

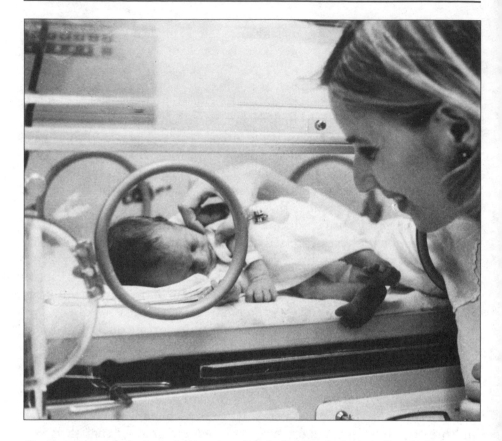

Even a preterm baby in an isolette can often be fed his mother's milk, which is especially suited for his growth needs. It's also vital for mothers to touch their tiny babies, as this mother is doing.

the nose into the stomach) for several weeks until they become strong enough to nurse. Ideally, the doctor in your hospital's preterm unit will graduate your baby directly from gavage to breast. In the United States this often happens when an infant reaches a weight between three and four pounds. Some hospitals, however, still require preterm babies to suck first from a bottle to demonstrate their ability to feed; only when they're taking a bottle at every feeding are they permitted to nurse at the breast.

Neonatologists disagree on the best milk for the very small preterm baby. Small preemies grow fastest when fed special, high-protein formulas. This, however, taxes their bodies' capacities to dispose of the end products of the high-protein intakes. Furthermore, this route deprives them of the protective factors in breast milk. In many hospitals, preterm babies receive human milk fortified with protein, calcium, and sodium in amounts that would meet intrauterine needs.

Whether your baby will be fed your own breast milk or a special high-protein formula depends, again, on your baby's size and strength, and also on your doctor's and your hospital medical staff's philosophy. You may want to offer your health care providers literature on the benefits of breast milk for preterm babies.* Ultimately, of course, you will follow the procedures recommended by your doctor.

Why Your Milk Is Best

Because of recent research findings, more physicians now favor feeding preterm babies their own mothers' milk. This is because we now know that the milk of women who bear preterm babies differs in several ways from the milk produced by women who deliver at term. Mothers of preterm babies produce milk specifically designed for their own babies at the infants' stage of development.

Your milk is better for your baby than the milk he could get from a milk bank, which pools the milk from different women (usually mothers of older full-term babies, who are producing more than their own babies need). It is also better for a preterm baby than a standard formula. As we said earlier, however, if your baby is very tiny, a specially fortified formula may be required until he gains some weight.

Compared to the milk of a mother of a full-term baby, the milk of a mother of a preterm baby is easier to digest and better constituted for developing the preterm baby's brain and nervous system. Milk from mothers of preemies has higher levels of nitrogen, protein, sodium, and chloride than full-term milk, and lower lactose content than full-term milk. It provides more energy for the preterm infant's growth needs than mature milk. It also has a high level of *lipase,* an enzyme that aids in fat absorption. In some studies, preemies who received a combination of low-birthweight formula and their own mothers' fresh, unheated milk absorbed fat better than those fed heat-sterilized human milk or formula alone. Since preterm babies need to put on fat, this is an important advantage.

In fact, one way of helping low-birthweight babies gain weight on breast milk involves having the mother pump her milk, and then dividing that milk into the fore milk and the hind milk. The fore milk, which is expressed first, is frozen for later use, while the baby gets the hind

---

*Such literature is available from La Leche League International. See the Resource Appendix.

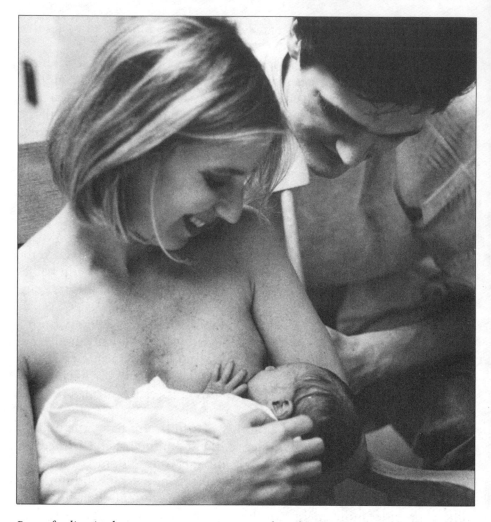

Breastfeeding in the preterm nursery is easier when there's a comfortable chair and a privacy screen for mother and a welcoming attitude toward father.

milk, which is three to four times higher in fat and thus also higher in calories.

If your baby will not be able to receive your breast milk right away—whether for a few days or several weeks—you should begin expressing your milk as soon as possible after the baby's birth. Arrange to rent a hospital-grade electric pump so that you can continue pumping after you go home. This will enable you to build up your milk supply toward the day your baby will be able to nurse, and will provide a supply of breast milk to be given to your baby either now or as supplemental feedings in the future. See Chapter 17 for suggestions on pumping your milk.

Why Breastfeeding Is Good for You, Too

Parents of preterm babies experience a jumble of upsetting emotions. You're likely to be disappointed, worried, confused, and exhausted until the day you feel your baby is out of danger and will survive, healthy and happy. All these feelings are normal. It will be easier for you to get through these early, difficult times if you get as much support as you can, take as good care of yourself as you can, remind yourself that medicine can do more today for preterm babies than ever before, and look forward to the day when your baby will have made up for his hurry to come into this world.

Many women find that offering their milk to their babies makes them feel like better mothers, knowing they're providing a special resource that no one else can give. And you don't need to make a long-term commitment to breastfeed. Even if your preterm baby gets breast milk for only a week or two, she will benefit, and you'll know that you contributed something very special to this small life. All the time, keep your ultimate goal in mind— mothering a healthy, happy baby and enjoying the relationship.

If you want to breastfeed, tell your baby's doctor right away and ask for help in doing it. She or he is the one who makes arrangements for your baby to receive your expressed milk or for you to come in to nurse your baby. The two of you will be in close daily touch about your baby's progress. You'll find it easier to nurse your preterm baby if you follow the guidelines given below.

Link Up with a Support System

As soon as possible, contact your childbirth educator, an organization for parents of babies with special needs, a local La Leche League leader, or another mother who has breastfed a preterm baby. Your doctor or nurse may be able to put you in touch with a support person.

Let your family and friends know that you plan to breastfeed your baby because you believe that breast milk is the best thing for a preemie. Surround yourself with people who will help and encourage you; stay as far away as you can from those who question and doubt.

Before Your Baby Is Able to Nurse

Ask hospital personnel what arrangements can be made to feed your baby your own expressed milk—where and how you should bring it, how it will be stored, both at home and in the hospital, and so forth.

• Rent an automatic, hospital-grade electric breast pump, which is the most efficient and comfortable way to express milk (see Chapter 17).

• Begin to express or pump milk on the day after your baby is born. Even though your mature milk will not yet be in, your colostrum will be, with its special immunity-boosting properties.

• Try to express your milk every two and a half to three hours. This will build up your production now and in the future. You can freeze any extra milk for use later on (see Chapter 17).

• If the hospital is feeding your baby a special high-calorie formula and you're expressing only to maintain your milk supply until he will be able to nurse, a pumping frequency of every four hours may be enough. You can freeze this milk for use later on. If you are supplying most or all of your baby's milk, you will want to pump oftener.

• Find out your own best way to manage nighttime expression. Some women produce more milk if they sleep longer at night, while others do better if they wake up once or twice during the night to pump.

• Don't be discouraged if you're not producing as much milk as you would like. Once your baby begins to nurse, he will stimulate your breasts to help you make more. Meanwhile, whatever you're giving him contains precious antibodies, nutrients, and enzymes.

• Don't be alarmed about ups and downs in your milk supply. Every woman has them; women who express their milk are more aware of the variations.

• Expect a drop in your milk supply if you're still pumping after several weeks, because no pump stimulates the breasts the way a baby does. Your production will rise again once your baby begins to nurse.

• If your baby is being fed by bottle, she should be using the kind of soft rubber nipple made especially for preterm babies.

• You may begin to ovulate and menstruate during the time you're pumping your breasts, since pumping does not stimulate the breasts as much as a baby's suckling. Once your baby is nursing regularly, your menses may stop again, not to resume for several months. Either way, you need to be aware that it is possible to get pregnant at this time (see Chapter 13).

Breastfeeding Your Preterm Baby in the Hospital

Nursing your very small baby is not that different from nursing a baby delivered at term, although you may need to adjust your nursing positions to accommodate her small size and to help her a little more than you would if she were bigger.

If your hospital will not let your baby leave the nursery to breastfeed, ask whether there's a special place where you can nurse in privacy. Many hospitals now have separate rooms for this purpose; others will provide

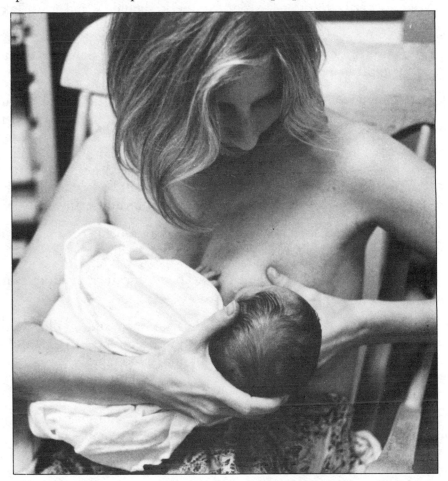

This mother is helping her preterm baby by the way she holds him and her breast. She keeps his head steady as she supports and guides her breast. She is using the "transition position," described in Chapter 6.

screens in the nursery. Ideally, this place will protect the baby from distracting sounds, lights, and activity.

• Choose a time when your baby is awake and alert, but is not yet crying from hunger. It's also best if she has not just come from a stressful and tiring experience like having blood drawn.

• Ask for a comfortable armchair, with support for your back, arms, and feet.

• Get into a comfortable position. Put one or two pillows on your lap to raise your baby to breast height.

• Make a special effort to relax your face, neck, shoulders, and arms. Take a few slow, deep breaths before you begin.

• Ask a nurse or lactation consultant to help you position your baby and to sit with you the first few times.

• Experiment with different positions. You will need to support your baby's entire body, and especially his head. The clutch (football) hold is good for tiny babies. So is the transition position. Another good position involves extending your arm (the one opposite the breast you're nursing) under your baby's back and neck and holding his head steady with your hand. Then move him to a half-upright position. His body should not be flexed; his spine should be straight so that he can breathe easily.

• Make your nipple as easy as possible to grasp, pinching it to make it longer. (If necessary, wear breast shells before the feeding.)

• Use your thumb and forefinger to keep the breast away from your baby's nose and to support your breast.

• If you're not sure whether your baby can suck and swallow well enough, offer a breast from which milk has just been expressed so that the flow of liquid into your baby's mouth will not be too rapid.

• Express a few drops of milk into your baby's mouth to whet her appetite.

• Consider the first few nursings "practice feeds," and give your baby plenty of time. If your baby does no more than lick the nipple a few times, count this as a good beginning. Even full-term babies often take a while to learn how to suck; preterm babies need extra learning time.

• If your baby falls asleep at your breast, try burping him and switching to the other breast. Or offer the other breast after an hour or two.

• Expect the first few feedings to be short, possibly only two or three minutes, since a small baby tires easily. Feeding activity is likely to vary from day to day, and if your baby does not nurse long, you can use the rest of your time together to hold her and to be available if she does express interest in nursing more.

• Push to stay with your baby as much as possible. If the hospital is far from your home, try to find temporary lodging nearby so you can visit your baby frequently every day. This will also give you more opportunities to give your baby that energizing, growth-enhancing special ingredient— your loving touch.

• If your baby has to stay in the hospital much longer than you do, try to obtain permission to stay overnight for a few nights just before his discharge. This will help you learn his rhythms and begin to establish breast-feeding while you still have the nurses to help you. If there are no regular facilities, ask whether you can sleep on a portable cot or a reclining chair in a room not used in the evening and night, such as an office or a conference or treatment room.

• A growing number of hospitals are letting parents stay with their babies, either before initial discharge or upon a child's later admission to the hospital. If this is impossible, you may still be able to visit several times a day and nurse your baby at those times, and pump or express your milk at the times of any missed feedings.

• If your baby needs supplements to your milk, ask whether they can be given by gavage or by cup instead of bottles, to minimize nipple confusion.

When Your Baby Comes Home

This is an exciting—and often scary—day, especially if the two of you have been separated for some time. Remember, though, that the hospital would not have discharged your baby if the physicians who were caring for him did not believe that he was ready to go home. He will have some catch-up growing to do, and his parents are the ones who can help him do this, in their own home.

You can do a number of things to make this period easier:

• Keep your rented breast pump for at least a month after the homecoming, and maybe longer. If your baby has too weak a suck to give your breasts enough stimulation, pumping after feedings will help you build your milk production. It will also give you additional milk to supplement nursings if you need to.

• Nurse frequently—every one and a half or two hours for the first day or two, then every two to three hours (eight to ten times a day).

• See a lactation specialist for careful assessment of your baby's abilities.

• If you need to supplement, use a nursing supplementer (see Chapter 15), a teaspoon, a cup, or an eyedropper. Or put some milk on your clean finger and let your baby suck it off. If you can avoid giving your baby a bottle, both you and he will be better off. If you do need to give him a bottle, offer one and a half to two ounces of milk in a separate feeding, not immediately after a nursing. (Giving a bottle immediately after a nursing conditions the baby to wait for the bottle.) Gradually eliminate these supplementary bottles.

• Take good care of yourself. Sleep when your baby does; get as much help as possible with the housework; take as long a leave from work as you can. Try not to do anything but feed your baby until he is stronger and the breastfeeding is well established (which may not be until your baby's actual due date, or later).

• Be patient. As your baby gets closer to his originally expected due date or to a weight considered healthy for a full-term baby, he will become a more eager and efficient nurser. When this happens, you will be able to stop supplementing and pumping.

Kangaroo Care

Over the past couple of decades, more and more preterm infants have benefited from research showing that they thrive from a kind of care that is physically and psychologically sound—and simple and cost-free. This care involves skin-to-skin contact between baby and parent in a position similar to that of the joey in the mother kangaroo's pouch. In "kangaroo care," an infant, clad only in a diaper and hat, is held against his breastfeeding mother's bare skin. The baby's body and the mother's exposed skin are covered by a blanket or loose-fitting shirt or gown to maintain body heat.

In the most complete version of this care, the mother serves as the infant's "incubator," as well as his main source of food and stimulation. She keeps her baby for many hours a day in an upright position, skin-to-skin against her chest, until he shows he wants to move by crying and moving his arms and legs.

This kind of care produces almost magical results, especially with regard to breastfeeding and infant development. The mothers produce more milk and breastfeed longer, and the babies have more oxygen in their blood, are calmer, and breathe better. Although most of the research has involved preterm babies, the bonding and closeness that result from this intimate contact would be good for babies of any size.

More and more hospitals are integrating some form of kangaroo care for their preterm babies, and fathers often participate as well. As one father said, "When you hold a baby in a blanket, you can hardly see the baby. In the kangaroo technique it's not just a bundle; it's a baby!"

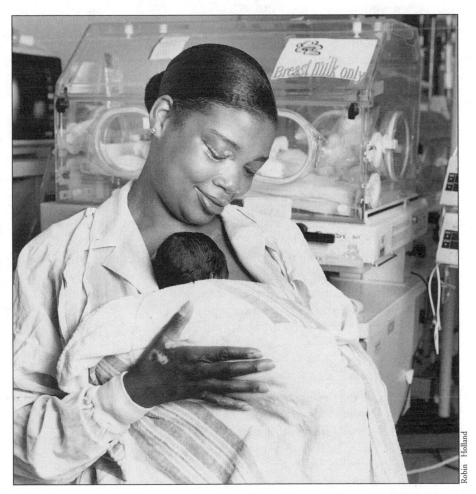

Robin Holland

With the skin-to-skin contact permitted by "kangaroo care," preterm babies breast-feed better and also enjoy other health benefits.

SEPARATION OF MOTHER AND BABY

Prematurity is not the only time when mother and baby may be apart for a while. Occasionally emergencies come up that separate a breastfeeding mother and her baby for a period of days or weeks. If you want to continue nursing past this separation, it can be done. During the separation, pump or express your milk at about the time that your baby would ordinarily be nursing. When you get together again, it may take a week or more before you resume the kind of schedule you had before. You may need to nurse more frequently for a while to build up your supply and to comfort your baby.

If you want to wean your baby before the separation, plan ahead, if possible, so that you can do it gradually. If you do wean, you may be able to relactate later, as described at the end of this chapter.

IF YOUR BABY GETS SICK

In most cases, breastfeeding is the best thing you can do for your sick baby. For one thing, it will provide her with protective antibodies. And because breast milk is extremely digestible, it is the ideal nutritional substance for a baby with a gastrointestinal disorder. Breast milk is probably the best fluid to give a baby with diarrhea, since the fat, carbohydrates, and proteins in your milk can be easily broken down in your infant's digestive tract, and its nutrients and antibodies quickly absorbed into your infant's bloodstream.

If your baby has to be hospitalized, obtain permission to stay with him and to nurse him in the hospital. If your baby needs surgery, you should be able to nurse him up to three hours before the operation. If it's impossible for you to nurse your baby, see whether you can rent an electric pump so that you can express your milk and resume breastfeeding when your baby returns home. See Chapter 17 for suggestions for pumping your milk and feeding it to your baby.

If your baby needs to be in the neonatal intensive care unit right after birth, many of the suggestions given for preterm babies at the beginning of this chapter may also apply to your situation.

IF YOU GET SICK

If you have some condition that raises questions about your ability to nurse, or the advisability of your nursing, ask your doctor and your baby's doctor if they think it's all right for you to breastfeed. You might also check with La Leche League International (see the Resource Appendix), which is apt to have the most current information on medical issues.

If you must be hospitalized, and if your condition permits, you may be able to have your baby come to stay with you in your room or at least visit you in the hospital. If this is impossible, ask your doctor to leave orders and make arrangements so that you can pump your breasts regularly during your hospital stay. Meanwhile, your baby can be fed by bottle or cup, either with your own breast milk that you have previously expressed and frozen or with formula.

Women with colds, flu, pneumonia, urinary tract or respiratory tract infections, or intestinal upsets can nurse their babies. In fact, doing so helps to protect their babies from the organisms causing the mother's illness. In addition, as of this writing, recommendations can be made for the following conditions.

Herpes

Two kinds of herpes virus that can be passed from mother to baby during vaginal delivery are cytomegalovirus (CMV) and herpes simplex virus (HSV). CMV, the commoner, less harmful kind, can also be transmitted through breast milk. This does not pose a problem to the typical full-term newborn; in fact, it may help the baby develop antibodies to the virus. However, CMV can pose a problem for preterm infants.

HSV, which carries more risks for a baby, does not seem to be transmitted through breast milk, but it can be passed to a baby who comes into direct contact with a herpes sore on the mother's breast. The herpes simplex virus can cause cold sores or fever blisters on the lips, face, mouth, or breast, or the same type of sore in the genital area. It can be spread through sexual relations with someone who has an active infection, or from an infected person's mouth to her own genitals or eyes if she touches the sores with her fingers, or from an infected baby to the mother if the baby has a lesion in the mouth.

While much research still needs to be done on this condition, at this time the following guidelines seem useful:

- If you do not have herpes, don't have sexual relations with anyone in an active stage of the disease, especially while you're pregnant or breastfeeding.

- If you have already contracted herpes, get periodic exams and cultures before delivery. If you have an active outbreak, or are in the stage just before sores are apt to break out, tell your doctor. It may be safest for you to have a cesarean birth.

- If you're having an outbreak right after delivery, be careful that your baby does not come into contact with any sores or with clothing that has been worn over them. Wash your hands very carefully after you use the toilet, after you touch your sores, and before you hold your baby. When you hold your baby, drape a clean towel or robe over your lap. You do not need to wear gloves while you nurse.

- If you have sores on your breast, postpone nursing your newborn on that breast until they are fully healed. Until then, express or pump your milk (to maintain your supply) and throw it away; in the meantime feed your baby on the other breast or by bottle or cup.

- If you have a sore on your mouth, do not kiss your baby—or anyone else.

- Your doctor may prescribe an antiviral drug like acyclovir or vidabarine. You may continue to nurse while taking either of these medications—provided you do not have active lesions on your breast.

- If you have an active outbreak when your baby is older, continue to nurse, as long as you can keep your baby's mouth from touching any sores.

Hepatitis B

This virus, which affects about 150,000 Americans each year, appears in breast milk, but there is no evidence that it has ever been passed to a nursing infant. Therefore, there is no reason for mothers who carry this virus not to breastfeed. The chances are that the baby of a mother who has hepatitis B will have already been exposed to the virus during pregnancy or delivery.

In any case, all newborns now receive immunization against hepatitis B immediately after birth to protect them from contracting the condition. The baby of a hepatitis B carrier should receive both the active vaccine and the passive hepatitis B hyperimmune globulin. However, even if the infant was not immunized, there is no reason for a mother who is a carrier not to breastfeed. Since each case is different, however, if you suspect or know that you have been exposed to hepatitis B, you should discuss your situation with your baby's doctor.

Hepatitis C

This virus may begin with a mild infection and flu-like symptoms, or it may carry no symptoms at all for years. Then a person carrying the infection may feel tired all the time, lose her appetite, become jaundiced, and suffer abdominal pain, nausea, and/or vomiting. Breastfed babies of mothers with hepatitis C have about the same incidence of the virus as do formula-fed infants. There is no evidence that breastfeeding increases the risk of an infant's acquiring the infection from the mother.

However, when a mother is feeling ill due to an active outbreak of the infection, her pediatrician may advise her to interrupt nursing and to pump her milk until her symptoms go away.

Human Immunodeficiency Virus (HIV) or Acquired Immune Deficiency Syndrome (AIDS)

There is strong evidence that a mother who is HIV-positive—that is, who has been infected with the virus that can cause AIDS—can pass the virus to her child through her milk. Although some research suggests that the risk of a child's contracting at least one type of human immunodeficiency virus (HIV-1) by breastfeeding is low even if the mother was infected with it prenatally, most public health advocates (including the American Academy of Pediatrics, the World Health Organization, and the United States Centers for Disease Control) advise against an HIV-infected mother's breastfeeding when a safe alternative is available.

Breast Cancer

A number of research studies have tried to find a correlation between breast cancer and breastfeeding. The best available evidence follows:

• Women who breastfeed are less likely to develop breast cancer before menopause (see Chapter 1). In China, where women routinely breastfeed for three years, breast cancer is also less common among older, postmenopausal women who nursed their babies.

• There is no evidence that women transmit any cancer-causing factors to their babies through breast milk.

• If a malignant tumor is found in a pregnant or lactating woman, its surgical removal should be carried out immediately. Waiting can be dangerous for the mother. Breastfeeding can safely continue through most diagnostic tests—including mammograms, ultrasound, and biopsy. However, if radioactive isotope testing is performed, nursing will have to be interrupted. The mother should express her milk and discard it until the radioactive elements are gone from her body. If a biopsy is performed, the mother should ask her surgeon to avoid cutting the milk ducts.

• It is more difficult to get a good image in a mammogram during lactation and for four to six weeks after weaning, although a skilled radiologist can often achieve good results. If your doctor urges you to wean your child so you can get a mammogram, you have a decision to make.

If there is a sound medical reason (for example, if you have a suspicious lump on your breast), you will probably want to wean, or at least interrupt, breastfeeding. However, if your doctor just wants you to have a baseline mammogram because of your age or family history, you will want to consider your child's readiness for weaning or need for continued nursing, and discuss this with your doctor so that you can come to the wisest decision for you and your child.

• A woman who has had a breast surgically removed because of a diagnosis of breast cancer may continue to nurse from the other breast, with no apparent risk to her child. However, if she is receiving chemotherapy, she will have to wean the baby, since the drugs used in this treatment may be dangerous for the baby. Fortunately, breast cancer rarely occurs in pregnant or nursing women.

At one time physicians advised women who had breast cancer not to get pregnant and not to breastfeed, because both these activities were thought to stimulate hormones that seemed to activate cancer cells. Several large studies have shown, however, that pregnancy after diagnosis of breast cancer does not increase the chance of the cancer's recurrence and does not affect the woman's survival rate.

• Although breast cancer is extremely rare in nursing women, it can occur. The danger of missing a diagnosis of breast cancer during lactation is that lumps in the breast may be attributed to nursing-related causes and may not be sufficiently investigated to determine whether they are malignant. It is important to check with a physician any lump that remains unchanged for more than three days.

• Research performed to date suggests that if there is any relationship at all between breastfeeding and breast cancer, it is in the direction of lactation's offering protection to the mother.

• One type of breast lump that is benign and does not require surgery is a galactocele, or milk-retention cyst, described in Chapter 15.

BREAST SURGERY

If you have had surgery to make your breasts either larger or smaller, you may be able to breastfeed, depending on the kind of procedures that were followed. In recent years more plastic surgeons have made efforts not to sever or block the milk ducts. For specific information, ask the physician who performed your surgery. Even if you're doubtful, go ahead and try to breastfeed. It can't hurt your baby. Lactation may well proceed normally, and if it doesn't, you can always switch to formula. Meanwhile, watch your baby closely to be sure she is getting enough milk and gaining weight appropriately.

Breast Augmentation

If you had silicone or saline implants to make your breasts larger and if the implants do not come into contact with mammary tissue, as most do not, and if the duct system in your breasts remains intact after the surgery, you can most probably breastfeed. The procedures in common use today do not damage the milk ducts, since the implant is usually placed beneath the mammary gland or the gland and muscle and is therefore far away from the ducts.

There is no published research showing the presence of silicone in human milk, but even if some of the silicone did leak into the milk, this should not be harmful, since the substance is very similar to the main ingredient in a medication often given to babies who are troubled by excess stomach gas. There is no evidence that any babies have been harmed by nursing at breasts that contain implants.

If you have implants, you should ask your surgeon what kind you received, who manufactured it and when, and whether any complications have shown up with this type of implant.

Breast Reduction

If you have had surgery to make your breasts smaller and if the nipple/areola complex has not been severed during the operation, you can probably breastfeed. While the newer procedures are more likely to permit breastfeeding than previous techniques did, there's still a significant chance that any breast reduction may interfere with your ability to nurse. If, for example, your nipple has been removed and replaced on the reconstructed breast, the milk ducts and nerves will have been cut and breastfeeding may be impossible. If you're considering this surgery, it's safest to wait until after your childbearing years if you want to be sure you can nurse your babies.

PIERCED NIPPLES

If you had one or both nipples pierced, you should still be able to breast-feed your baby. There might, however, be a problem if there was any scar-ring, either internal or external, if an infection occurred at the time of piercing or during the initial healing. Occasionally some milk leaks through the site of the piercing, but since the hole is usually quite small, this should not interfere with nursing. If there is any question at all about whether your baby is nursing well (check signs of suckling and adequate milk intake in Chapter 6), consult a lactation specialist.

If you wear a nipple ring, you should remove it for as long as you are breastfeeding. This is especially important if the ring is large, since a very large ring can prevent a baby from being able to get his mouth around the nipple and areola as fully as he needs to to latch on properly. Removal of even a smaller ring will make nursing easier for your baby, and of course will eliminate any possibility of your baby swallowing the ring.

TWINS AND MORE

When Bobbi McCaughey of Carlisle, Iowa, told the doctors caring for her septuplets, who were born November 19, 1997, that she wanted to pro-vide breast milk for them, the neonatalogist in charge said, "We are com-mitted to providing as much milk as she is able to come up with to all of the babies." This indeed showed confidence in the benefits of breast milk! Even though it would be a major challenge for this mother to breastfeed all seven septuplets, whatever breast milk these tiny babies received would be a bonus.

But what about twins? If you deliver two babies, one question is moot: You don't have to wonder if you should offer one or both breasts at a feed-ing. You have been designed with perfect efficiency for just this possibility. Furthermore, since breastfeeding operates on a supply-and-demand princi-ple, your breasts will produce ample supplies of milk for both babies. Since babies born in multiples are likely to be small, they derive special benefits from breast milk.

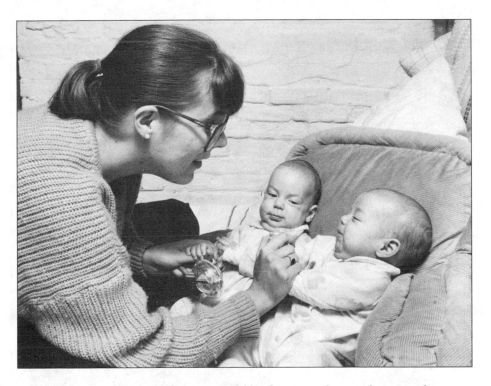

When both twins are about the same size, like these two, they can be on similar schedules, leaving more time free just for play.

You'll probably find it easiest to nurse both babies simultaneously for most early feedings (see the box on page 330). However, you'll want to nurse them individually occasionally, so that each one will have a chance from time to time to enjoy your undivided attention. Then there will be times when one twin is desperately hungry—and the other sound asleep. As a general rule, you can try letting the hungrier twin set the pattern. When you're about to feed him, wake his twin at the same time. This works best, of course, if both babies are about the same size.

Try to alternate breasts and babies, so that the same twin doesn't always drink at the same fount. This way, if one baby nurses more vigorously than the other, both your breasts will be stimulated.

You'll have to work out your own individual schedule. Some mothers nurse twins or even triplets totally, never giving any of the babies a bottle. Others alternate bottles of formula right from the start, rotating between breast and formula. Thus, baby A gets the breast at one feeding, baby B the bottle; they switch at the next feeding. You need to weigh the benefits of breast milk for your babies with the demands on your own energy and time,

Nursing Two Babies at the Same Time

When breastfeeding two babies simultaneously, position is everything. Ask someone to help you get the babies set for the first few times, as in the positions described below. Experiment until you and the babies are comfortable. Find a comfortable armchair and a couple of pillows. Then try one of these:

• Half-recline and lay each baby on his or her side or stomach lengthwise along your body.

• Sit up and tuck each baby under an arm, heads resting on firm pillows on your lap and feet by your back (the clutch hold).

• Hold baby A on your lap and crisscross baby B across baby A's body.

• Hold baby A on your lap and tuck baby B under your arm.

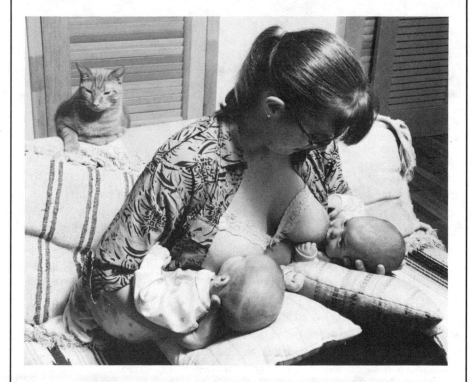

Some mothers prefer to nurse both twins at the same time; others find it easier and more satisfying to feed one baby at a time. This mother is nursing both babies in the clutch hold.

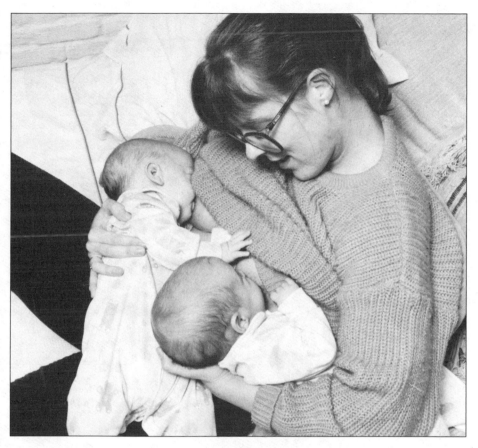

Here, the mother combines the clutch and transitional positions.

and do what's best. For special sources of help for mothers of multiples, see the Resource Appendix.

NURSING THROUGH A PREGNANCY AND TANDEM NURSING AFTERWARD

If you become pregnant while you're nursing, your baby may decide to wean, either because your milk tastes different or because there's less of it. Or you may take the initiative in weaning your nursling because of breast or nipple pain, because you're tired, or because you're uncomfort-

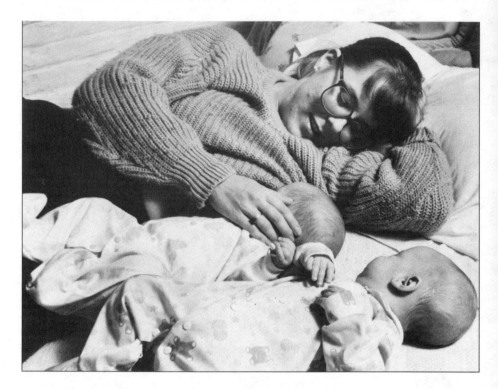

Sometimes one twin is hungrier than the other; if either develops a preference for one breast, this may result in temporary lopsidedness, but the mother eventually resumes her symmetry.

able with the idea. Around the world, a new pregnancy is among the commonest reasons for weaning. Some women do, however, continue to breastfeed throughout pregnancy, and continue to nurse both the older child and the infant afterward. This latter practice is known as "tandem" nursing.

Why do mothers do this? They cite the continued needs of the older child, whose emotional need for nursing is heightened rather than lessened by the arrival of the new baby. Then, the mothers themselves sometimes find that they're not ready to sever the nursing tie. Still, tandem nursing mothers often have ambivalent feelings, sometimes resenting the older child, questioning the wisdom of what they're doing, and dealing with the doubled demands on their body.

Some of the challenges facing such a mother include the need for extra nutrition and extra rest, which she needs first because of the pregnancy and then because of the nursing infant. While she's pregnant, she needs to find comfortable nursing positions and maternity clothes compatible with nursing. Women with a history of miscarriage are often advised to wean their nursing babies before becoming pregnant again, since some reports have indicated that nipple stimulation can induce labor.

After the new baby is born, the mother needs to ensure that the new baby gets his rightful share of the colostrum and the milk and she needs to be aware of the danger of cross-infection between both children. Most women who nurse a baby and a toddler take pains to nurse the infant first. Many use explanations, agreements, and delaying tactics to lessen the number of times the older child nurses. (Some of these are suggested in Chapter 18.)

Tandem nursing is not a decision to be undertaken lightly, and it is not for everyone. There's no evidence, however, that the practice is harmful to the new baby, either while in the womb or after birth, if his needs are kept paramount.

RELACTATION AND NURSING AN ADOPTED BABY

Sometimes a woman decides, or is advised, not to breastfeed her newborn infant; or she begins to nurse and then stops for one reason or another. Then, as soon as one week or as late as several months later, she wants to nurse—either because her baby has grown stronger and is now able to nurse, because he has a digestive or allergic problem that makes it difficult for him to take formula, or for some other reason. In such a case, it is often possible to initiate breastfeeding. This process is known as *relactation.*

In other cases, women who have adopted babies have been able to lactate, even if they have never been pregnant or have not been pregnant for years. This process is called *induced lactation.*

Neither of these endeavors is easy; both call for a great deal of time, effort, and dedication. Both also require very close observation of the baby to be sure he is gaining weight properly. Many women who have made the effort, however, have been happy with their decision, especially if they look at it not for its value as a feeding method, but for how it can enhance the mother-baby relationship. This is the most important aspect of this kind of nursing. If you hold up quantifiable measures like the amount of milk you produce, the ability to provide *all* of your baby's milk, or the length of time you nurse your baby, you may be disappointed and frustrated. Based on several studies of women who have done this, the

Succeeding at Induced Lactation or Relactation

- Ask yourself *why* you want to do this. If you'll be happy with the experience of nurturing your baby *at* your breast, and not necessarily nourishing him *from* your breast, you're likely to have a more positive experience than if you have your heart set on providing a set amount of milk. It's very rare for all of a baby's nutritional needs to be met with induced lactation and may even be difficult with relactation.

- Be prepared for a stressful first few weeks, during which time your baby may resist suckling at the breast, your milk may be slow in coming in, and you'll be nursing almost constantly around the clock and supplementing your baby's diet with formula.

- Find a support system, consisting of people who will encourage and help you through the difficult days. These people can include your husband, doctor, lactation consultant, La Leche League leader, and, most important, another woman who has done what you want to do, either relactated or nursed an adopted baby.

- You'll find it easiest to relactate if your baby is under three months old.

- Expect initial resistance from your baby, who is used to getting milk some other way. It may take ten days or longer for him to nurse well, but after that he is very likely to become an avid nurser. Don't give up too soon.

- Nipple stimulation is the most important mechanism for bringing in your milk. The best kind of stimulation is your baby's suckling. Other techniques include breast massage and hand-expression or breast pumps. (Expressed milk can be fed through a nursing supplementer.)

- Nurse your baby frequently, whenever she shows any signs of hunger, such as increased alertness or activity, smacking her lips, making sucking motions, or moving her head around in search of the breast. Do not wait until your baby begins to cry, which is a late sign of hunger. In one study, most of the relactating babies nursed eight times a day, at intervals of two to three hours, with two

guidelines given in the box above should help you and your baby to achieve a happy nursing relationship.

For some of the situations in this chapter—the ones that require separation from your baby—you will want to collect your milk to give to her.

night feedings. (This is an average; some babies need to nurse more often than this at the beginning.) The average duration of each feeding was about twenty to twenty-five minutes.

• The most popular form of supplementing the baby's diet is the use of a nursing supplementer (see Chapter 15 and the Resource Appendix). This ensures your baby of adequate nutrition while providing stimulation to your nipples. Many women who considered their experience highly successful continued to use a supplementer throughout the course of breastfeeding.

• It is extremely important to have your doctor follow your baby carefully for adequate weight gain. The suggestions given in the section beginning on page 118 will help you and the doctor assess whether your baby is being well enough nourished for healthy development.

TECHNIQUES THAT ARE HELPFUL INCLUDE:

• Increasing your fluid intake and the amount of protein in your diet;
• Resting as much as possible, and lying down to nurse when you can;
• Asking your doctor to prescribe a drug like metoclopramide, chlorpromazine, or theophylline for the first week or so, which sometimes helps to increase milk supply;
• Stroking your baby while she's nursing to help you relax and let down your milk; and
• Providing as much skin contact as possible between you and your baby. (See the description of "kangaroo care" earlier in this chapter.)
• Also see the suggestions given on page 308 for encouraging a baby who's gone "on strike" to nurse.

TECHNIQUES THAT ARE NOT HELPFUL INCLUDE:

• Keeping the baby hungry to try to encourage him to nurse;
• Using nipple shields; and,
• For adoptive mothers, trying to stimulate the breasts with the nursing infants of friends (the babies usually refuse to suckle at a breast that's not producing milk).

The next chapter describes the different ways you can do this and offers a number of suggestions for making it easier for you to give your baby the benefits of breast milk even during those times when she cannot nurse directly.

Expressing and Storing Breast Milk

At first the idea of collecting my milk to feed to my baby seemed like an insurmountable obstacle. When I first tried to express I was so frustrated I burst into tears. But I got the knack of it in a little while, and now both my baby and I are grateful for this "liquid gold."

PATRICIA, ANCHORAGE, ALASKA

T hroughout this book we have talked about situations in which you might want to express or pump your milk to give to your baby. This chapter provides practical, "how-to" suggestions that have worked for other nursing mothers, which you can adapt for yourself. Working nursing mothers will find specific suggestions for their situation in Chapter 12; mothers of premature or sick babies will find help in Chapters 15 and 16.

There are several ways of collecting breast milk—by electric pump, by manual (handheld) pump, and by hand-expression (using your hands to get your milk flowing and into a container). The method you decide on will depend on your own individual needs and preferences, based on your own unique situation, as well as on your comfort, convenience, and pocketbook.

In recent years manufacturers have responded to the double trend of rising breastfeeding rates and rising numbers of working mothers by producing a wide variety of pumps. Although many women still prefer to express their milk by hand (and this is a valuable skill to learn), the pumps are often quicker and more efficient for working nursing mothers, as well as for women in other situations calling for temporary collection of breast milk. First we'll talk about the different kinds of pumps; then we'll offer guidelines for hand-expression.

There are a bewildering number of different pumps to choose from, and although we provide a general overall view of the most popular types, it is impossible for any book to remain completely up to date on the available products.

To help you decide on the type of pump to use, see the box on page 338 and the information that follows.

CHOOSING A PUMP

Let's look at the three basic types of pumps: the electric, the battery-operated, and the manual or hand-operated.

The best way to decide on the particular model to use is to find out which pumps women seem to be happiest with. Ask a lactation consultant, other nursing mothers, or your local La Leche League leader, or contact the companies listed in the Resource Appendix. When speaking to their representatives (some have lactation consultants on staff), ask them to send information about their products. To locate up-to-date information, you can search the Internet (a good combination of words is "breastfeeding *and* pump"). Start your research a few weeks before you plan to pump, if possible.

If you will be pumping your milk every day to be given to your baby while you are at school or work, you will want to see the suggestions in Chapter 12 about the equipment you'll need and the pumping schedule you may want to follow.

Electric Pump

Hospital-grade fully automatic electric pumps, which allow you to collect milk from both breasts simultaneously, are the easiest, fastest, most comfortable, and most efficient way to collect breast milk. They control suction to simulate a baby's suckling action, and while they're doing the work, you can read, watch television, or do paperwork.

If you are collecting your milk for a premature or sick baby who cannot yet nurse, if you plan to collect milk to be fed to your baby while you are at work, or if you plan for some other reason to collect your milk for longer than a couple of weeks, this is by far the best way to do it.

What Kind of Pump Do You Need?

The following guidelines* may help you choose the type of pump you use. However, every woman is different, and some women who would fit into the electric-pump category may do just fine with a manual type, whereas others who, according to these guidelines, would fit into the manual category, may prefer a battery-operated or electric pump. Only you can decide which type of pump is right for you and your situation.

YOU PROBABLY WANT TO BUY OR RENT A HOSPITAL-GRADE ELECTRIC PUMP IF:

- You are working or going to school full-time;
- Your baby is preterm or in the hospital for several weeks;
- Your baby has a physical or neurological impairment interfering with her ability to nurse;
- You are trying to increase your milk supply;
- You are trying to relactate or nurse an adopted baby; or
- You are pumping at least half of your baby's daily feedings.

YOU PROBABLY WANT A SMALL ELECTRIC PUMP IF:

- You are working or going to school part-time;
- You are preparing for a brief separation from your baby; or
- You are pumping about one-third of your baby's daily feedings.

YOU CAN PROBABLY GET BY WITH HAND-EXPRESSING OR USING A HAND-OPERATED PUMP IF:

- You are caring for your healthy baby at home; or
- You want to pump milk for an occasional missed feeding.

*These guidelines are based on those developed by White River Concepts.

The biggest drawback is expense. The most popular hospital-grade electric pumps cost about $1,200 to buy. However, they can be rented on a weekly or monthly basis from pharmacies, medical supply houses, hospitals, and childbirth education and La Leche League groups.* It may be well worth the expense to rent an electric pump for a while; it's sometimes possible to get a lower price if you contract to rent over a period of several months. Also, remember that the price of renting is less than the cost of formula for an equivalent time period—and also, the happier you are with your pump, the likelier you are to breastfeed for a longer time.

Smaller (and therefore portable) and less expensive semiautomatic electric pumps are also available. With these pumps the mother regulates the suction and release herself, aided by an electric motor. These models are often the choice of working mothers who will be pumping for several months. One small-size electric breast pump has five settings for suction control. Another has such optional accessories as a carrying case, rechargeable battery, and cable adaptation for use in a car or boat.

Choosing an Electric Pump   How do you know which pump to choose? Two criteria are the number of cycles in a minute and the strength of the suction. The best pumps mimic a baby's suckling very closely.

The most efficient electric pumps, the fully automatic ones that hospitals use and that you can rent, cycle about fifty times a minute, which is comparable to a baby's rhythm. These pumps also mimic a baby's nursing pattern: suck, release, and relax. These high-grade pumps apply strong suction to the breast, comparable to the suction a baby applies.

Lighter-weight pumps, which work by a small motor powered by electricity or batteries, cycle less often. They can sometimes cause sore nipples because they keep the nipple extended for a longer time. Also, since they apply less suction, they require more time to collect milk. However, some women find them satisfactory.

Manual Pump

There are several different types of hand-operated pumps. Some of the most important features to look for include:

• *Gentleness:* It should not hurt your nipples. The pump's breast shield should fit comfortably, so that your nipple does not rub against it.

• *Comfort:* The pumping motions should not put stress on your elbow or forearm muscles.

• *Effectiveness:* It should drain your breast *almost* as well as your baby does and stimulate further production of milk, and it should do this fairly quickly.

• *Safety:* It should be easy to clean so that bacteria do not accumulate to spoil your milk.

---

*For information on purchasing or renting electric pumps, see the Resource Appendix.

• *Portability:* If you plan to carry the pump to and from work, it should be easy to carry.

• *Convenience:* The fewer separate parts, the better. Additional parts should be available without having to buy a new pump or kit.

Types of Hand-Operated Pumps   The following evaluations are based on research, professional opinion, and the comments of women who have used these pumps.

• *Cylinder-type:* Also called a piston- or syringe-type pump, this kind is the most popular handheld nonelectric pump. It's easy to operate, easy to clean, and easy to carry around. It consists of two cylinders, one of which fits inside the other; the pumping is accomplished by moving the outer cylinder up and down; the piston action creates suction. The end of the smaller cylinder fits over the breast, and milk is collected in the larger cylinder, which can then be fitted with a nipple and used as a feeding bottle. Some of these models can be used in conjunction with an electric pump, so that a woman can switch back and forth between manual and electric pumping.

Cylinder-type pumps are relatively inexpensive, and shopping around (by phone or in person) often pays off.

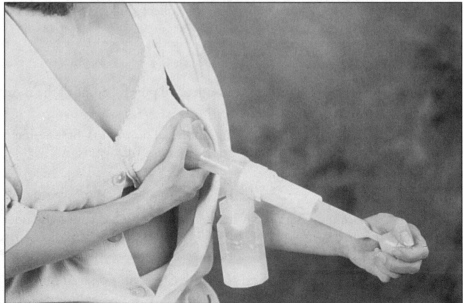

Medela, Inc.

The most popular handheld pump is the cylinder-type, which is available from several different manufacturers.

• *Trigger-type:* The Loyd-B pump, which has been around for years, is shaped like a gun. You put it to the breast and pull a trigger, which creates suction on the breast, making the milk flow into a small baby-food jar. You can control the amount of suction by the force you use to squeeze the trigger. Some women like the pump because they find that it does the job and although bulky, it's small enough to carry to work, easy to clean, and comfortable.

However, it has drawbacks. Because it requires a fair amount of dexterity, the breast opposite the dominant hand (the left breast for right-handed women) gets emptied more efficiently; thus plugged ducts may develop in the other breast. Also, it's hard to use on one breast while you're nursing from the other, and women with small hands have difficulty working it.

• *Bulb-type:* Do *not* buy or use one of these small "bicycle horn" pumps consisting of a glass cup attached to a rubber bulb. They're sold in some drugstores and are the least expensive kind, but are highly unsatisfactory. They are potentially dangerous, because they're so hard to clean that drops of milk cling to them, and mold and bacteria grow. Furthermore, they're hard to use and often uncomfortable since the cup that's supposed to fit over the nipple doesn't press down on the areola. *Stay far away from them.*

Battery-Operated Pumps

With these pumps, you press on a bar or a lever to activate an alternating suction action designed to imitate a baby's suckling. The milk goes into a small nursing bottle that can be refrigerated or frozen. Since these pumps can be operated with one hand, they can be used while nursing. Some can also be adapted to use household current.

Battery-operated pumps sound like a good idea but so far these pumps have not fulfilled their promise. They provide neither the power of an electric nor the control of a hand-operated pump; they're less efficient than the electric and more expensive than the hand-operated; they may be annoyingly noisy; and the high rate at which they use up batteries can drive the cost up considerably. If you need to pump regularly, the battery-operated pump is probably not for you. If you do use one, you should keep two sets of rechargeable batteries on hand so you can always be sure of having fresh batteries.

Hand-Expression

Manual expression is a valuable skill to have since you can do it at any time, without any equipment other than your own body and something to catch the milk. Many mothers prefer it above other methods because it's more natural, and, of course, it doesn't cost anything. However, it requires practice to become proficient, and some women never get milk from this method. Others get so good at it that they wouldn't express any other way. Here's how to do it:

• Wash your hands and be sure your fingernails are clean.

• Before proceeding, massage, stroke, and shake your breasts (see the instructions in the box on page 346).

• Position a clean cup, wide-mouthed jar, or thermos bottle under your breast.

• Hold your breast with your thumb above and your first two fingers below, about an inch or an inch and a half behind the nipple. For most women this is the edge of the areola, but if your areola is narrower or wider, it's the distance from the nipple that counts.

• Push your thumb and fingers together, back toward the chest wall.

• Very gently roll the thumb and fingers forward to empty the milk pools. Do not apply pressure down the breast, since this can bruise your breast tissue.

• Repeat the push-roll sequence a few times until no more drops come out.

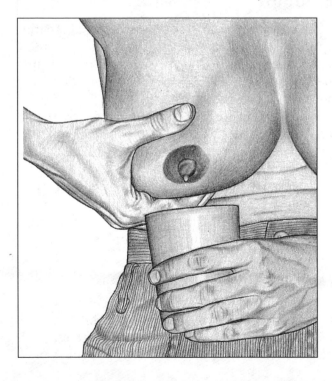

Women who become skillful at expressing milk by hand usually prefer it to any other method.

- Repeat this at several different locastions on your breast. Some places may be better for you than others.

- Do not squeeze or cup the breast, slide your fingers, or pull out the skin on the breast.

- Be sure the milk does not run over your fingers as it flows from your breast.

- If you don't get any milk the first few times, keep trying.

Breast Shells (Milk Cups)

The same kind of breast shells that are sometimes used to bring out inverted nipples (as described in Chapter 4) are marketed as a way to collect milk from one breast while you're nursing or pumping on the other. We do *not* recommend this method for collecting milk, since the milk is too easily contaminated.

PRINCIPLES THAT APPLY TO ALL METHODS OF COLLECTING MILK

1. *Cleanliness.* Before you express or pump by any method, wash your hands with soap and water and clean your fingernails with a good nail brush. Germs on your hands can contaminate the milk you're preparing for your baby.

Rinse your breasts with clean water (no soap, alcohol, or other drying agents) and pat them dry with a clean paper towel. Dry the nipple first and then the rest of the breast; do not let your clothes touch your nipple until after you have finished collecting your milk.

Follow the manufacturer's instructions for keeping your pump clean, and before using the pump for the first time, sterilize the parts as the manufacturer directs. Be sure your containers are clean as well. (See the section "Containers.")

2. *Time and practice are needed to master all the methods.* If you can plan ahead (for example, for going back to work), practice at home for a while before you need to express regularly. Consider the first few times practice sessions, just like an infant's first few feedings. Practice once or twice a day, five minutes on each breast. If you don't get the amount of milk you'd like at first, keep it up. The more you do it, the more efficient you'll become.

At first it may take you up to thirty minutes each session to drain both breasts; eventually you may be able to get it down to eight minutes each time; some women continue to need fifteen to twenty minutes. And the amount of time needed may vary from time to time. The more you practice, the better you'll do.

3. *Effect of timing.* You'll most likely produce more milk early in the day and early in the week. Most women's milk supply tends to drop at about 6:00 P.M. Between 7:00 A.M. and 1:00 P.M. is the best time for the first sessions; late afternoon and early evening are the worst. If you're currently nursing your baby, wait for about an hour after the first morning feeding.

Working women often find that their milk supply diminishes during the week, so that by Friday they're giving less than they did on Monday, when they had the weekend to take things a little easier. Knowing this may help you plan your schedule and accept your body's ability to yield milk.

4. *Taking advantage of your milk-ejection reflex.* Even if you don't pump *during* your baby's feeding, your let-down reflex will help you produce more milk. Some of the suggestions in the box on page 346 will help stimulate your let-down. Give it a chance to get going; don't pump harder or increase the suction in the pump if you don't see any milk coming out. This will just make you uncomfortable and will not produce more milk. Time and practice will improve your efficiency.

5. *Collecting your milk according to your baby's feeding schedule.* Once you've learned the basics of expressing or pumping, try to schedule these sessions at about the times your baby would ordinarily nurse. This will help keep up your supply of milk.

6. *Amount of milk collected.* It is normal for the amount of milk you collect to vary from time to time. Quantity will depend on many factors, including how much time has elapsed since your last nursing or pumping session, what time of day it is, how established your milk supply is, and how proficient you have become.

At first you may get no more than an ounce at a time, but as you increase the frequency of pumping, you will increase your milk yield. The amount of milk pumped does not necessarily reflect how much milk you can give your child, since your nursing baby is more efficient than the best pump. See the suggestions in the box on page 346 for increasing the amount of milk you collect.

7. *Experimenting with breast inserts.* If your pump comes with inserts that fit into the breast shield portion, see which size feels best. You might try pumping with the smaller size first, and then switch to the larger one.

PRINCIPLES THAT APPLY TO ALL PUMPING METHODS

1. *The cost of buying or renting a pump.* Hospital-grade electric pumps are quite expensive, but there are ways to reduce the cost. If your doctor says that breastfeeding is essential for some medical reason (such as your baby's prematurity or allergy to cow's milk) and if pumping is necessary, your medical insurance may cover the cost of buying or renting a pump. Or you may be able to join with other nursing mothers to ask your employer to buy a pump to keep at your place of work. Or you and a friend may rent one that you can share. Although you can share the pump itself with other mothers, you each need your own attachable kit and tubing so that your milk will not come into contact with any surface touched by another mother's milk.

2. *Choosing a pump.* To find the type of pump you like the best, see whether you can borrow different models, either from a friend who isn't using hers at the moment, or from a local hospital, lactation consultant, childbirth education group, or La Leche League chapter. Decide which features are important for you and evaluate the pumps based on your own needs. Take the time to carefully read the manufacturer's instructions for each pump.

3. *Mimicking your baby's suckling action as much as possible.* High-grade electric pumps do this automatically. You can do this to some degree with a manual pump by beginning your pumping with a rhythm of fast, short bursts. Once you feel your milk flowing, you can slow your pace.

4. *Pumping while nursing.* You can take advantage of the ejection of milk that occurs from one breast while the other is being stimulated. Instead of wasting this milk, or looking on it as a nuisance, you can build your milk-collecting program around it. Doing this has another advantage: It tends to increase your milk supply. This double-duty nursing can fool your body into thinking that you're nursing twins; operating by the law of supply and demand, it will produce more milk.

To pump while nursing, first get your baby started at your breast. Prop her on a pillow under the nursing breast. For the first few times, when

Enhancing Milk Production When Expressing or Pumping

You may want to try one or more of the following methods to increase the amount of milk you can collect for your baby. Different ones work well for different women in different situations. If you're pumping at work, for example, some of these suggestions will not apply. As with the rest of this book, take the suggestions that make sense to you, see which ones work, and stick with them.

- First, take care of yourself: Get as much rest as possible, and be sure you're drinking enough liquid throughout the day.
- For two to five minutes before you begin, do deep breathing or some other relaxation exercise.
- Drink a cup of hot tea before beginning. If your baby is not sensitive to cow's milk products that you eat or drink, you might try warm milk or cocoa.
- Make yourself as comfortable as possible. If you can, sit with your feet up.
- If you have time, massage your breasts. Just before you begin, if possible, lay a warm towel on your breasts for a minute or two. (The towel is helpful, but not essential.) Then massage your breasts gently, one at a time, starting from the top and moving around the sides and the bottom, moving your fingers in a circular motion. With your fingertips, stroke yourself lightly from the armpit, from above and below the breast, and from the middle of the chest toward the nipple. You don't need to massage or stroke the nipples themselves. (If necessary, you can massage your breasts even while you're dressed.)

you're ready to pump, ask a helper to hold the pump in position. Then you can use both your hands to hold your baby. After you do this several times, you'll get the hang of it and will be able to do it by yourself.

5. *Getting started.* The first time you express or pump, try to choose a quiet time when you're not likely to be distracted or interrupted. Give yourself as much help as you can. Ask someone to be with you, if possible someone who's done this herself. It's wonderful to have someone to answer the telephone or doorbell, take care of an older child, provide another pair of hands in any way you need them. This person can help you maneuver both the pump and your baby (if your initial pumping is done on the non-baby side while you're nursing on the other side). Then get yourself comfortable—in a chair or couch, with pillows for support. And do whatever you can to relax.

• Pump both breasts at the same time, using a good electric pump.

• If you are expressing one breast at a time, switch breasts at least once during each session and preferably twice to ensure maximum draining. Usually the second expression on each breast is briefer than the first.

• Pump frequently. It's better to schedule three pumping sessions of no more than ten minutes each than to schedule two for fifteen minutes each. It yields more milk, it's more efficient, and it's also more comfortable, since it will cut down the likelihood of trauma from too much pressure exerted for too long a time. Some women get sore nipples from pumping more than seven or eight minutes on a breast.

• Prop a photo of your baby in front of you. Look at it and remember what it feels like (or imagine what it will feel like) to have him at your breast. (Or use a photo of you nursing your baby.)

• Visualize your baby in your mind. Imagine what she looks like, sounds like, feels like, smells like when she nurses.

• Make the time go faster while you're expressing or pumping by talking with a friend, listening to the radio, reading something light, or watching television.

• If your baby is present but cannot suckle and is not nursing, and if you don't need two hands to express, hold him while you're pumping.

• Wear comfortable clothes that open up or pull up but still cover your shoulders, so you don't get chilled.

• Listen to music that you associate with nursing. This works best if you play the tape or CD initially during actual breastfeeding sessions; then when you're expressing, hearing the same music may help evoke the memory and the sensations you felt then. (Handel's "Water Music" gets high marks from women who enjoy classical music.)

STORING COLLECTED BREAST MILK

Containers

The best containers for storing your breast milk are four-ounce plastic nursing bottles or disposable plastic milk storage bags, depending on your preference.

• Plastic has an advantage over glass. For one thing, of course, plastic doesn't break when dropped, and you don't want to waste that liquid gold. In addition, if you are going to store your milk for less than twenty-four hours, you want plastic bottles, since some research suggests that some of the leukoyctes (white blood cells) in breast milk cling to glass, making them unavailable to your baby. They don't cling to plastic. However, the cells detach from glass after about twenty-four hours. So if you will be storing your milk that long or longer, the composition of the container doesn't matter.

• You want the small four-ounce bottles rather than the eight-ounce ones, so that you can defrost small amounts of milk at a time. Once thawed, milk should not be refrozen.

• Some women like the disposable milk storage bags made especially for storing breast milk. These bags lie flat in a freezer, are easy to stack, and thaw quickly. However, other mothers find them hard to handle and easy to puncture. The bags do need careful handling to avoid spillage and puncture, they sometimes split when frozen, and they absorb odors from nearby foods (although babies don't seem to mind milk that smells like the garlicky sausages in the next container). Double-bagging helps to overcome some of these difficulties. Some of these bags have a layer of nylon in addition to the plastic to prevent contamination of milk should the bags split or be punctured. At this point, then, it seems a matter of personal preference.

Cleaning and Sterilizing

If you're collecting milk to be given to your own baby within one week, you don't need to sterilize your bottles, rubber nipples, and pumping equipment. Wash everything thoroughly with a bottle brush and nipple brush to remove any milk scum, and then wash in a dishwasher or a basin of hot soapy water. Be sure to rinse out all the soap.

If you are going to take milk to the hospital for a sick or premature baby or for donation to a milk bank, the hospital will probably give you instructions. If not, or if you want to freeze the milk for your own future use, sterilize your containers and equipment. If you have a dishwasher that uses 180° water, this will sterilize everything well enough. (Check to be sure all the pump parts can be safely washed in the dishwasher.)

To sterilize just a few things, pad the inside of a large soup pot with a clean towel and fill it with enough water to completely cover the items you're sterilizing (bottle, cup, bottle caps, nipples, funnel, etc.). Bring the water to a boil over high heat; then turn down the heat just enough so that the water continues to boil gently. After five minutes of boiling, remove the nipples with sterile tongs. Place them on a clean dry towel. Allow the other items to boil fifteen minutes longer. Do not touch the rims of the bottles or the insides of the caps.

Helpful Suggestions

• Use a nontoxic marker to label each container of frozen milk with the date so you'll be able to use the oldest milk first. If you're taking it to a baby-sitter, child-care center, or hospital, put your baby's name on it.

• Don't fill bottles or storage bags to the top. Milk expands as it freezes, so no more than three and a half ounces should go into a four-ounce bottle.

• You can collect milk a little at a time, chill it in the refrigerator, and add the cold milk to milk that's already frozen. It will have an interesting layered look that will not affect its quality. Be sure to chill the milk first; adding warm milk can defrost the top layer of the frozen milk.

• You can also freeze milk in a plastic ice cube tray covered by plastic wrap. The frozen cubes (about half an ounce to an ounce each, depending on the size of the compartments) can then be transferred to an airtight plastic or glass container. When you or your sitter is ready to feed your baby, put the number of cubes you need into a feeding bottle and defrost as described below. This way you have more flexibility, since you can defrost only what your baby needs. Since the cubes defrost quickly, it's easy to add another one if your baby still seems hungry.

Transporting Expressed Milk

Although milk will keep at room temperature for several hours, it's always safest to keep the milk cold. You can do this whatever way is most convenient for you—in a thermos, in an insulated bottle bag, in an ice chest, or in an insulated bag filled with ice cubes or ice packs. Check the method you're using to be sure that the milk is still cold when it arrives at its destination and that frozen milk is still frozen.

OFFERING EXPRESSED MILK TO YOUR BABY

Both you and anyone else who feeds your baby your collected breast milk need to know the following information, so you may want to photocopy these pages to have them handy.

Don't be alarmed by the appearance of stored breast milk. It often separates or turns yellow, either of which may be perfectly normal. If you're not sure about the quality of the milk, taste it. If it tastes sweet and good, it's fine. If there is any hint of an "off" flavor, you should throw it out. It's pos-

Storage Times for Collected Milk

Basically, your collected breast milk will keep for several hours at room temperature if it's covered; it will keep in the refrigerator for about two days; and if you want to keep it longer than that, you should freeze it.

The following guidelines should assure safety and maximum benefit to your healthy, full-term baby. If you are expressing and storing milk for a preterm infant or a baby hospitalized for some other reason, you need to follow the recommendations of the institution where your baby is being cared for. Otherwise, you risk failing to have your milk given to your baby.

• *To be given to baby within 30 minutes:* No special storage needed. Can be kept at room temperature.

• *To be given to baby within 6 to 10 hours:* Pour into a clean container; cap tightly. If it's convenient, refrigerate the milk. This is the safest course, even though human milk kept in a capped clean container does not grow bacteria at normal room temperature (66° to 72°F) because of its ability to slow the growth of bacteria. If the room temperature is higher than 72°, be sure to refrigerate it.

• *To be given to baby within 48 hours (2 days):* Pour into a clean container; cap tightly. Refrigerate at 40°F (4°C) or below.

• *To be given to baby within 1 to 2 weeks:* Pour into a clean container; cap tightly. Quick-cool in the refrigerator for 30 minutes. Then freeze in refrigerator-freezer unit.

• *To be given to baby after 2 weeks:* Pour into a sterile container; cap tightly. Quick-cool in the refrigerator for 30 minutes. Then freeze in refrigerator-freezer unit.

sible that the milk has just picked up some odor or taste from other strong foods in your refrigerator or freezer. However, you don't want to take any chances of giving your baby spoiled milk. So trust your senses and your own good sense: If you feel worried or uneasy, don't give the milk to your baby.

Defrosting Your Milk and Feeding Your Baby

• Avoid overnight thawing of milk.

• Do not leave frozen milk out at room temperature.

• About half an hour before feeding time take the container from the

- *To be given to baby within 3 to 6 months:* Pour into a sterile container; cap tightly. Quick-cool in the refrigerator for 30 minutes. Then freeze at 0°F (–18°C) or below in the freezer of a two-door refrigerator or a deep freeze that is not opened often. Not all freezers stay cold enough for long-term storage. Check the temperature with a freezer thermometer at different places in the unit. The freezer should maintain a constant temperature of 0°F. If it keeps ice cream very solid, it is probably cold enough.

If your freezer does not get this cold but does keep other frozen foods hard, keep the milk in the center of the freezer and use within three to four months. Frost-free refrigerators, which have a warming element, generally do not maintain 0°.

To find out whether your milk thaws and then refreezes in your freezer, check by keeping an ice cube in a little jar; if you check it a day later and find that it has melted and refrozen, you'll know that this has probably happened to your milk, too. If so, you'll have to discard the milk.

It's best to use milk soon after collecting it. Ideally, you will not keep it longer than three months. For one thing, milk collected when your baby is two months old will not meet her needs as effectively when she is six months old.

- *Keeping breast milk longer than 6 months:* This is not a good idea. While instructions are sometimes given for keeping frozen milk up to two years, long-term freezing alters the chemical composition of the milk. (Some of the fats break down, and the milk loses some of its ability to fight harmful organisms.) Furthermore, you run the risk of contamination if you lose electrical power during that time and the milk thaws and refreezes.

- *Do not refreeze milk that has defrosted:* If frozen milk has started to thaw, refrigerate it immediately and use it within twelve hours.

freezer and hold it under tepid running water. Gradually increase the temperature of the water to hot. Shake the bag or bottle *gently* as you warm it; this remixes the cream that has separated. (Since your milk is not homogenized, the fat rises to the top on standing. If you shake the milk too vigorously, you might turn this fat to butter.) It should take about four minutes to thaw four ounces of frozen milk. This method can also be used to heat refrigerated milk.

- Do not heat either breast milk or formula in a microwave oven. Vitamins and other components in the milk may be destroyed, glass bottles may crack or explode, and hot spots may occur, which could cause severe burns to your baby's mouth or esophagus.

• Do not heat milk on the stove if you can avoid it. First, there's a danger of overheating and destroying antibodies and nutrients. Second, there's the chance that frozen milk will curdle. And then there's the all-too-common scenario of the mother or baby-sitter warming milk in a pan of water on the stove, running to answer the phone or the door—and coming back to find the bottle or bag melted and the milk boiled into the bottom of the pan. No way to treat that liquid gold—or the baby waiting for it.

However, if you do not have running warm water, put a bottle in a pan with warm water. Heat on medium heat, do not let the water boil, and do not leave the kitchen. Test the milk on the inside of your elbow; you should barely be able to feel it. If it feels warm, let it cool down to body temperature before feeding your baby.

• Roll or shake the bottle again gently before feeding.

• Use milk that has been defrosted but not heated within twelve hours. If the milk has been heated, use within thirty minutes.

• Discard any milk in the bottle that your baby does not finish at one feeding.

• Do not refreeze defrosted milk. If you can't use it within the suggested time limit, throw it away. It's painful to have to discard what seems like such a precious resource, but this milk is no longer the liquid gold it was before. There is a possibility that it might make your baby sick.

• If you have both fresh and frozen milk, give your baby the fresh milk and save the frozen for supplements and emergencies since freezing causes some loss of antibodies.

The above measures sound complicated, but most women who express milk for their babies find that once they establish a routine, they are able to carry it off. If all the steps involved with expressing or pumping your milk do become too burdensome, it's always possible, of course, to switch to formula. If you do make this switch, don't be hard on yourself for the change. Instead, congratulate yourself for the efforts you have made and for your contributions to your baby's health and well-being.

Weaning Your Child

18

How do I wean my one-year-old without making her feel abandoned? Kaylee eats three meals a day and drinks cups of juice and water, but she finds the breast her security and protection. We have both loved the nursing, but now I need to go back to work, which will mean being away from her for days at a time, and I feel it's time to wean her. But she has never been able to fall asleep without nursing, so I don't know what to do now.

OLIVIA, FLEMINGTON, NEW JERSEY

You've known from the first time you nursed your beautiful new-born that breastfeeding would not last forever—even though sometimes over these weeks, or months, or years, you may have felt that it would. You've known that one day this child who depended on you for all her nourishment and all her comforting would reach a stage when she—and you—would leave your breastfeeding days behind.

Weaning can take many different forms, depending on when it's begun, how it's begun, and who initiates it—the mother or the child. This chapter is about making the transition of weaning as easy as possible for both of you.

What exactly is weaning? The most global definition involves the process by which your child stops depending on your milk for nourishment and eventually stops nursing at the breast completely. This process starts the minute you give your baby something besides your breast milk and ends when you are no longer nursing at all. The usual progression includes four phases: (1) accustoming your baby to small amounts of foods other than breast milk before they are needed for nutrition; (2) adding foods when breast milk can no longer meet your child's nutritional needs; (3) replacing breast milk with other foods; and, finally, (4) stopping breastfeeding completely. (Sometimes this progression is short-circuited because of the need to wean abruptly, a situation we talk about later in this chapter.)

Weaning has an emotional meaning, too, one that is just as important as the nutritional one. Weaning is one of the first steps in a child's becoming independent of his mother. It's hard to look at your infant or toddler, who still needs so much care, and think of his moving toward independence. But this is only the beginning of a long path that every child must take to achieve maturity. And it's a path that must be walked by every mother, too.

Many babies accept gradual weaning fairly easily, but others love nursing so much that they want to continue long past the time their mothers think it's time to stop. On the other hand, it's sometimes harder for the mother to wean than it is for the child.

The end of breastfeeding is bittersweet: Together with the relief and the freedom of not being tied to your child's nursing needs—which even the happiest nursing mother is apt to feel when she stops breastfeeding—comes the sadness you may experience of giving up this precious way of relating to your child and of no longer being needed in the same unique way. But even as you feel the end of one era, you know that you are ushering in others, in which your relationship with your child will develop in innumerable ways.

Now let's talk about the when and the how of weaning.

WHEN SHOULD YOU WEAN FROM THE BREAST?

While you'll probably be asked more times than you care to think about how long you plan to breastfeed, there's no reason why you have to set an advance deadline on the duration of breastfeeding, any more than you set a date well ahead of time for the length of time you plan to wheel your baby in a stroller. You'll stop nursing when the time seems right for both you and your child.

This is a topic on which many people have strong opinions (which they don't hesitate to voice), but few have any evidence to base them on. There's no single optimal time for weaning, as we can see from the great range of weaning ages around the world.

The 1997 policy statement of the American Academy of Pediatrics (AAP) on breastfeeding (its most recent) recommends nursing ideally for at least a year and as long thereafter as mother and child want to continue. Both the World Health Organization and UNICEF recommend breastfeeding for at least two years. In many countries babies are routinely nursed well into the second or third year of life, and in its statement the

AAP cited a study that discusses the normality of extended breastfeeding as late as age seven.

(Anthropologist Katherine Dettwyler cites criteria for weaning in non-human primates, the animal class that includes chimpanzees and gorillas. These include tripling or quadrupling of birth weight, attaining one-third adult weight, and appearance of the first permanent molars. Extrapolating these measures to human beings would set a weaning age somewhere between two and a half to seven years of age.)

However, even if you cannot or do not want to nurse for many months, whatever breastfeeding you do offer your baby will go far to provide a good start in life.

During the first couple of days after birth, infants get the immunological advantages of colostrum; they continue to receive immunological benefits from breast milk at least through the toddler years. During the first six months, babies can satisfy all their nutritional needs from breast milk; at some time after this the combination of breast milk and various other foods will provide their essential nutrients. By nine months they usually have enough teeth and the intestinal maturity to handle a wide variety of foods. They are still, of course, dependent on their parents for many of the essentials of life, but from a nutritional aspect, they need no longer be dependent solely on their mothers' milk.

The emotional benefits that a mother and child derive from breastfeeding are just as valid, however, at two months, six months, nine months, one year, or later. You are still maintaining a special intimate relationship with your child, still able to comfort her at your breast when she's sick, unhappy, or in an unfamiliar situation. You're still able to forget the cares of the day for those peaceful minutes while the two of you are a nursing couple.

If you want to continue nursing for emotional reasons rather than nutritional ones, there's no need to stop at any specified time. Your decision will depend on your own unique situation. If you have a challenging child who gets upset easily and nursing is the most reliable way to calm her, or if your child finds it hard to get to sleep and stay asleep, or if you have to be at work all day and want to offer your child something that your caregiver can't give, you may want to nurse longer. Also, if you or your husband have any food allergies, you may want to hold off giving your baby any foods other than breast milk for at least six to eight months.

But what if you decide, for one reason or another, to stop nursing after three months? Even if you have nursed only a few weeks and you have to, or want to, stop breastfeeding, you are still a successful nursing mother. You have given your baby a good start in life and you yourself have known the special joy of the nursing relationship. Some breastfeeding is better than none at all.

How to Decide When to Wean

How, then, do you set a time for weaning? You and your child together constitute the nursing couple; either one of you may begin the process. Under child-led weaning, you continue to nurse until your child loses interest. This may happen toward the end of the first year, or when your baby begins to walk, or at about a year and a half.

Babies sometimes reject the breast completely and refuse to nurse, no matter how hard you try to hold their interest. One may make a big joke of biting: He gets into a nursing position, laughs, and then bites the breast that feeds him. Another may nurse eagerly for a minute or two and then—just as soon as her mother's milk lets down—pull away and show no further interest. Or you may have a jolly gymnast on your hands (and your lap)—a baby who starts to stand up while nursing, then shows off some of his other acrobatic tricks.

If you think that your baby may be on a temporary nursing strike,

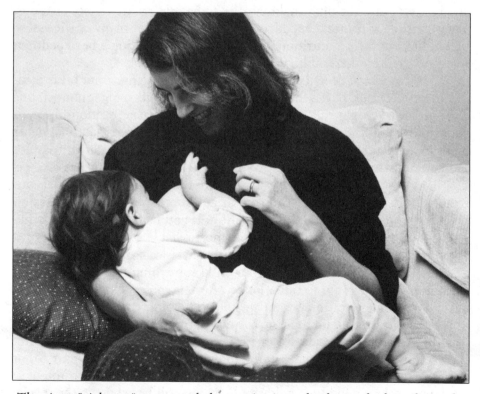

There's no "right age" to wean a baby; nursing is good as long as both mother and child want it to continue.

try the suggestions in the box on page 308. If none of these work, and if your baby is more than eight months old, he may be letting you know that he is ready to say good-bye to his nursing days.

But suppose that your baby or toddler has shown no signs of giving up the breast, but *you* are restless. Your child eagerly takes an occasional bottle, eats healthy portions of solid food, and drinks from a cup. You have gone back to work or are busy caring for your older children or have resumed other activities. You look at your nursling and, with some annoyance, wonder, "Is he *ever* going to stop?"

At this point you have options. You can continue to breastfeed, accepting the fact that your child still benefits from the experience and making efforts to be more patient. But if you find yourself resenting your nursing child, you may be doing both of you a favor by taking a gentle initiative toward weaning. Otherwise, your child will sense your annoyance and impatience. It seems a shame to spoil months of happy breastfeeding by continuing to nurse out of a sense of duty, when you can be a better mother when you feel happy and comfortable about what you're doing. It's better for a child to drink a bottle happily than to nurse at a grudging breast, just as it's better for a child to be cared for by a warm, affectionate baby-sitter than by a restless, unhappy mother who would rather be at work. Sometimes just knowing that you have begun the process of weaning will enable you to continue to nurse happily for another few months.

On the other hand, suppose you would really like to continue breastfeeding past your child's first, second, or even third birthday, but are embarrassed by the idea. (Somehow friends, relatives, and perfect strangers criticize a late nurser more than they do the toddler or preschooler of the same age who carries a bottle around.) In our society, women who nurse babies older than a year are often "closet" nursers, who feel they need to hide what they're doing to avoid having to defend the practice.

You may also wonder whether nursing beyond infancy harms your child psychologically. Your concern may stem partly from media attention to occasional cases over the past few years charging mothers nursing older children with abuse. However, virtually all of these cases were resolved favorably. This is because there is no evidence at all that extended breastfeeding makes children more dependent on their parents or harms them in any other way.

Although we have not found any scientific research comparing children weaned at different ages, our own observations and those of many other child-care professionals suggest that children who were nursed as toddlers or preschoolers seem no different psychologically from children who were weaned earlier. Provided the mother-child relationship is warm

---

"When Are You Going to Stop Nursing?"

You can toss off this question with a good-natured smile and a light response. Some of our favorite answers among those we've heard:

- "Oh, in about five minutes."

- "When she grows breasts of her own."

- "When he finds breasts he likes better than mine."

- "When his mustache gets in the way."

- "When she'd rather have a chocolate milkshake."

- "Till she starts dating."

- "Well, I plan to accompany him to college, so I can continue to breastfeed there—especially before his exams."

---

and loving, the length of breastfeeding—or even the fact of breastfeeding itself—does not seem to be an all-important factor in a child's healthy psychological development.

One problem that your child may encounter if she or he is still nursing at a later age than is typical in our society is teasing or ridicule from relatives, neighbors, or even strangers. If this happens, you can speak to the people doing the teasing, asking them to talk to you and not your child about any feelings they have about the appropriateness of your child's nursing. You can also speak to your child directly, reassuring her that you feel it's perfectly fine for her to continue nursing, but that some other people don't understand how important this is to children. You can also give her the option of nursing in private to avoid public comment. If she wants to give up nursing, you can let her know that this is fine with you, that this is a decision she can certainly make.

Whatever your choice, when people ask you, "What? *Still* nursing?" or exclaim, "You gave up *already?*" feel free to answer that you think this is a decision every nursing couple needs to make for themselves and that you feel that this is the best choice for you. You might also point out that the average age of weaning worldwide is between two and four years and that the World Health Organization and UNICEF both recommend nursing until age two or later. If you had not expected to nurse this long, you might add that and explain your reasons for doing so.

If you don't want to go into all of this, you can always use humor. The box above lists some retorts some women who practice extended breastfeeding have come up with. They represent ways to end a conversation you don't want to be having.

HOW SHOULD YOU WEAN?

There may not be a right time to wean, but there is definitely a right way—gradually if possible, sympathetically, and with a positive attitude. Weaning is a natural process; the natural way to help it along is to do it little by little, over a period of some weeks, or even months.

Weaning represents a positive growth experience for both you and your child. It's a sign that your child is able to become independent of you in one important way and, as such, is the first step in a series of independent steps. It's best accomplished slowly, bit by bit. Gradual weaning is best for both of you. If you wean slowly, for example, you should have little or no discomfort from milk pressure. If you can possibly avoid the physical and emotional discomfort for both of you of doing it "cold turkey," do so. If there is no alternative, see the section "Sudden Weaning."

You'll want to make yourself as available as possible to your child during the weaning process. Since she's losing something she has valued greatly—the pleasure of suckling at your breast—she needs the reassurance of your love and comforting. If you can devote extra time to her now, this should be heartening. While you don't need to feel guilty or apologetic, you do want to recognize the adjustment she's making and help her make it more smoothly through your loving understanding.

Child-Led Weaning

If you're still enjoying breastfeeding and are in no hurry to stop, but feel that weaning would be appropriate at this time in your child's life, you can let your nursing child lead the way. One phrase that governs the process for many mothers is "Don't offer, don't refuse."

This way, you nurse when your child asks to, but you don't suggest it at other times. While it sometimes seems hard to believe, even the most eager nurser will eventually find other activities and foods and comforts that are more interesting than nursing. No child nurses forever. With an older child, the end of nursing sometimes happens so gradually that you may not even think of it as weaning. One day you may suddenly realize that it's been several days since you've nursed. Typically, your child may ask to nurse a few more times, but by that time you may have no milk and the charm will be gone. Still a loving couple, you're no longer a nursing couple.

Mother-Led Weaning

If you're ready to wean, but your child hasn't shown any sign of losing interest, you may want to start the ball rolling yourself.

If possible, try to initiate weaning at a time when your child does not have to make other adjustments. If he's teething or has a cold, or you've just gone back to work, or there's a new baby-sitter, or you've just moved, or there's some other major disruption of routine, put off the weaning for a few weeks. It's always easier to manage only one change at a time.

Pinpoint the nursing session your child shows the least interest in, probably the early evening or noontime feeding. Eliminate this one first.

If your baby is under a year old, you may want to substitute a bottle. Most babies enjoy sucking on a bottle until they're well past a year, but not all find them appealing. If your baby doesn't seem interested in drinking from a bottle, don't try to force it on him. Instead, substitute something else, like a cup of milk (formula if your baby is under a year) or juice, or a few spoonfuls of applesauce.

For an older child, the substitution can be any of a number of things—a game, a cuddle, a walk to the park, a reading session with a favorite book, a piece of fruit or other healthful snack. Most important is your involvement with the activity, so that you show your child that you can show your love for him in many ways. For suggestions on weaning the older nursing child, see the following section.

Wait several days (up to two weeks) and then eliminate the next lightest feeding of the day. Keep doing this until you're down to one nursing a day, probably the first one of the morning or the last one at night. By now, you'll be producing very little milk and your child may give up this last feeding easily. Or you may decide to continue this one favorite feeding for a while longer. Many children wean easily during the day but want to continue nursing at bedtime for some time. Weaning this way should take from a couple of weeks to a couple of months or longer.

SUGGESTIONS FOR WEANING THE OLDER CHILD

• Make an agreement with your child about the places that nursing can take place. For example: only at home, in the car, or in a friend's house, but not in a restaurant or other public place.

• Make nursing sessions shorter.

- Use distraction. Before a child might ordinarily nurse or as you're bringing a brief nursing session to an end, involve her in an interesting activity.

- Offer something your child likes to eat just before he would ordinarily nurse. It's better to forestall a request to nurse than to deny it.

- Change your routine. At a usual nursing time, go out for a walk or a ride, or invite a playmate over, or bring out a new toy.

- Stay away from the places where you ordinarily nurse. If you're used to nursing in a special chair, hide it or move it out of your home temporarily.

- Don't sit down in front of your child, since many little ones associate sitting down with nursing time. Just keep on the move in the early days or weeks of weaning. Think of it as another opportunity to exercise!

- Do not uncover your breasts in front of your child. This will remind him of nursing when he may not have been thinking about it.

- Lavish physical affection on your child in activities not associated with breastfeeding, such as reading a picture book, telling stories, or singing.

- Enlist your child's favorite people. Ask her father, or grandmother, or an adored baby-sitter to get her up in the morning or put her to bed, or to go to her in the middle of the night, depending on which nursing session she asks for.

- Focus on eliminating the nursing sessions that are least important to your child and most inconvenient for you, and let the others continue for a while.

- Talk to your child about weaning as a definite occurrence in the future (after the next birthday, perhaps, or after Santa Claus comes). Even if there's some backsliding after these events, your child will think of nursing as ending someday. One mother told her three-year-old a story about a little rabbit whose mother said, "I love you and I love to nurse you, but my milk is going away and it's really special milk for babies."

- Emphasize what a big boy or girl your child is. Stress some of the benefits of getting older, like going to nursery school, having play dates, not wearing diapers anymore. Focus on the many things he can do for himself, like dressing himself and using the potty. Talk about nursing as something that's important for little children but not for big ones. One mother told her three-year-old that if she was old enough to chew gum, she was too old to nurse. The little girl was not about to give up her sugar-free bubble gum and never asked to nurse again.

- If your child is over three, you might be able to make a contract—to promise some special "big boy (or girl)" outing or treat one week (or whatever time period you set) after the last nursing. A child younger than this won't be able to keep his end of the bargain—and even a three-year-old might not be able to.

• Ask your child to postpone a nursing; this will sometimes lead to his forgetting it. A child who asks to nurse in public, for example, can often accept waiting "until we get home." At some times he'll dash into the door and climb onto your lap to collect what's been promised; at other times he'll become interested in something else.

• While you're weaning, continue to be willing to nurse your child at times when she's especially needy. If she hurts herself or is sick or unhappy, depriving her of the comfort she's used to will only create more unhappiness for both of you. Once she's weaned, you'll be able to comfort her in other ways.

• Stay away from traumatic techniques like painting your breasts with pepper, soot, or evil-tasting substances. Allow your child to keep his happy memories and his trust in you. The best way to end this stage in your child's life is through an agreement between the two of you—even if that agreement originates with you rather than your child.

• Recognize those times when nursing is just what your child needs. As one mother said, "A lot of times when he asks to nurse I can distract him, but when he really needs it, I nurse—and then he's in a super mood and so it's good for both of us."

HOW WEANING AFFECTS YOU

Physical Changes

When you stop breastfeeding, your body will undergo a number of physiological changes as your hormonal balance reverts to what it was before you became pregnant. As soon as you added foods other than breast milk to your child's diet, it became easier for you to become pregnant again. If you have not already adopted a method of birth control and if you do not want to conceive right away, you will want to use some means of contraception now.

The most obvious change will be in your breasts. It may take several months for you to lose the bulk of your milk, even though none may be apparent within days after the last nursing session. Some women are able to express a drop or two of milk from their breasts up to several years after weaning. Remember that nipple stimulation promotes milk production, so if you are always checking for milk, you are likely to find some. Also, consistent nipple stimulation during sexual activity can result in slight milk secretion for some time.

It may also take several months for your breasts to return to their former size. They will most likely be less firm than they were before you became pregnant, but this is the result of childbearing, not breastfeeding. They will probably seem to be the same size they were before your pregnancy, although some women feel that their breasts become larger or smaller after nursing. This may have something to do with the amount of weight gained or lost or with their having become accustomed to having larger breasts.

If you wean slowly, you should have little or no discomfort from milk pressure. You'll gradually produce less and less milk until there's virtually none at all to speak of. If at any point during weaning your breasts become overfull, you can express just enough milk to ease your discomfort, or you can put your child to the breast for a minute or two (if she's willing to stop at that). Don't overdo it or you'll just encourage your breasts to continue producing copious amounts of milk. If you're uncomfortably full most of the time, slow down the pace of weaning.

Two once popular remedies are no longer recommended. One, binding your breasts, can actually make you feel worse and cause a plugged duct besides. And medicine to dry up your milk usually didn't work and often had unpleasant side effects; it has been taken off the market for this purpose.

Emotional Responses

Your emotional reactions to weaning may be even more apparent than your physical ones. Much of your feeling about weaning will depend on your particular circumstances. If your baby is setting the pace for weaning earlier than you had expected, you may be feeling sad, surprised, and rejected. Rejoice, instead, in your child's push for independence and in his demonstration that he can take the initiative toward a new chapter in his life. This is only the first of many steps toward self-reliance that he will take in his lifetime. One of the primary goals of parenthood is to help our children become as self-sufficient as possible, in small stages appropriate to their level of development.

While it can be a blow to realize that your child does not need you in this particular way as much as she did before, you shouldn't lose sight of the fact that she will need you even more in other ways. Right now, for example, she may have special needs for the comfort of your arms and the reassurance of your love. Parenthood involves learning what our children need at different stages in their lives—and being willing to give it.

If you have to wean abruptly, earlier than you had expected or wanted to, you will most likely feel the grief of unrealized expectations, of having to give up a joyful activity, and of depriving your child of something that means so much to him. As you mourn what you both have lost, however, you need to tell yourself that you have done the best you could for your child, and that you will have many opportunities throughout his life to show your love for him in an infinite number of ways.

Even if you yourself initiated the weaning process and if it has gone smoothly and gradually, you may be surprised to find that you feel more than a little sad as nursing draws to a close. This feeling is common and normal. The end of breastfeeding represents a loss to you both. No longer will you enjoy this close physical bond, this symbiosis between you and your child in which each of you needed the other in a very special way. The end of nursing, especially of a long-time nursing relationship, marks the beginning of a new phase in your child's life. And as much as we want our children to grow up and be independent, most of us have ambivalent feelings about our success.

You will probably have the same kind of mixed emotions the first time you leave each of your children playing happily in preschool or kindergarten, the day they go off to sleep-away camp, the day you leave them in the college dorm, or the day they say "I do" and go off to start their own nuclear families. A lump in the parental throat often accompanies our feelings of accomplishment for having helped our children to meet life's challenges with confidence and enthusiasm.

Sudden Weaning

Sometimes a circumstance comes up that requires abrupt weaning—a mother's need to be hospitalized or to take a medication incompatible with breastfeeding, a family crisis that involves travel without a child, or some other emergency.

In some cases, however, a situation that seemed to call for sudden weaning can be modified. You may, for example, be able to postpone a surgical procedure for a few weeks, which will give you a little time to cut down nursing sessions more gradually. Or you may be able to take a different medication, take your baby with you on a trip, or make some other change. It's worth exploring other options, since sudden weaning is hard on both mother and child.

If you have to wean suddenly, you are likely to be quite uncomfortable for several days unless you're producing very little milk. You can hasten the drying-up process and minimize discomfort in a few ways. You'll need to wear a firm, but not too tight, bra, perhaps in a size larger than the one you usually wear. You can also relieve discomfort by expressing just enough milk to ease the pressure on your breasts. And you may also get relief from ice packs applied to the breasts several times a day. Ask your doctor to prescribe a pain reliever, which can be relatively strong, since now that nursing has ended, you don't have to worry about the medication reaching your child.

Occasionally, a mother under stress will make a spur-of-the-moment decision: "Okay, this has gone on long enough. Today's the day!" and will go the "cold turkey" route. This is almost always a mistake. If you don't have to wean abruptly, reconsider your decision. Are you doing it because of criticism by other people, because you think your child will sleep better at night (she probably won't), or because you're just tired of breastfeeding? Even after reconsideration, if you decide to begin the process, do it gradually, if at all possible. Both you and she will benefit.

YOUR CHILD'S DIET NOW

As part of the weaning process, and while he is still breastfeeding, your child will be eating some other foods and getting nutritional elements from some other sources. So what else should your baby be eating or drinking while you're still breastfeeding? Let's take a look at some of these other sources of nutrients.

Vitamin Drops

Most of your child's vitamins will come through your milk, and later through the food he eats, rather than from vitamin drops or pills. Some elements, however, cannot always be obtained in the diet. Considerable controversy exists in the medical community about the extent of vitamin supplementation needed by breastfed babies, and you and your doctor may hold different opinions from ours. It's our judgment, however, that the recommendations summarized in the box on page 366 are wise to follow.

All babies, no matter how they are fed, should receive *vitamin K* immediately after birth. During the next six months, your totally breastfed baby may receive enough vitamins from your milk if your own intake is high enough. If, however, you're not sure whether you're eating enough fruits and vegetables, your baby should receive a multiple vitamin preparation that includes *vitamins A and C.* This, of course, is a superb time for you to improve your own diet by increasing the amount of fruits and vegetables you eat. Not only will this be good for you and your baby now, but it is also important for setting a good example to your child as she grows up.

Vitamin D is especially important to help your child absorb calcium

Recommended Vitamin and Mineral Supplementation

BREASTFED CHILD	MULTIVITAMIN/ MULTIMINERAL	VITAMINS A, C, D	MINERALS	
			IRON[1]	FLUORIDE[2]
Full-term Infant	No	Sometimes	No	No
Preterm Infant	Yes	No	Yes	No
Healthy Baby (over 6 months)*	No	Sometimes	No	Yes‡
High-risk Baby (over 6 months)*	Yes	No	Yes	Yes‡
Healthy Child (over 2 years)*	No	No	No	Yes‡
High-risk Child (over 2 years)*	Yes	No	Sometimes	Yes‡

[1] Iron-fortified cereal is the preferred form of supplementation.

[2] If child drinks water with a fluoride content over 0.3 parts per million, additional supplement is not needed.

*These recommendations apply if the child is eating a well-balanced diet of solid foods at this time.

‡A fluoride supplement is recommended if the child is not drinking water with a fluoride content over 0.3 parts per million.

and phosphorus, essential elements for bone and tooth growth and development. Both you and your child need this vitamin, which appears in only tiny amounts in any food, including breast milk. Vitamin D is called the "sunshine" vitamin, since it's manufactured by our bodies when we spend a great deal of time outdoors and expose our bodies to sunlight.

Many mothers and children can get enough vitamin D from sunshine, but some do not. Dark-skinned people do not absorb as much from the sun because of their deeper pigmentation; high levels of air pollution block transmission of vitamin D to residents of some urban areas; and mothers and babies who do not go out of doors often, or who are bundled up by layers of clothing or covered with sunblock when they do, lessen their exposure to the sun, and thus to vitamin D.

People in the above categories may need extra vitamin D. If you're not in any of these categories, you probably don't need it, but again it can't hurt to be on the safe side. The drops are harmless, inexpensive, and convenient. You should be sure of getting adequate vitamin D throughout pregnancy and lactation, and if your baby's doctor recommends it for her, she can begin taking it from the seventh to tenth day of life.

If your community's water supply contains less than 0.3 ppm (parts per million) of *fluoride,* your older baby will benefit from a fluoride supplement. If he doesn't drink much water, a fluoride supplement is beneficial even if your water contains a higher level than this. You can find out the level of fluoride in your water by calling your local health department. The fluoride in the water that a nursing mother drinks probably does not pass through her milk in sufficient amounts to help her child develop decay-resistant teeth. Since research has shown that children who get extra fluoride (either in the water or in drops) develop fewer cavities, you'll want your child to have this advantage. The fluoride may be included in your baby's vitamin drops and should be offered starting at six months of age.

Although breast milk contains little *iron,* what there is is present in a very easily absorbable form. This iron, plus the stores your baby is born with, will see him through his first six months. After this time, he'll need extra iron. One way to get this is by feeding an iron-fortified baby cereal, which is normally the first solid food your pediatrician will suggest. After that, meats and other iron-rich foods can be added to his diet.

If you do offer an iron supplement, it will be absorbed best if given with a fruit juice rich in vitamin C.

Other Milk

If you offer any milk other than breast milk in the first year of life, you should be giving your baby a specially constituted infant formula. Most infant formulas consist of modified cow's milk, but if your baby has special needs (for example, an allergy to cow's milk), the baby might need a goat's milk or soybean base formula.

You should not offer plain cow's milk before one year of age for several reasons. For one thing, babies fed on whole milk before this time sometimes suffer from iron-deficiency anemia. Cow's milk contains very little iron and sometimes causes intestinal bleeding, which contributes further to iron loss. Also, early ingestion of cow's milk may contribute to cow's milk protein allergy. And the high intake of sodium, potassium, chloride, and protein from cow's milk can burden a baby's system.

Also, you should not offer skim milk or reduced-fat milk (1 or 2 percent) until your child is over two years. These milks do not provide the necessary fatty acids that babies need for brain growth and for the development of hormones and enzyme systems. Furthermore, since such milks are too high in protein concentration for the baby's digestive system to handle easily, they can overload the baby's kidney excretory capacity.

A baby who is several months old before being offered a bottle will probably be mystified by the strange contraption the first time around and may absolutely refuse to try sucking the rubber nipple. If you plan to wean your baby before six to eight months of age, you may begin offering an occasional bottle or cup by about three months of age, to let him get used to this way of getting food.

If you have not fed your baby anything from a cup by the time she is about five months old, you can begin now to offer a few sips of expressed breast milk or water this way. By the time she's really ready for it, she'll be quite proficient at draining it to the last drop.

If you have a family history of allergy, avoid cow's milk as long as

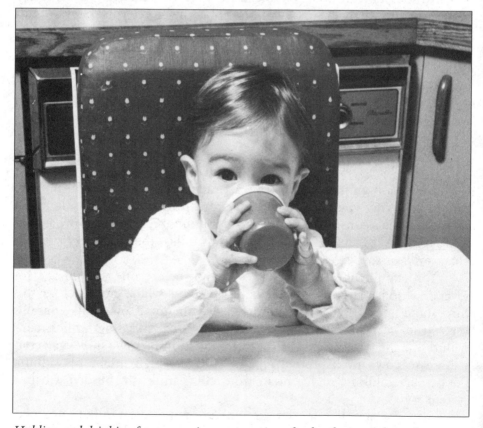

Holding and drinking from a cup is one more sign of a developing independence.

possible. The later a baby is given a potentially allergenic food, the less likely he is to react to it. Don't try formula till about six months, and then watch your baby closely. If he vomits, has diarrhea, or shows other unusual reactions, don't give any milk other than breast milk and be careful about any other additions to the diet.

Water and Juice

While breastfed babies don't *need* water, even in hot and dry climates, some enjoy it. If you want to give your baby an occasional sip of water *after* breastfeeding is well established, try offering it in a cup. To prevent nipple confusion, it's best not to give any bottles of anything before six to eight weeks.

Some babies like fruit juice, which can be offered after six months of age, preferably by cup. It isn't necessary, though, and if you have a family history of allergy, it's better to wait until after eight months of age to lower the chances of your child's developing an allergy to fruit. If you do feed your baby fruit juice, be sure that it has been pasteurized and offer only small amounts. One study of toddlers who had failed to grow normally found that they had been drinking large quantities of juice, which filled them up so much that they had too little appetite for higher-calorie, more nutritious foods. Also, some had diarrhea. Children two or three years old should drink no more than four to eight ounces of juice a day, and younger babies should have less. Letting babies take a bottle of juice to bed with them or walk around sucking from it for a long period of time can also lead to tooth decay.

Solid Foods

Breast milk is an ideal total food for the young infant, but older babies need additional foods to meet their growing nutritional requirements. Sometime between four and eight months of age, your baby will probably signal her readiness to add solid foods to her diet. Advantages to starting on the early side—about six months—include both the openness to new experience that is more characteristic of younger rather than older babies and the extra time your baby will have to learn how to handle these new foods before she needs them for nourishment.

Furthermore, while the average baby does not need any food other than breast milk until about six months of age, a rapidly growing baby may need more iron than the amount present in human milk. You may, there-

---

Offering Solid Foods

- Nurse your baby first before you offer her food by spoon. She'll be more open to trying a new experience if she isn't wildly hungry.
- Pick a time when there are few distractions, and both you and your baby are relaxed.
- Sit her on your lap, where she will feel secure.
- Introduce a single-ingredient food first. If your baby develops a rash or any other symptom, you'll be able to identify a possible cause.
- The first serving should be between one-half and one teaspoon of food.
- Use a spoon—the kind with a small bowl and a long handle works best. Do not feed solids from a bottle, since that can release too much food at once, causing a baby to choke.
- Start spoon-feeding by putting a little food into the bowl of the spoon, turning the spoon upside down, and scraping the food onto the top of the baby's tongue. He will easily propel the food to the back of his mouth where he will swallow it. He'll probably like it and will want more.
- Introduce new foods one at a time, over a fairly long period of time: There's no need to rush in with a cornucopia of new foods.
- One good first food is iron-fortified rice cereal mixed with expressed breast milk, water, or formula; after your baby is a year old you can use homogenized milk. Rice is a good starter, since babies are least likely to be allergic to it.
- A good progression after iron-fortified rice cereal includes other cereals,

---

fore, want to add iron-fortified cereal to your baby's diet at about six months of age. Babies absorb the iron in cereal better than the iron in drops.

Some years ago, possibly when you yourself were a baby, mothers (including one of the authors of this book) were advised to begin feeding their babies solid foods when they were only a couple of weeks old. We now know that this is not only unnecessary but unwise (as well as a waste of time and money). Such foods may strain a baby's immature digestive system. Furthermore, they can fill a baby up so much that she doesn't nurse as vigorously, thereby not getting enough breast milk, or becomes too fat from the solid foods. The nutrients in them often go right through the baby's system, exiting in the stool. In addition, they may predispose a baby to allergies.

How, then, will you know when to offer your baby solid foods? Look for signs of readiness in your baby. Teeth are not necessary, but the following aspects of development are:

fruits, vegetables, and meats. Among babies' most enjoyed flavors are those of applesauce, bananas, pears, peas, carrots, and squash.

• Do not feed your baby directly from a jar of baby food. Take out the amount you plan to feed, and refrigerate the rest. If the baby doesn't eat all of the food you removed, throw away whatever is left. The saliva that goes back into the food can foster the growth of bacteria.

• Do not heat food in a microwave; it may heat unevenly and make food too hot.

• Consider these first few feedings of solid foods "practice feeds," just like those first few nursings so many months ago. Your baby now has to learn how to master a completely new set of muscle movements to take the food from a spoon and to swallow it. At first she'll get more food on her face, her bib, and you than she will in her mouth. You'll be surprised, though, at how quickly she'll catch on, and how soon she'll be ready to start eating foods she can pick up with her fingers.

• Ask your pediatrician which finger foods are safe for your baby. Some, like raw carrot or even zwieback, can cause choking if they're given to a baby who cannot properly chew and swallow small enough amounts.

• Avoid, as much as possible, foods that contain added sugar, salt, and starch. You can make your own baby foods (which can be as easy as using a fork to mash a ripe banana or cooked peas). Or you can buy organic baby foods. Jarred foods may be more convenient when you are traveling, or when your table food is not appropriate for your baby.

• In any case, read the labels and graduate your child to table food as soon as she is ready. Commercial "stage 3," "junior," or "toddler" foods are unnecesssary and costly.

First, he should be able to sit up with support and should have good control of his head and neck muscles. This way, he'll be able to show you when he wants food by leaning forward and opening his mouth, and to show when he doesn't by leaning back and turning away. If he can't do this, pushing food into his mouth will be a kind of forced feeding.

Then, be sure that she is not pushing the spoon out of her mouth with her tongue. This tongue-extrusion reflex is usually no longer operative by about five months. To test this, give your baby a quarter-teaspoon of a simple food (like mashed ripe banana, an excellent first food, which most babies love). If the food goes from the front of her mouth to the back of her throat, and if she swallows it, she's clearly ready for solids. But if she spits it out, you may want to wait a few days and try again. A little gagging is part of the learning process; just watch your baby carefully to be sure she doesn't choke.

And finally, your baby may be giving you very clear signals of readi-

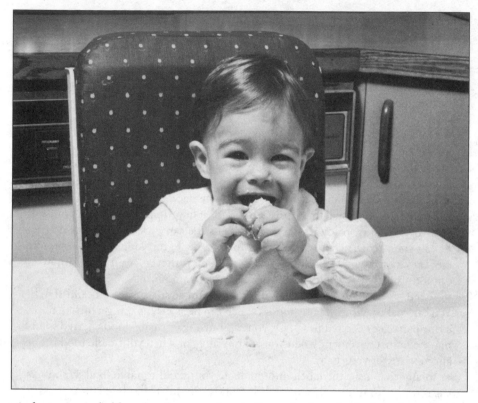

A chewy unseeded bagel makes a good early finger food, as this little girl's smile shows.

ness for solid food by reaching for the food on your plate, making noises, or pointing.

Just as you learned to read your baby's cues for hunger and readiness for nursings, you can now pay attention to the signals that mean, "Hey, Mom, I want some of that!" For suggestions on the first few "meals" of solid foods, see the box on page 370.

STAYING CLOSE WITH YOUR CHILD

When you wean your child and help her take this first big step toward independence, you will very likely look back over her young life. You think of the months you carried her under your heart, nourishing her through your body, wondering who she was, what kind of a person she would be. You remember the exertion on both your parts as she burst into the world as an individual human being, breathing through her own lungs, making her own efforts to draw nourishment, learning how to cope with a strange world. You dwell on the time you spent together as a nursing couple, re-living the many happy moments you knew as you held your child in your arms and gave deeply of yourself.

And then you look forward. You think of the many other ways you will give of yourself to this child: the guidance you will provide to help him find his way in life, the love that will support him, the courage you will give him to let go of you and be his own person, the happy hours you'll spend enjoying each other's company, playing together, having fun. You accept the fact that as a mother you will know tears and anger, as well as laughter and delight. But just as you now remember, not the minor set-backs or worries about breastfeeding, but its heartfelt joys, so too will you balance out the stresses and demands of motherhood with the love and the warmth and the personal growth that you gain from your relationship with your children.

Resource Appendix: Helpful Organizations and Sources of Information

FOR INFORMATION AND HELP ABOUT BREASTFEEDING

- **La Leche League International**
1400 N. Meacham Road, P.O. Box 4079
Schaumburg, IL 60168-4079

La Leche League is the largest organization in the world devoted specifically to promoting and providing information and help related to many different aspects of breastfeeding. Phone (800)LALECHE (525-3243) for a short answer to your question about breastfeeding, a catalog, and/or a referral to your local La Leche leader. For general information, phone: (847) 519-7730, write, fax: (847) 519-0035, or e-mail: LLLHQ@llli.org. For recorded information about common problems at $1.99 a minute, call (900) 448-7475, ext. 92. Or go to the League's website on the Internet to ask questions (www.lalecheleague.org) or to America Online (keyword: Parent Soup) to join a chat group.

- **International Childbirth Education Association (ICEA)**
P.O. Box 20048
Minneapolis, MN 55420-0048
Phone: (612)854-8660 or (800)624-4934
Fax: (612)854-8772
E-mail: info@icea.org; Website: www.icea.org

ICEA promotes family-centered maternity care, offers professional certification and training programs for educators and health care providers, publishes a quarterly journal and many smaller publications, many of which deal with breastfeeding. It also has a wonderfully comprehensive mail-order catalog of books and pamphlets related to pregnancy, birth, breastfeeding, and other family issues.

• **World Alliance for Breastfeeding Action (WABA)**
Secretariat, P.O. Box 1200
10850 Penang, Malaysia
Fax: 60-4-657-2655
E-mail: secr@waba.po.my; Website: www.elogica.com.br/waba

This international umbrella organization advocates for breastfeeding and serves as a liaison among various agencies and individuals around the world. In connection with its annual World Breastfeeding Week (August 1–7), it distributes an action folder with information and ideas for actions that individuals and organizations can take in their own communities to support the year's theme (for example, in 1998 it was "Breastfeeding: The Best Investment").

TO FIND PROFESSIONALS IN A FIELD

• **OBSTETRICIAN**

American College of Obstetricians and Gynecologists (ACOG)
409 12th Street, S.W.
Washington, DC 20024
Website: www.acog.com

ACOG can refer you to an obstetrician in your area. The association does not want to be contacted by telephone.

• **FAMILY PHYSICIAN**

American Academy of Family Physicians
8880 Ward Parkway
Kansas City, MO 64114-2797
Phone: (816)333-9700
Fax: (816)822-0580
E-mail: fp@aafp.org; Website: http://www.aafp.org

Family physicians are medical specialists who are trained to care for everyone in your family and can therefore see you through your pregnancy and then care for your newborn, while continuing to care for other family members. To find a family doctor, you can ask family and friends to recommend the doctor they use and like, ask a hospital you like for a list of family practitioners, or write to the Academy and ask for a list of family physicians in your area. The Academy's reference manual makes a strong statement in favor of breastfeeding.

• NURSE-MIDWIFE

American College of Nurse-Midwives
818 Connecticut Avenue, N.W., Suite 900
Washington, DC 20006
Phone: (202)728-9860
Fax: (202)728-9897
E-mail: info@acnm.org; Website: www.midwife.org

By phoning the toll-free number 888-MIDWIFE (888-643-9433), you can learn the name, address, and phone number of Certified Nurse Midwives (CNMs) in your area.

• CERTIFIED PROFESSIONAL MIDWIFE OR DIRECT-ENTRY MIDWIFE

North American Registry of Midwives (NARM)
Phone: (888)84-BIRTH (842-4784)
E-mail: narmcpm@aol.com

Through examination and assessment of skills and experience, NARM certifies midwives who have entered the profession by varied routes.

Midwives Alliance of North America (MANA)
Phone: (888)923-MANA (923-6262)
E-mail: manainfo@aol.com; Website: www.mana.org

MANA is a membership organization of practicing and student midwives, supportive health-care providers, and consumers. Both NARM and MANA can provide referrals to a midwife in your area.

• PEDIATRICIAN

American Academy of Pediatrics (AAP)
141 Northwest Point Boulevard
Elk Grove Village, IL 60007
Phone: (800) 433-9016
Fax: (847) 228-5097 or (847) 228-7320
E-mail: kidsdocs@aap.org; Website: www.pediatrics.org

For help in finding a qualified general pediatrician or pediatric subspecialist near you, send the name of your town and state and a business-size, self-addressed, stamped envelope (SASE) to: Physician Referral Service, American Academy of Pediatrics, Box 927, address listed above.

For a list of free brochures for parents (such as "Allergies in Children," "Child Care," or "Starting Solid Foods"), send a business-size SASE to AAP, Dept. C, Box 927, address listed above. Then, request the brochures you want by title, sending a separate request and SASE for each one.

The AAP's 1997 policy statement on breastfeeding urges exclusive nursing for six months and continued nursing until at least one year of age. For information about current breastfeeding initiatives, e-mail: BCrase@aap.org.

• NUTRITIONIST

The American Dietetic Association
216 West Jackson Boulevard
Chicago, IL 60606-6995
Phone: (800)366-1655 or (312)899-0040
Fax: (312)899-1772
Website: www.eatright.org

Members of the ADA are nutritionists who have met stringent requirements entitling them to put the letters R.D. (for Registered Dietitian) after their names. The organization can help you find a nutritionist in your area. It also can provide a wealth of information on food and nutrition by phone or by mail. Customized answers to individual questions can be obtained by phoning (900)225-5267 (per-minute charges assessed).

• CHILDBIRTH EDUCATOR

ASPO/Lamaze (American Society for Psychoprophylaxis in
Obstetrics, Inc.)
1200 19th Street, N.W., Suite 300
Washington, DC 20036-2422
Phone: (202)857-1128 or (800)368-4404
Fax: (202)223-4579
E-mail: ASPO@sba.com; Website: www.lamaze-childbirth.com

One of the oldest childbirth education organizations, ASPO/Lamaze was founded in 1960 to encourage birthing experiences in which the mother is awake and aware, supported by her family and friends, and is not separated from her baby. The organization trains and certifies childbirth educators and "breastfeeding support specialists" and publishes a magazine for parents.

• LACTATION CONSULTANT

International Lactation Consultant Association (ILCA)
4101 Lake Boone Trail, Suite 201
Raleigh, NC 27607
Phone: (919)787-5181
Fax: (919)787-4916
E-mail: ilca@erols.com

ILCA conducts ongoing education programs and publishes a peer-reviewed journal, among its other activities. It has affiliate groups in many countries and localities and can refer you to a lactation consultant in your area who has been certified by the International Board of Lactation Consultant Examiners.

International Board of Lactation Consultant Examiners (IBLCE)
P.O. Box 2348
Falls Church, VA 22042-0348
Phone: (703)560-7330
Fax: (703)560-7332
E-mail: iblce@erols.com

IBLCE is the professional accrediting association for lactation consultants, recognized by the International Lactation Consultant Association (ILCA). IBLCE sets standards by developing yearly certifying examinations, which are given in several languages. Lactation consultants who have met IBLCE's requirements may add the letters *IBCLC* after their names.

• DOULA

National Association of Postpartum Care Services, Inc. (NAPCS)
P.O. Box 1012
Edmonds, WA 98020
Phone: (800)45DOULA (800-453-6852).

NAPCS is an association of national and international professionals concerned with the practical responsibilities and personal needs of families during the postdelivery period or during pregnancy when special help is needed. It makes referrals to certified doulas who can provide emotional and practical support around infant care, breastfeeding, and other postpartum needs like household chores and caring for older siblings.

Doulas of North America (DONA)
1100 23rd Avenue
East Seattle, WA 98112
Phone: (206)324-5440
E-mail: askDONA@aol.com

DONA makes referrals to certified birth doulas in various areas, principally for help during pregnancy and childbirth but also for postpartum help.

• INFANT MASSAGE PRACTITIONER

The International Association of Infant Massage
1720 Willow Creek Circle, Suite 516
Eugene, OR 97402
Phone: (800)248-5432 or (541)431-6280
Fax: (541)485-7372

This membership organization trains instructors to work directly with parents and babies in small classes, private lessons, or with community agencies. It will refer you to an instructor in your area, and will send you a catalog featuring books, videos, audiocassettes, and other products for sale.

• NATURAL CHILDBIRTH TEACHER

The Bradley Method of Natural Childbirth
P.O. Box 5224
Sherman Oaks, CA 91413-5224
Phone: (818)788-6662 or (800)4ABIRTH (800-422-4784)
Fax: (818)-788-1580
Website: www.bradleybirth.com

This organization will send out a free national directory of teachers who help couples who want to avoid childbirth drugs and want their babies to be breastfed.

FOR MOTHERS OF MULTIPLES

• **National Organization of Mothers of Twins Club,** P.O. Box 23188, Albuquerque, NM 87192-1188. Phone: (800) 243-2276 or (505) 275-0955. E-mail: nomotc@aol.com. Website: nomotc.org. This is a network of some 475 local clubs representing parents of twins, triplets, and quadruplets. It fosters development of local support groups, participates in research projects, and will put you in touch with local chapters.

• **The Center for Study of Multiple Birth** will send out a reference and resource list of books and other helpful information if you write to the Center at Suite 463-5, 333 East Superior Street, Chicago, IL 60611; (312) 266-9093.

HUMAN MILK BANKS

• **The Human Milk Banking Association of North America, Inc.,** c/o Mothers' Milk Bank, P/SL Medical Center, 1719 East 19th Avenue, Denver, CO 80218. Phone: 919-250-8599. At this writing only nine human milk banks exist in North America: seven in the United States, one in Canada, and one in Mexico. These banks carefully screen volunteer donors; collect, screen, and process milk; and dispense it to critically ill infants and children. Recipients pay a processing fee on a per-ounce basis, but no one is denied access for inability to pay. Clinical uses of donor milk have included prematurity, failure to thrive, immunodeficiencies, chronic renal failure, infant botulism, and management of chronic diarrhea.

THE INTERNET

The Net is an invaluable source of information about breastfeeding and child care and a route to networking with professionals and other parents. In addition to the websites of the organizations listed here, you can find a wealth of information by using your search engine to find "breastfeeding" or "lactation."

LEGAL HELP

If you are in a situation with legal ramifications, you may find answers to your questions by contacting La Leche League International (contact information on page 374). Through its Legal Advisory Council, your questions can be routed to a knowledgeable attorney in your state.

Two members of the council who are in private practice are:
• Elizabeth N. Baldwin, Esq., 2020 N.E. 163rd Street, Suite 300, North Miami Beach, FL 33162. Phone: (305) 944-9100. Fax: (305) 949-9029. E-mail: baldwin@icanect.net. Ms. Baldwin has written and coauthored numerous articles about legal issues involving breastfeeding, including jury duty and how to come up with visitation plans in custody cases. Some of these articles can be reached through La Leche League's webpage, under www.lalecheleague.org/Law/Main.html. Others may be obtained from Ms. Baldwin.
• Mary Ann Kerwin, Esq., 5130 Nassau Circle West, Cherry Hills Village, CO 80110. Phone: (303) 639-9581. E-mail: makerwin@aol.com.

HELP IN THE WORKPLACE

- **Healthy Mothers, Healthy Babies Coalition (HMHB),** 409 12th Street, S.W., Suite 309, Washington, DC 20024-2188. Phone: (202) 863-2458. Fax: (202) 484-5107. This consortium of public and private organizations, employers, policymakers, and consumers works to promote and improve community-based services on behalf of healthy mothers, babies, and families. It publishes newsletters for professionals, maintains committees (including one on Breastfeeding Promotion), and holds local and national meetings. Its publications include the free pamphlet *Working and Breastfeeding: Can You Do It? Yes, You Can!*

- **Sanvita Corporate Lactation Programs,** P.O. Box 660, McHenry, IL 60051-0660. Phone: (800) 435-5557. Fax: (815) 363-1246. These programs, sponsored by Medela, Inc., manufacturer of breast pumps and other equipment for nursing mothers, work with employers to promote maternal and child health, with the point of view that supporting employees as parents benefits the entire organization. Sanvita's managed care program includes prenatal and breastfeeding education by lactation professionals, maternity leave support, and worksite centers where mothers can express milk.

- **Washington Business Group on Health,** 777 North Capitol Street, N.W., Suite 800, Washington, DC 20002. Phone: (202) 408-9320. Fax: (202) 408-9332. E-mail: traylor@wbgh.com. This national nonprofit organization analyzes health policy and related worksite issues from the perspective of large employers. It promotes employer-sponsored services and benefits that support the health and well-being of workers as an investment in the company's productivity. Its publication, *Business, Babies & the Bottom Line: Corporate Innovations and Best Practices in Maternal and Child Health*, offers case histories of successful family-oriented programs.

SOURCES FOR ELECTRIC AND HAND-OPERATED BREAST PUMPS

- Hollister Inc. (Ameda/Egnell), 2000 Hollister Drive, Libertyville, IL 60048-3781. Phone: (800) 323-4060. In Canada: (800) 665-9533. Call for information on where to rent or buy a variety of breast pumps and other products, and where to purchase Lansinoh® for Breastfeeding Mothers.

• Medela, Inc., P.O. Box 660, McHenry, IL 60051-0660. Phone: (800) 835-5968 (800-TELL YOU). Call for information on where to rent or buy a variety of breast pumps and other products and how to find lactation consultants in your area, and for the *Breastfeeding Information Guide,* a free catalog of products, with helpful tips.

• White River Concepts, 924 C Calle Negocio, San Clemente, CA 92673. Phone: (800) 342-3906. Mother's Helpline: (800) 824-6351. Fax: (714) 366-1664. Website: www.whiteriver.com. Call for information on where to rent or buy a variety of breast pumps and other products.

• Omron Healthcare, Inc. (for Comfort Plus breast pump, formerly called the Marshall/Kaneson pump, the battery-operated Mag-Mag pump, and other products), 300 Lakeview Parkway, Vernon Hills, IL 60061. Phone: (800) 231-3434 or (847) 680-6200. Fax for orders: (800) 637-6763. Website: www.omronhealthcare.com

• Lopuco, Ltd. (for Loyd-B pump), 1615 Old Annapolis Road, Woodbine, MD 21797. Phone: (800) 634-7867 or (410) 489-4949.

• Bailey Medical Engineering (for Nurture III double electric breast pump), 2216 Sunset Drive, Los Osos, CA 93402. Phone: (800) 413-3216 or (805) 528-5781. Fax: (805) 528-1461. E-mail: folks@baileymed.com. Website: www.baileymed.com

SOURCES FOR NURSING SUPPLEMENTERS

See Chapter 15 for descriptions of nursing supplementers. Both companies listed below sell direct, can refer you to local outlets, and offer consultation on the use of their products.

• Lact-Aid®International, P.O. Box 1066, Athens, TN 37303. Phone: (423) 744-9090. Fax: (423) 744-9116. E-mail: info@lact-aid.com. Website: www.Lact-Aid.com. First introduced in 1971, the Lact-Aid Nursing-Trainer™ System is the company's major product; other accessory items for nursing mothers are also offered. Executive director Jimmie Lynne Avery publishes a quarterly newsletter directed principally to health practitioners, institutions, and businesses. The company also maintains a network of volunteers who have used the Lact-Aid system and are willing to speak with mothers in similar situations.

• Medela, Inc. See page 382 for contact information. Medela makes a number of different nursing supplementers: the Supplemental Nursing System (SNS)™ and the Starter SNS (meant for short-term disposable use), and the Haberman and the mini-Haberman feeders designed for babies with cleft palate or other special feeding problems. The smaller feeders are especially suited for premature babies. The company also makes a specially designed flexible silicone cup designed for cup-feeding of infants.

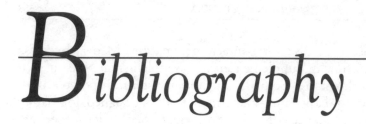

Bibliography

ADA Reports. (1997). Position of The American Dietetic Association: Promotion of breast-feeding. *Journal of the American Dietetic Association,* 97(6):662–666.

ADA Reports. (1997). Position of The American Dietetic Association: Vegetarian diets. *Journal of the American Dietetic Association,* 97(11):1317–1321.

Ahmed, F. et al. (1992). Community-based evaluation of the effect of breast-feeding on the risk of microbiologically confirmed or clinically presumptive shigellosis in Bangladeshi children. *Pediatrics,* 90(5):406–411.

American Academy of Pediatrics. (1997). Human milk. In: Peter, G., ed. *Red Book: Report of the Committee on Infectious Diseases,* 24th ed. Elk Grove Village, IL: American Academy of Pediatrics, pp. 74–79.

American Academy of Pediatrics Committee on Drugs. (1994). The transfer of drugs and other chemicals into human milk. *Pediatrics,* 93(1): 137–150.

American Academy of Pediatrics, Committee on Environmental Health. (1994). PCBs in breast milk. *Pediatrics,* 94(1):122–123.

American Academy of Pediatrics, Committee on Nutrition. (1992). The use of whole cow's milk in infancy. *Pediatrics,* 89(6):1105–1109.

American Academy of Pediatrics, Committee on Pediatric AIDS. (1995). Human milk, breastfeeding, and transmission of human immunodeficiency virus in the United States. *Pediatrics,* 96(5):977–979.

American Academy of Pediatrics Work Group on Breastfeeding. (1997). Breastfeeding and the use of human milk. *Pediatrics,* 100(6):1035–1039.

American Academy of Pediatrics, Work Group on Cow's Milk Protein and Diabetes Mellitus. (1994). Infant feeding practices and their possible relationship to the etiology of diabetes mellitus. *Pediatrics,* 94:752–754.

Amir, L., Hoover, K., & Mulford, C. (1995). *Candidiasis & Breastfeeding,* Lactation Consultant Series. Garden City Park, NY: Avery Publishing.

Angelou, Maya. (1974). *Gather Together in My Name.* New York: Random House.

Angier, N. (1994, May 24). Mother's milk found to be potent cocktail of hormones. *New York Times,* pp. C1, C10.

Angier, N. (1997, Sept. 16). Theorists see evolutionary advantages in menopause. *New York Times,* pp. F1, F8.

Arnon, S.S., Damus, K., Thompson, B., Midura, T.F., & Chin, J. (1982). Protective role of human milk against sudden death from infant botulism. *Journal of Pediatrics,* 100:568–573.

Auerbach, K. (1984). Babies, breasts, and bosses: Providing practical help for the employed breastfeeding mother. In: *Breastfeeding and Women Today: Conference Proceedings.* Washington, DC: National Center for Education in Maternal and Child Health, pp. 37–55.

Auerbach, K.G. & Avery, J.L. (1980). Relactation: A study of 366 cases. *Pediatrics,* 65(2):236–242.

Auerbach, K.G. & Avery, J.L. (1981). Induced lactation: A study of adoptive nursing by 240 women. *American Journal of Diseases of Children,* 135:340–343.

Auerbach, K.G. & Gartner, L.M. (1987). Breastfeeding and human milk: Their association with jaundice in the neonate. *Clinics in Perinatology,* 14(1):89–107.

Auerbach, K.G. & Guss, E. (1984). Maternal employment and breastfeeding: A study of 567 women's experiences. *American Journal of Diseases of Children,* 138:958–960.

Bachu, A. (1993). *Fertility of American Women: June 1992* (Current Population Report P24-470). Washington, DC: U.S. Government Printing Office.

Baldwin, E.N. (1993, Spring). Extended breastfeeding and the law. *Mothering,* pp. 88–91.

Baldwin, E.N. & Friedman, K.A. (1997, July 7). A current summary of breastfeeding legislation in the U.S. http:/www.lalecheleague.org/LawBills.html.

Baldwin, E.N., Kerwin, M.A., & Elder, J. (1997, July 4). Legal issues for breastfeeding families. Paper presented at La Leche League International Conference, Washington, DC.

Barros, F.C., Victora, C.G., Semer, T.C., et al. (1995). Use of pacifier is associated with decreased breast-feeding duration. *Pediatrics,* 96:495.

Berkowitz, H. (1993, Nov. 22). Some stores are refusing to market magazine with breast-feeding cover. *Newsday,* p. 31.

Berlin, C.M., Jr. (1997, July 2). Maternal medications: Are they a threat to the breastfeeding infant? Paper presented to the 25th Annual Seminar for Physicians on Breastfeeding, sponsored by La Leche League International, the American Academy of Pediatrics, and the American College of Obstetricians and Gynecologists, Washington, DC.

Bier, J.A. et al. (1996). Comparison of skin-to-skin contact with standard contact in low-birth-weight infants who are breast-fed. *Archives of Pediatric and Adolescent Medicine,* 150:1265–1269.

Blaauw, R. et al. (1994). Risk factors for development of osteoporosis in a South African population. *South African Medical Journal,* 84:328–332.

Børresen, H.C. (1995). Rethinking current recommendations to introduce solid food between four and six months to exclusively breastfeeding infants. *Journal of Human Lactation,* 11(3):201–204.

Brazelton, T.B. (1983). *Infants and Mothers: Differences in Development.* New York: Delacorte Press.

Briggs, G.G., Freeman, R.K., & Yaffe, S.J. (1994). *Drugs in Pregnancy and Lactation: A Reference Guide to Fetal and Neonatal Risk.* Baltimore: Williams & Wilkins.

Brown, A. B. & McPherson, K., eds. (1998). *The Reality of Breastfeeding: Reflections by Contemporary Women.* Westport, CT: Greenwood Publishing Group.

Burros, M. (1997, June 4). Eating well: Testing calcium supplements for lead. *New York Times,* p. C6.

Calvo, E.B., Galindo, A.C., & Aspres, N.B. (1992). Iron status in exclusively breast-fed infants. *Pediatrics,* 90(3):375–379.

Cant, A., Marsden, R.A., & Kilshaw, P.J. (1986). Egg and cows' milk hypersensitivity in exclusively breast fed infants with eczema, and detection of egg protein in breast milk. *British Medical Journal,* 291:932–935.
Carlson, S.E. (1997). Functional effects of increasing omega-3 fatty acid intake.
Journal of Pediatrics, 131:173–175.
Charpak, N., Ruiz-Peláez, J.G., Figueroa de C., Z., & Charpak, Y. (1997). Kan-
garoo mother versus traditional care for newborn infants ≤ 2000 grams: A
randomized, controlled trial. *Pediatrics,* 100(4):682–688.
Children's Nutrition Research Center. (1991). *Guidelines for Collection, Storage
and Home Use of Human Milk.* Houston, TX: Baylor College of Medicine.
Cohen, R. & Mrtek, M. (1994). The impact of two corporate lactation programs
on the incidence and duration of breast-feeding by employed mothers.
American Journal of Health Promotion, 8(6):436–441.
Cohen, R., Mrtek, M.B., & Mrtek, R.G. (1995). Comparison of maternal absenteeism and infant illness rates among breast-feeding and formula-feeding
women in two corporations. *American Journal of Health Promotion,*
10(2):148–153.
Cooney, K. (1994). Assessment of nine-month Lactational Amenorrhea Method
in Rwanda. Occasional paper, Institute of Reproductive Health, Washington, DC.
Corbett-Dick, P. & Bezek, S.K. (1997). Breastfeeding promotion for the employed mother. *Journal of Pediatric Health Care,* 11:12–19.
Cumming, E. et al. (1993). Breastfeeding and other reproductive factors and the
risk of hip fractures in elderly women. *International Journal of Epidemiology,*
22(4):684–691.
Cunningham, A.S., Jelliffe, D.B., & Jelliffe, E.F.P. (1991). Breastfeeding and
health in the 1980s: A global epidemiologic review. *The Journal of Pediatrics,*
118(5):659–666.
Dettwyler, K.A. (1995). Beauty and the breast: The cultural context of breastfeeding in the United States, Chapter 7. In: Stuart-Macadam,
P. & Dettwyler, K.A., eds. *Breastfeeding: Biocultural Perspectives.* New York:
Aldine De Gruyter.
Dewey, K.G. (1994, August). Aerobic exercise for breast-feeding moms. *Health-
line.* Reprinted June 23, 1997, on www.health-line.com/
articles/hl940801.htm.
Dewey, K.G. et al. (1992). Growth of breast-fed and formula-fed infants from 0
to 18 months: The DARLING study. *Pediatrics,* 89(6):1035–1041.
Dewey, K.G. Lovelady, C.A., Nommsen-Rivers, L.A., McCrory, M.A., & Lön-
nerdal, B. (1994). A randomized study of the effects of aerobic exercise by
lactating women on breast-milk volume and composition. *New England
Journal of Medicine,* 330(7):449–453.
Dewey, K.G., Heinig, M.J., & Nommsen-Rivers, L.A. (1995). Differences in
morbidity between breast-fed and formula-fed infants. *Journal of Pediatrics,*
126(5,1):696-702.

Dewey, K.G. et al. (1995). Growth of breast-fed infants deviates from current reference data: A pooled analysis of US, Canadian, and European data sets. *Pediatrics,* 96:495–503.

Duffy, L. et al. (1997). Exclusive breastfeeding protects against bacterial colonization and day care exposure to otitis media. *Pediatrics,* http://www.pediatrics.org/cgi/content/full/100/4/e7.

Duncan, B. et al. (1993). Exclusive breast-feeding for at least 4 months protects against otitis media. *Pediatrics,* 91(5):867–872.

Dunn, J. & Kendrick, C. (1982). *Siblings: Love, Envy and Understanding.* Cambridge, MA: Harvard University Press.

Eiger, M.S. (1992). The feeding of infants and children, Chapter 2. In: Hoekelman, R.A., *Primary Pediatric Care,* 2nd ed., St. Louis: Mosby, pp. 182–194.

Eiger, M.S. (1994). Drugs and breastfeeding, Chapter 5. In: Mitchell, M.D., *The Pill Book Guide to Children's Medications,* New York: Bantam, pp. 247–267.

Eiger, M.S. (1995, April 11). Helping breastfeeding mothers during the early weeks. Presentation to American Academy of Pediatrics, spring session, Philadelphia.

European Collaborative Study. (1992). Risk factors for mother-to-child transmission of HIV-1. *Lancet,* 339:1007–1012.

Eyer, D.E. (1992). *Mother-infant Bonding: A Scientific Fiction.* New Haven, CT: Yale University Press.

Farnsworth, C.H. (1994, Apr. 5). Quebec bets on subsidized milk, mother's kind. *New York Times,* p. A4.

Fischman, S.H., Raskin, P.H., & Raskin, E.A. (1983). Changes in intimate and sexual relationships in postpartum couples. Presentation given at conference of The Society for the Scientific Study of Sex, Eastern Region, University City Holiday Inn, Philadelphia, April 15.

Fisher, W. & Gray, J. (1983, Nov. 18). Erotophobia-erotophilia and couples' sexual behavior during pregnancy and after childbirth. Paper presented at the annual meeting of the Society of the Scientific Study of Sex, Chicago.

Folic acid fortification: Is it enough? (1998). *Harvard Women's Health Watch,* V(6):1.

Folley, S.J. (1969). The milk-ejection reflex: a neuroendocrine theme in biology, myth and art. *Journal of Endocrinology,* 44:x–xx.

Foreman, J. (1998, Jan. 5). Making a place for nursing mothers. *Boston Globe,* p. C1.

Fox, K. et al. (1993). Reproductive correlates of bone mass in elderly women. *Journal of Bone & Mineral Resorption,* 8(8):901–908.

Freudenheim, J. et al. (1994). Exposure to breastmilk in infancy and the risk of breast cancer. *Epidemiology,* 5(3):324–331.

Gartner, L.M. (1994). Neonatal jaundice. *Pediatrics in Review,* 15(11):422–432.

Gielin, A.C., Faden, R.R., O'Campo, P., Brown, C.H., & Paige, D.M. (1991). Maternal employment during the early postpartum period: Effects on initiation and continuation of breast-feeding. *Pediatrics,* 87(3):298–305.

Goldman, A.S. (1993). The immune system of human milk: Antimicrobial, anti-inflammatory and immunomodulating properties. *Pediatric Infectious Disease Journal,* 12(8):664–671.

Gould, S.J. (1993, Nov.). The sexual politics of classification. *Natural History,* pp. 20–29.

Grams, M. (1985). *Breastfeeding Success for Working Mothers.* Sheridan, WY: Achievement Press.

Gregory, R.L., Wallace, J.P., Gfell, L.E., Marks, J., & King, B.A. (1997). Effect of exercise on milk immunoglobulin A. *Medicine & Science in Sports & Exercise,* 29(12):1596–1601.

Greiner, T. (1996). The concept of weaning: Definitions and their implications. *Journal of Human Lactation,* 12(2):123–128.

Grulee, C.G. & Sanford, H. N. (1936). The influence of breast and artificial feeding on infantile eczema. *Journal of Pediatrics,* 9:223.

Gruskay, F.L. (1982, August). Comparison of breast, cow, and soy feedings in the prevention of onset of allergic disease: A 15-year prospective study. *Clinical Pediatrics,* 486–491.

Guay, L. et al. (1996). Detection of human immunodeficiency virus type 1 (HIV-1) DNA and p24 antigen in breast milk of HIV-1-infected Ugandan women and vertical transmission. *Pediatrics,* 98(3):pt1:438–444.

Guidelines for Perinatal Care, 4th ed. (1997). The American Academy of Pediatrics and the American College of Obstetricians and Gynecologists. Washington, DC: ACOG and AAP.

György, P. (1971, August). Biochemical aspects, in symposium, The uniqueness of human milk. *American Journal of Clinical Nutrition,* pp. 970–975.

Hamosh, M., Ellis, L.A., Pollock, D.R., Henderson, T.R., & Hamosh, P. (1996). Breastfeeding and the working mother: Effect of time and temperature of short-term storage on proteolysis, lipolysis, and bacterial growth in milk. *Pediatrics,* 97(4):492–498.

Hatcher, R. A., Rinehart, W., Blackburn, R., & Geller, J.S. (1997). *The Essentials of Contraceptive Technology.* Baltimore: Johns Hopkins School of Public Health, Population Information Program.

Hayssen, V. (1995, Dec.). Milk: It does a baby good. *Natural History,* pp. 36–42.

Heird, W.C., Prager, T.C., & Anderson, R.E. (1997). Docosahexaenoic acid and the development and function of the infant retina. *Current Opinion in Lipidology,* 8:12–16.

Hide, D.W. & Guyer, B.M. (1985). Clinical manifestations of allergy related to breast- and cow's milk-feeding. *Pediatrics,* 76(6):973–974.

Hill, P.D., Aldag, J.C., & Chatterton, R.T. (1996). The effect of sequential and simultaneous breast pumping on milk volume and prolactin levels: A pilot study. *Journal of Human Lactation,* 12(3):193–199.

Hofmeyer, G.J. et al. (1991). Companionship to modify the clinical birth environment: Effects on progress and perceptions of labor and breastfeeding. *British Journal of Obstetrics and Gynecology,* 98:756–764.

Horwood, L.J. & Fergusson, D.M. (1998). Breastfeeding and child achievement. *Pediatrics,* 101(1):e9.

Hrdy, S.B. (1995, Dec.). Natural-born mothers. *Natural History,* pp. 30–34.

Hrdy, S.B. (1995, Dec.). Liquid assets: A brief history of wet-nursing. *Natural History,* p. 40.

Hrdy, S.B. & Carter, C.S. (1995, Dec.). Hormonal cocktails for two. *Natural History,* pp. 34–36.

Human Nutrition Information Service. (1992). *The Food Guide Pyramid.* Hyattsville, MD: U.S. Dept. of Agriculture, Home and Garden Bulletin, No. 252.

Humenick, S.S. & Hill, P.D. (1996). Salespeople and the lactation army: Taking a stand for health and human milk. *Journal of Human Lactation,* 12(1):5–8.

Institute of Medicine, National Academy of Sciences. (1991). *Nutrition During Lactation.* Washington, DC: National Academy Press.

Institute of Medicine, National Academy of Sciences. (1992). *Nutrition During Pregnancy and Lactation.* Washington, DC: National Academy Press.

Isabella, P.H. & Isabella, R.A. (1994). Correlates of successful breastfeeding: A study of social and personal factors. *Journal of Human Lactation,* 10:257–264.

Jarosz, L. (1993). Breastfeeding versus formula: A cost comparison. *Hawaii Medical Journal,* 52:14–17.

Jelliffe, D.B. and Jelliffe, E.F.P., eds. (1971, August). The uniqueness of human milk. A symposium. *American Journal of Clinical Nutrition,* pp. 968–1024.

Jensen, C.L., Prager, T.C., et al. (1997). Effect of dietary linoleic/alpha-linolenic acid ratio on growth and visual function of term infants. *The Journal of Pediatrics,* 131:200–209.

Kelsey, J.L. & John, E.M. (1994). Lactation and the risk of breast cancer. *New England Journal of Medicine,* 330(2):136–137.

Kemper, K., Forsyth, B., & McCarthy, P. (1989). Jaundice, terminating breastfeeding, and the vulnerable child. *Pediatrics,* 84(5):773–778.

Kendall-Tackett, K.A. (1997, July 2). Postpartum depression and the breastfeeding mother. Paper presented to the 25th Annual Seminar for Physicians on Breastfeeding, sponsored by La Leche League International, the American Academy of Pediatrics, and the American College of Obstetricians and Gynecologists, Washington, DC.

Kendall-Tackett, K.A. & Sugarman, M. (1995). The social consequences of long-term breastfeeding. *Journal of Human Lactation,* 11(3):179–183.

Kennedy, K.I. & Visness, C.M. (1992). Contraceptive efficacy of lactational amenorrhoea. *Lancet,* 339:227–30.

Kennell, J., Klaus, M., McGrath, S., Robertson, S., & Hinckley, C. (1991). Continuous emotional support during labor in a U.S. hospital. *Journal of the American Medical Association,* 265:2197–2201.

Kinsey, A.C., Pomeroy, W.B., Martin, C.E., & Gebhart, P.H. (1953). *Sexual Behavior in the Human Female.* Philadelphia: Saunders.

Kitzinger, S. (1985). *Woman's Experience of Sex.* New York: Penguin.

Klaus, M.H. (1987). The frequency of suckling: A neglected but essential ingredient of breast-feeding. *Obstetrics and Gynecology Clinics of North America,* 14(3):623–633.

Klaus, M.H. & Kennell, J.H. (1982). *Parent-Infant Bonding,* 2nd ed. St. Louis: C.V. Mosby.

Koetting, C.A. & Wardlaw, G.M. (1988). Wrist, spine, and hip bone density in women with variable histories of lactation. *American Journal of Clinical Nutrition,* 48:1479–1481.

Kramer, F., Stunkard, A.J., Marshall, K.A., McKinney, S., & Liebschutz, J. (1993). Breast-feeding reduces maternal lower-body fat. *Journal of American Dietetic Association,* 93:429–433.

Kritz-Silverstein, D. et al. (1993). Pregnancy and lactation as determinants of bone mineral density in postmenopausal women. *American Journal of Epidemiology,* 136(9):1052–1059.

Kruell, K. (1995, Fall). Running after children. *FootNotes,* pp. 14–15.

La Leche League International. (1997). *The Womanly Art of Breastfeeding.* Schaumburg, IL: La Leche League International.

La Leche League International. *New Beginnings* (bimonthly newsletter). Schaumburg, IL: La Leche League International.

Labbok, M.H. (1997, July 4). Cost effectiveness of breastfeeding in the U.S.: The forgotten women's and children's preventive health issue. Paper presented to the 15th international conference of La Leche League International, Washington, DC.

Labbok, M.H. & Hendershot, G.E. (1987). Does breastfeeding protect against malocclusion? An analysis of the 1981 child health supplement to the National Health Interview Survey. *American Journal of Preventive Medicine,* 3:4.

Labbok, M.H. et al. (1997). Multicenter study of the Lactational Amenorrhea Method (LAM): I. Efficacy, duration, and implications for clinical application. *Contraception,* 55(6):327–336.

Lang, S., Lawrence, C.J., & Orme, R.L'E. (1994). Cup feeding: An alternative method of infant feeding. *Archives of Disease in Childhood,* 71:365–369.

Lanting, C.I., Fidler, V., Huisman, M., Touwen, B.C.L., & Boersma, E.R. (1994). Neurological differences between 9-year-old children fed breast-milk or formula-milk as babies. *Lancet,* 344:1319–1322.

Lawrence, R.A. (1994). *Breastfeeding: A Guide for the Medical Profession,* 4th ed. St. Louis: C.V. Mosby.

Lawrence, R.A. (1997, October). *A Review of the Medical Benefits and Contraindications to Breastfeeding in the United States* (Maternal and Child Health Technical Information Bulletin). Arlington, VA: National Center for Education in Maternal and Child Health.

Levine, B. (1997, Oct. 22). Recent research on docosahexaenoic acid (DHA) in health and disease. *Current Concepts and Perspectives in Nutrition,* 8(3).

Lindberg, L.D. (1996). Women's decisions about breast feeding and maternal employment. *Journal of Marriage and the Family,* 58:239–251.

Lozoff, B. et al. (1977). The mother-newborn relationship: Limits of adaptability. *Journal of Pediatrics,* 91(1):1–12.

Lucas, A. et al. (1992). Breast milk and subsequent intelligence quotient in children born preterm. *Lancet,* 339:261-64.

Lucas, A., Fewtrell, M.S., Davies, P.S.W., et al. (1997). Breastfeeding and catch-up growth in infants born small for gestational age. *Acta Paediatrica,* 86:564–569.

Lumpkin, M.D., Samson, W.K., & McCann, S.M. (1983). Hypothalamic and pituitary sites of action of oxytocin to alter prolactin secretion in the rat. *Endocrinology,* 112(5):1711–1717.

Makrides, M., Neumann, M.A., & Gibson, R.A. (1996). Effect of maternal docosahexaenoic acid (DHA) supplementation on breast milk composition. *European Journal of Clinical Nutrition,* 50:352–357.

Makrides, M., Neumann, M.A., Simmer, K., Pater, J., & Gibson, R.A. (1995). Are long-chain polyunsaturated fatty acids essential nutrients in infancy? *Lancet,* 345:1463–1468.

Marmet, C. (1981). Manual expression of breast milk: Marmet technique. Franklin Park, IL: La Leche League (Reprint No. 107).

Marmet, C. & Shell, E. (1984). *How to Solve Neonatal Sucking Problems: A Key to Overcoming Sore Nipples, Slower Gain and Failure to Thrive.* Los Angeles: Lactation Institute.

Marmet, C. & Shell, E. (1984). Training neonates to suck correctly. *Maternal & Child Nursing,* 9(6):401–407.

Masters, W. H. & Johnson, V. E. (1966). *Human Sexual Response.* Boston: Little, Brown.

McClelland, D., Constantian, C., Regalado, D., & Stone, C. (1978, January). Making it to maturity. *Psychology Today,* pp. 42–53, 118.

McKenna, J.J. & Mosko, S. (1993). Evolution and infant sleep: An experimental study of infant-parent co-sleeping and its implications for SIDS. *Acta Paediatrica,* 389(Supplement):31–36.

McKenna, J.J., Mosko, S., & Richard, C.A. (1997). Bedsharing promotes breastfeeding. *Pediatrics,* 100(2):214–219.

Melton, L.J. III, Bryant, S.C., et al. (1993). Influence of breastfeeding and other reproductive factors on bone mass later in life. *Osteoporosis Int.,* 3(2):76–83.

Mennella, J.A. (1997, July 2). The transfer of flavors from mother's diet to breast milk: Effects on the recipient infant. Paper presented to the 25th Annual Seminar for Physicians on Breastfeeding, sponsored by La Leche League International, the American Academy of Pediatrics, and the American College of Obstetricians and Gynecologists, Washington, DC.

Mennella, J.A. & Beauchamp, G.K. (1996). The early development of human flavor preferences. In Capaldi, E.D., ed. *Why We Eat What We Eat: The Psychology of Eating.* Washington, DC. American Psychological Association, pp. 83–112.

Mennella, J.A. & Beauchamp, G.K. (1991). Maternal diet alters the sensory qualities of human milk and the nursling's behavior. *Pediatrics,* 88(4):737–744.

Mennella, J.A. & Beauchamp, G.K. (1991). The transfer of alcohol to human milk: Effects on flavor and the infant's behavior. *Pediatrics,* 325(14):981–985.

Mestecky, J. et al., eds. (1991). *Immunology of Milk and the Neonate.* New York: Plenum Press.

Mohrbacher, N. & Stock, J. (1997). *The Breastfeeding Answer Book.* Schaumburg, IL: La Leche League International.

Montague, A. (1971). *Touching: The Human Significance of the Skin.* New York: Columbia University Press.

Morelli, G.A., Rogoff, B., Oppenheim, D., & Goldsmith, D. (1992). Cultural variation in infants' sleeping arrangements: Questions of independence. *Developmental Psychology,* 28:604–613.

Nash, J.M. (1997, Feb. 3). Fertile minds. *Time,* pp. 49–56.

National Center for Environmental Health. (1996, Nov.). U.S. Public Health Service recommends that women consume 400 mcg of the vitamin folic acid daily to prevent serious and common birth defects. Atlanta: Centers for Disease Control and Prevention.

National Institutes of Health. (1997, March 24–26). Management of hepatitis C. *NIH Consensus Statement,* 15(3):1–41.

Neifert, M. (1996). Early assessment of the breastfeeding infant. *Contemporary Pediatrics,* 13(10):142–166.

Neifert, M.R., Seacat, J.M., & Jobe, W.E. (1985). Lactation failure due to insufficient glandular development of the breast. *Pediatrics,* 76(5):823–828.

Neville, M. C. and Neifert, M.R., eds. (1983). *Lactation: Physiology, Nutrition, and Breast-Feeding.* New York: Plenum Press.

New York Times. (1995, Feb. 12). Baby formula counterfeited; man is held. *New York Times,* 29.

Newburg, D.S. (1996). Oligosaccharides and glycoconjugates in human milk: Their role in host defense. *Journal of Mammary Gland Biology and Neoplasia,* 1(3):271–283.

Newburg, D.S., ed. (1998). *Bioactive Substances in Human Milk.* New York: Plenum Publishing.

Newburg, D.S. & Sweet, J.M. (1997). Bioactive materials in human milk: Milk sugars sweeten the argument for breast-feeding. *Nutrition Today,* 32(5):191–201.

Newburg, D.S., Peterson, J.A., et al. (1998). Role of human-milk lactadherin in protection against symptomatic rotavirus infection. *Lancet,* 351:1160–1164.

Newcomb, P.A. et al. (1994). Lactation and a reduced risk of premenopausal breast cancer. *New England Journal of Medicine,* 330(2):81–87.

Newman, J. (1995). How breast milk protects newborns. *Scientific American,* 273(6):76–79.

Newton, N. (1955). *Maternal Emotions.* New York: Paul B. Hoeber, Inc. (Harper & Row).

Newton, N. (1971, February 5). Interrelationship between various aspects of the female reproductive role: A review. Paper presented to the annual meeting of the American Psychopathological Association, New York.

Newton, N. (1971). Psychologic differences betwen breast and bottle feeding. *American Journal of Clinical Nutrition,* 24:993–1004.

Olds, S.W. (1985). *The Eternal Garden: Seasons of Our Sexuality.* New York: Times Books.

Olds, S.W. (1989). *The Working Parents' Survival Guide.* Rocklin, CA: Prima Publishing.

Oski, F.A. (1997). What we eat may determine who we can be. *Nutrition,* 13:220–221.

Papalia, D.E. & Olds, S.W. (1996). *A Child's World: Infancy Through Adolescence,* 7th ed. New York: McGraw-Hill.

Papalia, D.E., Olds, S.W., & Feldman, R.D. (1998). *Human Development,* 7th ed. New York: McGraw-Hill.

Paradise, J.L., Elster, B.A., & Tan, L. (1994). Evidence in infants with cleft palate that breast milk protects against otitis media. *Pediatrics,* 94(6):853–860.

Pear, R. (1992, June 12). Top infant-formula makers charged by U.S. over pricing. *New York Times,* pp. A1, D6.

Perez, A., Labbok, M., & Queenan, J. (1992). Clinical study of the Lactational Amenorrhea Method for family planning. *Lancet,* 339:968–970.

Picciano, M.F. (1994). The folate status of women and health. *Nutrition Today,* 29(6):20–27.

Picciano, M.F. (1995). Folate nutrition in lactation. In: Bailey, L.B., ed., *Folate in Health and Disease,* New York: Marcel Dekker, pp. 153–169.

Pickering, L.K., Granoff, D.M., et al. (1998). Modulation of the immune system by human milk and infant formula containing nucleotides. *Pediatrics,* 101(2):242–249.

Pisacane, A., Graziano, L., Mazzarella, G., et al. (1992). Breast-feeding and urinary tract infection. *The Journal of Pediatrics,* 120:87–89.

Popkin, B.M. et al. (1990). Breast-feeding and diarrheal morbidity. *Pediatrics,* 86(6):874–882.

Queenan, J.T. (1997, July 2). The obstetrician's role in successful breastfeeding. Paper presented to the 25th Annual Seminar for Physicians on Breastfeeding, sponsored by La Leche League International, the American Academy of Pediatrics, and the American College of Obstetricians and Gynecologists, Washington, DC.

Quindlen, A. (1994, May 25). To feed or not to feed. *New York Times,* p. A21.

Raphael, D. (1973). *The Tender Gift: Breastfeeding.* New York: Schocken Books.

Raphael, D. & Davis, F. (1985). *Only Mothers Know.* Westport, CT: Greenwood Press.

Righard, L. & Alade, M.O. (1997). Breastfeeding and the use of pacifiers. *Birth*, 24:116–20.

Rimm, E.B. et al. (1998). Folate and vitamin B6 from diet and supplements in relation to risk of coronary heart disease among women. *Journal of the American Medical Association*, 279:359–364.

Riordan, J. (1997, July 3). Does epidural anesthesia influence successful breastfeeding? Paper presented to the 25th Annual Seminar for Physicians on Breastfeeding, sponsored by La Leche League International, the American Academy of Pediatrics, and the American College of Obstetricians and Gynecologists, Washington, DC.

Riordan, J.M. (1997). The cost of not breastfeeding: A commentary. *Journal of Human Lactation*, 13(2):93–97.

Riordan, J. & Auerbach, K.G. (1999). *Breastfeeding and Human Lactation*, 2nd ed. Boston & London: Jones & Bartlett.

Roberts, K.L., Reiter, M., & Schuster, D. (1995). A comparison of chilled and room temperature cabbage leaves in treating breast engorgement. *Journal of Human Lactation*, 11(3):191–194.

Rodriguez-Garcia, R. & Frazier, L. (1995). Cultural paradoxes relating to sexuality and breastfeeding. *Journal of Human Lactation*, 11:111–115.

Roepke, J.B. (1997, July 7). Breastfeeding and women's nutrition. Presentation at fifteenth international conference, La Leche League, Washington, DC.

Romieu, I. et al. (1996). Breast cancer and lactation history in Mexican women. *American Journal of Epidemiology*, 143(6):543–552.

Ross, M.W. (1987). Back to the breast: Retraining infant suckling patterns. Unit 15 in the Lactation Consult Series developed by La Leche League International. Series editor: Auerbach, K.G.

Rossi, A.S. (1971, Feb.). Maternalism, sexuality and the new feminism. Paper presented to the annual meeting of the American Psychopathological Association, New York City.

Ryan, A.S. (1997). The resurgence of breastfeeding in the United States. *Pediatrics*, 99(4). http://www.pediatrics.org/cgi/content/full/99/4/e12.

Ryan, A.S., Rush, D., Krieger, F.W., & Lewandowski, G.E. (1991). Recent declines in breast-feeding in the United States, 1984 through 1989. *Pediatrics*, 88(4):719–727.

Sauer, H.J. (1987). Physiology of lactation and factors affecting lactation. *Obstetrics and Gynecology Clinics of North America*, 14:615–622.

Scariati, P.D., Grummer-Strawn, L.M., & Fein, S.B. (1997). A longitudinal analysis of infant morbidity and the extent of breastfeeding in the United States. *Pediatrics*. 99(6):e5. Or http://www.pediatrics.org/cgi/content/full/99/6/e5.

Schulte, P. (1995). Minimizing alcohol exposure of the breastfeeding infant. *Journal of Human Lactation*, 11(4):317–319.

Sharp, D.A. (1992, Nov.). Moist wound healing for sore or cracked nipples. *Breastfeeding Abstracts*, 12(2):19.

Sinigaglia, L. et al. (1996). Effect of lactation on postmenopausal bone mineral density of the lumbar spine. *Journal of Reproductive Medicine*, 41(6):439–443.

Small, M. (1998). *Our Babies, Ourselves.* New York: Anchor Books/Doubleday.

Smith, M.E. (1995, May–June). Nursing the world back to health. *New Beginnings,* pp. 68–71.

Smith, M.M. & Lifshitz, F. (1994). Excess fruit juice consumption as a contributing factor in nonorganic failure to thrive. *Pediatrics,* 93:438–443.

Sowers, M. et al. (1995). Biochemical markers of bone turnover in lactating and nonlacting postpartum women. *J. of Clin. Endocrinol. Metab.,* 80:2210–2216.

Sowers, M. et al. (1995). A prospective study of bone density and pregnancy after an extended period of lactation with bone loss. *Obstetrics and Gynecology,* 85:285–289.

Specker, B., Tsang, R.C., & Hollis, B. (1985). Effect of race and diet on human-milk vitamin D and 25-hydroxyvitamin D. *American Journal of Diseases of Children,* 139:1134–1137.

Spock, B. and Parker, S.J. (1998). *Dr. Spock's Baby and Child Care,* 7th ed. New York: Pocket Books; Dutton.

Stuart-Macadam, P. & Dettwyler, K.A., eds. (1995). *Breastfeeding: Biocultural Perspectives.* New York: Aldine De Gruyter.

Sugarman, M. & Kendall-Tackett, K.A. (1995). Weaning ages in a sample of American women who practice extended breastfeeding. *Clinical Pediatrics,* 34:642–647.

Thoman, E.B., Connor, R.L., & Levine, S. (1970). Lactation suppresses adrenal corticosteriod activity and aggressiveness in rats. *Journal of Comparative and Physiological Psychology,* 70:364–369.

Thoman, E.B., Wetzel, A., & Levine, S. (1968). Lactation prevents disruption of temperature regulation and suppresses adrenocortical activity in rats. *Communications in Behavioral Biology,* Part A, 2:165–171, Abstract No. 10680066.

United Nations Children's Fund: Innocenti Declaration on the Protection, Promotion and Support of Breastfeeding, Florence, Italy. (1990, Aug. 1). UNICEF, Nutrition Cluster (H-8F), 3 United Nations Plaza, New York, NY 10017.

Valentine, C.J., Hurst, N.M., & Schanler, R.J. (1994). Hindmilk improves weight gain in low-birth-weight infants fed human milk. *Journal of Pediatric Gastroenterology and Nutrition,* 18(4):474–477.

Wade, K., Sevilla, F., & Labbock, M. (1994). The Lactational Amenorrhea Method as a family planning program component: Findings in an implementation study in Ecuador. *Studies in Family Planning,* 25(4).

Walker, M. (1997). Do labor medications affect breastfeeding? *Journal of Human Lactation,* 13(2):131–137.

Wallace, J.P., Inbar, G., & Ernsthausen, K. (1992). Infant acceptance of postexercise breast milk. *Pediatrics,* 89(6):1245–1247.

White River Concepts. (1997). Best methods for feeding: How to select a breast pump. www.whiteriver.com.

Wicssinger, D. & Miller, M. (1995). Breastfeeding difficulties as a result of tight lingual and labial frena: A case report. *Journal of Human Lactation,* 11(4):313–316.

Williamson, M.T. & Murti, P.K. (1996). Effects of storage, time, temperature, and composition of containers on biologic components of human milk. *Journal of Human Lactation,* 12(1):31–35.

Winikoff, B., Semeraro, P., Zimmerman, M., & Stein, K. (1997). *Contraception during Breastfeeding: A Clinician's Sourcebook,* 2nd ed. New York: Population Council.

Winikoff, B. et al. (1986). Dynamics of infant feeding: Mothers, professionals, and the institutional context in a large urban hospital. *Pediatrics,* 77(3):357–365.

Winikoff, B. et al. (1987). Overcoming obstacles to breast-feeding in a large municipal hospital: Application of lessons learned. *Pediatrics,* 80:423–433.

Wong, W., Hachey, D.L., Insull, W., Opekun, A.R., & Klein, P.D. (1993). Effect of dietary cholesterol on cholesterol synthesis in breast-fed and formula-fed infants. *Journal of Lipid Research,* 34:1403–1411.

Woodward, A. et al. (1990). Acute respiratory illness in Adelaide children: Breast-feeding modifies the effect of passive smoking. *Journal of Epidemiology and Community Health,* 44:224–230.

Woolridge, M.W. (1986). Aetiology of sore nipples. *Midwifery,* 2:172–176.

Woolridge, M.W. (1986). The "anatomy" of infant sucking. *Midwifery,* 2:164–171.

Woolridge, M.W. & Fisher, C. (1988). Colic, "overfeeding," and symptoms of lactose malabsorption in the breast-fed baby: A possible artifact of feed management? *Lancet,* 2:382–384.

Wright, A., Rice, S., & Wells, S. (1996). Changing hospital practices to increase the duration of breastfeeding. *Pediatrics,* 97(5):669–675.

Wright, A.L., Holberg, C.J., Taussig, L.M., & Martinez, F.D. (1995). Relationship of infant feeding to recurrent wheezing at age 6 years. *Archives of Pediatric Adolescent Medicine,* 149:758–763.

Wright, A.L., Bauer, M., Naylor, A., Sutcliffe, E., & Clark, L. (1998). Increasing breastfeeding rates to reduce infant illness at the community level. *Pediatrics,* 101(5):837–844.

Yalom, M. (1997). *A History of the Breast.* New York: Knopf.

Yamauchi, Y. & Yamanouchi, I. (1990). Breast-feeding frequency during the first 24 hours after birth in full-term neonates. *Pediatrics,* 86(2):171–175.

Yoo, K.Y., Tajima, K., Kuroishi, T., et al. (1992). Independent protective effect of lactation against breast cancer: A case-control study in Japan. *American Journal of Epidemiology,* 135:726–733.

Zavaleta, N., Lanata, C., Butron, B., et al. (1995). Effect of acute maternal infection on quantity and composition of breast milk. *American Journal of Clinical Nutrition,* 62:559–563.

*I*ndex

A

AA (arachidonic acid), 60
ABO incompatibility, 123, 123*n*
Acetaminophen, 174, 175, 192
Acyclovir, 174, 324
Adopted baby, 333–35
Advil, 174
Aerobic exercise, 148, 150, 151
Affirmations, 192
After-pains, 109
AIDS (Acquired Immune Deficiency
    Syndrome), 325
Alcohol, on nipples, 79, 292
Alcoholic drinks, 40, 138, 182–
    83
Allergies, 10, 15, 139, 369
Alpha-lactalbumin, 59
Alternative remedies, 167,
    180
Alveoli, 47, 48, *50*, 51, 52

American Academy of Pediatrics
    (AAP), 2, 10, 11, 29, 325
  breastfeeding recommendations,
    88, 90, 99, 204, 219, 354–55
  Committee on Environmental
    Health, 141–42
  policy on employment, 228
  sleeping recommendations, 117
American College of Nurse Midwives
    Certification Council (ACC),
    66
Amino acids, 56
Amniotic fluid, 9
Amphetamines, 183
Angelou, Maya, 20
Antianxiety drugs, 179
Antibiotics, 174
Antibodies, 12, 56, 57
Antidepressants, 167, 178, 179
Antiepileptic drugs, 174
Antihistamines, 174, 175

ABOUT THE AUTHORS

Marvin S. Eiger, M.D. is a nationally known pediatrician who practiced in New York City for 30 years; most of his patients were breastfed. Educated at Harvard University, Dr. Eiger received medical training at New York University School of Medicine and served his residency in pediatrics at Bellevue Hospital. A Fellow of the American Academy of Pediatrics, Dr. Eiger established the Comprehensive Lactation Program at New York's Beth Israel Hospital in 1987 and served as its Medical Director until 1991 helping to ensure the successful breastfeeding experience of hundreds of nursing mothers and babies.

Dr. Eiger frequently writes articles on breastfeeding topics for medical journals and magazines, lectures on breastfeeding to medical and lay groups, has been on the Editorial Review Board of the *Journal of Human Lactation,* and is a peer reviewer of papers submitted to *Pediatrics,* the Journal of the American Academy of Pediatrics. He also teaches breastfeeding basics to lactation consultants at various meetings and seminars.

Dr. Eiger is the father of two children and lives in Manhattan with his wife, Carol.

Sally Wendkos Olds has written extensively about relationships, health, and personal growth, and has won national awards for both her book and magazine writing. Her college textbooks on child and adult development, *A Child's World* and *Human Development,* co-authored with psychologist Diane E. Papalia, Ph.D., have been read by more than two million students and are the leading texts in their fields. She is also the author of *The Working Parents' Survival Guide* and *The Eternal Garden: Seasons of Our Sexuality,* and the co-author of *Helping Your Child Find Values to Live By, Psychology,* and *Raising a Hyperactive Child* (winner of the Family Service Association of America National Media Award).

A former president of the American Society of Journalists and Authors, Ms. Olds is also a member of La Leche League International, International Childbirth Education Association, the Authors Guild, and other professional and civic organizations.

Ms. Olds lives on Long Island with her husband, Mark. She nursed her own three daughters and is now the proud grandmother of four breastfed children.